Cancer Etiology, Diagnosis and Treatments

Hepatocellular Carcinoma in the 3rd Millennium

CANCER ETIOLOGY, DIAGNOSIS AND TREATMENTS

Additional books in this series can be found on Nova's website under the Series tab.

Additional e-books in this series can be found on Nova's website under the e-book tab.

CANCER ETIOLOGY, DIAGNOSIS AND TREATMENTS

HEPATOCELLULAR CARCINOMA IN THE 3RD MILLENNIUM

MASSIMILIANO BERRETTA
AND
BRUNO CACOPARDO
EDITORS

New York

NOTICE TO THE READER

Library of Congress Cataloging-in-Publication Data

ISBN: 978-1-63484-025-5

Library of Congress Control Number: 2015954516

Published by Nova Science Publishers, Inc. † New York

CONTENTS

PREFACE

HCC is the most common primary cancer of the liver and according to the WHO report, the fourth commonest cause of death. The estimated incidence of new cases worldwide is about 500,000-1,000,000 per year causing 600,000 deaths globally per year. Although there are large areas of the world where the incidence of HCC is still unknown, several countries in East Asia and some Sub-Saharan African regions are affected by a very high prevalence of HCC (over 20 cases/100,000 population). Areas with a moderately high risk (11-20 cases/100,000 population) include Italy, Spain and Latin America, while France, Germany and the United Kingdom have instead an intermediate risk (5-10 cases/100,000 population). A relatively low prevalence (less than 5 cases/100,000 population) is found in the United States, Canada and Scandinavia. The incidence of HCC has been rising in developed western countries in the last two decades, along with the emergence of the hepatitis C virus infection and due to the rise of immigration rates from HBV-endemic countries. In addition, even though the incidence of HCC reaches its highest peak among persons over 65 years, an increased incidence among younger individuals has been noted in the last two decades both in USA and Europe.

A multidisciplinary approach should be taken when assessing patients with HCC; stage of HCC and liver disease should always be taken into account and the best treatment should be offered. Liver resection and ablative treatments should never be denied to patients, and curative procedures should be performed in hepato-biliary-pancreatic centers. Each HCC patient has to be evaluated singularly, stratifying each time the risk for the procedure so as to determine which treatment is the best treatment. It is also important to analyze all the possibilities that can be offered. This similar approach showed a good efficacy and safety in all "frail" patient categories, such as elderly patients or patients with HCC and HIV infection. Early diagnosis of HCC and retreatment for HCC recurrence have a key role in the survival of patients. Therefore, regular screening programs for HCC should be extended to all patients according to proposed guidelines, together with a greater proclivity for treatment and retreatment options in cases of an HCC diagnosis or recurrence. This may be an important and needed breakthrough for this rising problem.

Chapter 1 – Hepatocellular carcinoma (HCC) is the most common primary malignancy of the liver and the second most common cause of death from cancer worldwide. The leading risk factor for HCC is cirrhosis due to chronic hepatitis B and hepatitis C. The incidence of HCC differs greatly according to the geographic area. Regions with the highest incidence rates of liver cancer include Eastern and Southeastern Asia as well as Northern and Western Africa, which are endemic for hepatitis B virus infection. In most developed countries, the incidence of HCC is at low (Northern Europe) or intermediate (Southern Europe and Northern America) levels. In Western countries, Egypt and Japan hepatitis C virus infection is the main risk factor for HCC. However, upcoming risk factors include obesity, diabetes and nonalcoholic fatty liver disease. Considering that these factors are rapidly increasing in prevalence, they might account for a growing proportion of HCC cases in the future.

In this chapter, the authors review the key aspects of HCC epidemiology, with a focus on the incidence and mortality rates in Western countries.

Chapter 2 – Hepatocellular carcinoma (HCC) is the second most common cause of death from cancer worldwide. The vast majority of cases occur in the setting of cirrhosis, usually due to hepatitis B virus (HBV) and hepatitis C virus (HCV) infection. In developed countries, chronic alcohol abuse is a significant risk factor for advanced liver disease and HCC; in addition, in Western countries obesity and diabetes are growing epidemics, which significantly contribute to the development of non-alcoholic fatty liver disease (NAFLD). NAFLD is an emerging risk factor for cirrhosis and HCC. Metabolic liver diseases, in particular hereditary hemochromatosis, account for a small number of liver cancers. In several regions of the world, including sub-Saharan Africa, Eastern Asia and parts of South America, aflatoxin exposure in food is a significant risk factor for HCC.

Unlike other cancers, risk factors for HCC can usually be identified at an individual level; moreover, the majority of risk factors are preventable. Vaccination against HBV is the most efficient primary prevention measure available in high-incidence countries, whereas antiviral treatment for HBV and HCV may reduce liver disease progression and the risk of HCC. Lifestyle modification, including weight loss and promotion of physical exercise, may have a significant impact in the management of NAFLD and its complications, including HCC.

Chapter 3 – Liver cancer is the sixth most commonly diagnosed cancer worldwide and the third leading cause of cancer death. The number of cases has also been rapidly increasing in Western countries, and globally, more than 700,000 new patients are diagnosed annually. HCC arising from hepatocytes, represents the most common histological subtype of liver cancers, accounting for approximately 70–85% of all cases. Multiple etiological factors for HCC have been identified. The most important risk factor is infection with hepatitis viruses, mainly HBV and HCV. Alcohol-induced liver damage also ranks high, especially in Western countries. Virus infection or metabolic stress results in liver damage including fatty change, hepatitis, and cirrhosis, which set premalignant conditions for HCC. Chronic inflammation, virus infection, and liver regeneration in cirrhosis have been reported to induce genetic and epigenetic damage to the host genome. Most HCCs gradually develop from these premalignant stages by the accumulation of these alterations. Accordingly, highly damaged livers are extremely susceptible to multiple tumors. The next-generation sequencing (NGS) era enabled whole-genome or exome sequencing of the cancer genome within a reasonable time frame and cost. This approach is rapidly and exhaustively identify potential key genetic events, including potential molecular therapeutic targets, in HCC. The current review summarizes the data about molecular pathogenesis and signal transduction pathways in hepatocellular carcinoma considering recent results in molecular research.

Chapter 4 – Hepatocellular carcinoma (HCC), the most common primary malignancy of the liver, represents 1 of the leading causes of cancer deaths in the world. The main risk factor for HCC is the presence of chronic liver disease, particularly when the disease has already resulted in liver cirrhosis. The constant process of destruction and repair within the parenchyma that is associated with cirrhosis increases hepatocyte metabolism and amplifies the risk of mutations in a multistep progression from hyper-plastic nodule to early HCC and finally to moderately/poorly differentiated HCC. Hepatitis B and C viruses (HBV and HCV) are known to have oncogenic potential, and the risk of HCC in HBV and HCV carriers is increased independently of the presence of cirrhosis.

The diagnosis of a hepatocellular carcinoma (HCC) strongly relies on imaging. Ultrasonography (US) plays a crucial role in surveillance, due to wide availability, relative inexpensiveness, and biological safety. According to the American Association for the Study of the Liver Diseases (AASLD) 2011 guidelines, US is recommended for surveillance of patients at risk of developing HCC; namely, US should be performed every 6 months in patients with chronic B hepatitis and cirrhotic patients, regardless of the cause. However, literature data indicate highly variable sensitivity rates for the US detection of HCC, ranging from 33% to 96%. Each suspected HCC discovered at US in a patient under surveillance must be therefore confirmed with multiphasic dynamic imaging. CT and MRI must be used for the non-invasive diagnosis of HCC in patients under surveillance; according to the AASLD 2011 guidelines and to the European Association for the Study of the Liver (EASL) and the European Organization for Research and Treatment of Cancer (EORTC), hyper-vascularity during hepatic arterial phase and wash-out on either portal venous or delayed phase are hallmark imaging features for the diagnosis of HCC. When present in patients under US surveillance, these features are sufficient for a non-invasive diagnosis.

Chapter 5 – The HCC has all the requirements to be considered a very affordable program of screening and surveillance. In fact, the incidence and prevalence of HCC is increasing in almost all regions of the world. The results obtained from most studies have confirmed that, in patients undergoing cancer surveillance, vascular invasion is less frequently present and, consequently, patients are more often eligible for curative treatment. As refers to target population, patients with cirrhosis in class A and B of Child-Pugh are the ideal candidates for a screening program, because of the high incidence of HCC and the possibility of treatment that is able to reduce the mortality. Nevertheless, there has been one main randomized clinical trial in literature that has demonstrated the benefit of surveillance (with by performing alphafetoprotein and ultrasound scan twice a year). All strategies are convenient in opposition to non-surveillance: the biannual surveillance with Ultrasound scan + Alphafetoprotein detection resulted as the most effective (irrespective of the etiology), being able to triple the number of the operable HCC diagnosis, and to reduce the tumor-related mortality. The evidence that a more aggressive ecographic surveillance program (3-4 months) allows the diagnosis of small tumors (<2 cm) in a high percentage of cases, was not confirmed subsequently. In literature there is no evidence that screening and surveillance with computerized tomography or magnetic resonance imaging present any cost-effectiveness advantages compared with US, with the exception of the patients in the transplant waiting list, and the cases where the ultrasonographic exploration is limited by physical and anatomic conditions.

Chapter 6 – Primary prevention of cancer consists in all the interventions that keep a cancerogenic agent from initiating the carcinogenic process. This is achieved by eliminating, avoiding, or neutralizing the carcinogen, or by stopping the *in vivo* conversion of a pre-carcinogen into a carcinogen. Prevention is the only realistic approach for reducing mortality rates associated with hepatocellular carcinoma (HCC) worldwide. Primary prevention of HCC is made through the prevention of its major risk factors, i.e., hepatitis B (HBV) and hepatitis C (HCV) infection. Vaccination against HBV and screening of blood donations are well-known and effective measures of primary prevention. Primary prevention also includes antiviral treatments, which may slow or definitively stop the progression of liver disease towards cirrhosis. Primary prevention seems to work successfully against HBV and its complications. In those areas where a nationwide HBV universal vaccination program was implemented, the incidence of HCC declined significantly. Also, in HBV-infected subjects, long-term suppression of HBV with antiviral therapies can slow the progression of liver disease or even reverse liver damage, therefore, preventing HCC formation. In HCV-infected subjects, a yet controversial strategy to reduce HCC incidence, is based on viral eradication by Interferon (IFN)-based or IFN-free treatments. In the latter case, the cost of new antiviral drugs for primary prevention of HCC remains a remarkable obstacle to such a strategy.

Chapter 7 – The natural history of Hepatocellular Carcinoma (HCC) is complex and severe because of the coexistence of liver inflammatory disease, often cirrhosis, which worsens the clinical progress causing the patient death and generally limiting the therapy choices. HCC natural history has been divided in 4 evolutionary stages, following Barcelona Clinic Liver Cancer classification, based on volume and number of tumor nodules, relationship of the tumor with portal vascular system, level of liver failure and presence/absence of general symptoms of neoplasm. Cirrhosis is the most important single risk factor for HCC. The risk for HCC differs depending on numerous factors such as sex, patients age, etiology and cirrhosis clinical stage, level of hepatocellular proliferation and presence/absence of hepatocellular dysplasia.

The understanding of HCC natural history has been possible because of perspective studies of patients at risk, in particular of patients with cirrhosis and chronic HBV infection. In most cases, HCC is unicentric, allowing clinically early diagnosis, with positive repercussion on treatment outcome. Since HCC is essentially a tumour that growths just inside the liver for years, it is successfully treatable with surgery resection or local ablation.

Dividing patients in different clinical stages with different prognosis levels, allowed different treatments and proven efficacy also for patients with intermediate and advanced tumour. Depending on geographic differences of HCC epidemiology and natural history, it is not clear if it would be necessary following a unique HCC staging system. Nevertheless, staging systems as BCLC, used by the most important international scientific society, allowed muticentric studies finalized to validating new therapeutic options.

Chapter 8 – Hepatocellular carcinoma (HCC) is a major health problem with a high incidence and mortality all over the world. The current ability to increase the survival of patients with HCC relies upon clinical surveillance, which allows HCC precursors and malignant tumors to be recognized at an earlier stage, making cure possible. In this report the authors describe the main histopathological criteria to discriminate between HCC precursors and well differentiated HCC, with attention to the role of immunohistochemical markers.

Over time, many staging and scoring systems have been proposed for the classification and prognosis of patients with HCC. A complete system for HCC classification nowadays should include multifunctional and phenotypic characteristics of the tumor, the general health of the patient and the potential therapeutic approaches available. The second part of the paper is devoted to an overview of the current staging systems for HCC.

Genetic studies of tumor samples and the use of newer molecular approaches such as non-coding RNA and genome-wide association studies, according to immunohistochemistry, proteomics and clinical criteria are highlighting the variability that exists among diverse

HCC. Identification of new target pathways for the treatment of HCC by more personalized and targeted regimens are the main goals of the current translational medical research.

Chapter 9 – Many options are available for the treatment of hepatocellular carcinoma (HCC). The selection among different treatment options varies in relation to the tumor stage and the degree of hepatic dysfunction. Treatments can be divided into curative treatments (liver transplantation, liver resection, local ablation) and palliative treatments (trans-arterial therapies and systemic chemotherapy). The best results have been reported after surgical resection in patients with single tumors and good liver function (no portal hypertension, normal bilirubin), after liver transplantation in single tumors ≤5 cm or three nodules ≤3 cm, and after ablative treatments for single tumors ≤3 cm in Child-Pugh A patients[1]. In these patients a 5-years survival of 50–70% can be achieved. Among the different treatments allocation algorithms described in literature, the Barcelona Cancer Liver Center (BCLC) is the most widely utilized in the Western Countries. Although this allocation system is criticized for the excessive decisional rigidity it is useful to give a guideline among the different treatments. This system divide HCCs in four different stages: very early stage; early stage, intermediate stage, advance stage and end stage.

Chapter 10 – In the recent years the management of locoregional and systemic symptoms of advanced Hepatocellular Carcinoma has improved. Although the mortality induced by the extrahepatic diffusion of the tumor is limited, treatment is necessary because of the severity of symptoms and the impact on quality of life. The therapeutic goal in patients with End-Stage Liver Disease is symptom control and maintenance of the best possible quality of life. In this setting, best supportive care consists of a broad spectrum of services and interventions aimed at improving patient's ability to tolerate treatments and better facing the impact with cancer. Active control of symptoms, by means of integrated medical interventions and multidisciplinary approaches (psychosocial, palliative, nutritional), must not be confined to the very end stage of the disease but must be part of a global approach to cancer patients.

Chapter 11 – The hepatocellular carcinoma (HCC) is the most common primary cancer of the liver and, according to the WHO report, the fourth commonest cause of death. The estimated incidence of new cases worldwide is about 500,000-1,000,000 per year, causing 600,000 deaths globally per year. The incidence of HCC has been rising in developed western countries in the last two decades, along with the emergence of hepatitis C virus infection and to the rise of immigration rates from HBV-endemic countries. In addition, even though the incidence of HCC reaches its highest peak among persons over 65 years, an increased incidence among younger individuals has been noted in the last two decades both in USA and Europe. In the last decades two kinds of HCC patients are more interesting, for clinical characteristics, than typical patients with HCC: elderly and HIV-positive patients. In fact due to the increase of the life expectancy in many countries, HCC represents a new challenge in this particular setting of patients.

In: Hepatocellular Carcinoma in the 3rd Millennium
Editors: M. Berretta and B. Cacopardo

ISBN: 978-1-63484-025-5

Chapter 1

THE EPIDEMIOLOGY OF HEPATOCELLULAR CARCINOMA

Marilia Rita Pinzone and Bruno Cacopardo*
Department of Clinical and Experimental Medicine,
Division of Infectious Diseases, University of Catania, Catania, Italy

ABSTRACT

Hepatocellular carcinoma (HCC) is the most common primary malignancy of the liver and the second most common cause of death from cancer worldwide. The leading risk factor for HCC is cirrhosis due to chronic hepatitis B and hepatitis C. The incidence of HCC differs greatly according to the geographic area. Regions with the highest incidence rates of liver cancer include Eastern and Southeastern Asia as well as Northern and Western Africa, which are endemic for hepatitis B virus infection. In most developed countries, the incidence of HCC is at low (Northern Europe) or intermediate (Southern Europe and Northern America) levels. In Western countries, Egypt and Japan hepatitis C virus infection is the main risk factor for HCC. However, upcoming risk factors include obesity, diabetes and nonalcoholic fatty liver disease. Considering that these factors are rapidly increasing in prevalence, they might account for a growing proportion of HCC cases in the future.

In this chapter, we review the key aspects of HCC epidemiology, with a focus on the incidence and mortality rates in Western countries.

INTRODUCTION

According to the GLOBOCAN database maintained by the International Agency for Research on Cancer (IARC), an estimated 782,000 primary liver cancer cases occurred worldwide in 2012 [1].

---

* Corresponding author: Bruno Cacopardo, Department of Clinical and Experimental Medicine, Division of Infectious Diseases, ARNAS Garibaldi Nesima, University of Catania, via Palermo 636, 95125 Catania, Italy. Tel: +39095 7598650, fax: +39 095 7598666, e-mail: cacopardobruno@inwind.it.

Liver cancer is the fifth most common cancer in men (554,000 cases in 2012) and the ninth in women (228,000 cases). In addition, it is the second most common cause of death from cancer worldwide, responsible for ~750,000 deaths annually [1]. Hepatocellular carcinoma (HCC) is the main histologic type of primary liver cancer, accounting for 70-85% of cases. In most cases, HCC develops in patients with cirrhosis, particularly those with chronic hepatitis B virus (HBV) or hepatitis C virus (HCV) infection. The burden of liver cancer mainly concentrates in developing countries, where chronic hepatitis B and C are highly prevalent. The prognosis of HCC generally is poor, with a 5-year survival rate of around 5% in the absence of any treatment [2]. In this chapter, we review the key aspects of HCC epidemiology, with a focus on the incidence and mortality rates in Western countries.

Primary Liver Cancer: A Global Epidemiological Overview

The incidence of HCC varies largely according to the geographical area: over 80% of cases occur in less developed regions (50% in China alone). Diagnostic confirmation of HCC is not routinely performed worldwide; as a consequence, it is easier to evaluate incidence rates of primary liver cancer rather than HCC. In fact, considering that HCC is the predominant subtype in most countries, primary liver cancer rates are an acceptable estimate of HCC rates. A notable exception is represented by countries with a high rate of intrahepatic cholangiocarcinoma, e.g., Thailand and Philippines [1].

In men, areas with the highest incidence rates of liver cancer include Eastern and Southeastern Asia (age-standardized rates (ASRs) 31.9 and 22.2 per 100,000 respectively). Northern and Western Africa have a moderately high incidence rate (11-20 cases per 100,000 male inhabitants).

In most developed countries, the incidence of liver cancer is at low (<5/100,000) or intermediate levels (5-10/100,000), with the lowest ASRs in Northern Europe (4.6 per 100,000) and intermediate rates in Southern Europe (ASRs 9.5 per 100,000) and Northern America (ASRs 9.3 per 100,000). An important exception in the developed world is represented by Japan, where the incidence of liver cancer is >20/100,000. In women, the highest incidence rates have been reported in Eastern Asia and Western Africa (ASRs 10.2 and 8.1 per 100,000 respectively) [1]. Incidence rates are 2- to 3-fold higher in men than in women. The reasons for this gender disparity are not completely understood: on the one hand, men have a higher prevalence of traditional risk factors for HCC, such as chronic HBV and HCV infection, alcohol abuse and smoking; on the other hand, the risk seems to be higher even after correcting for these confounders. The role of sexual hormones is still unclear: in nested case-control studies of HBV carriers in Taiwan and Shanghai, high serum levels of testosterone were associated with HCC risk [3]. In mouse models of HBV infection, the androgen pathway was reported to increase the transcription of HBV genes and conversely the HBV protein HBx was found to upregulate the transcription of androgen receptors [4, 5]. In other studies, estrogens were suggested to have a protective role against the progression of HBV infection. As for HCV, higher total serum levels of testosterone were associated with increased risk of advanced hepatic fibrosis in a small cohort of veterans with chronic HCV infection, although the authors did not report on the association with HCC [6].

HCC rarely occurs before the age of 40 years, except in populations where HBV is hyper-endemic. The mean age of diagnosis is 55-59 years in China and 63-65 years in Europe and North America. In low-risk populations, HCC reaches a peak among individuals aged 75 and older [2]. Unlike other cancers, HCC mortality rates are very close to the incidence rates, due to the poor prognosis associated with HCC. HCC incidence and mortality are slowly decreasing in high-risk countries, including China and Korea; the decrease is thought to reflect the reduction in HBV transmission through vaccine implementation and the reduction in food contamination with aflatoxins. In contrast to the decreasing trend in high-risk countries, the burden of HCC is increasing in several parts of the World, including the United States (US) and some European countries [2]. The epidemic of obesity and diabetes may contribute to the increasing trends observed in developed countries, because both obesity and diabetes are implicated in the development of nonalcoholic steatohepatitis (NASH), which may progress to cirrhosis and represents therefore a risk factor for HCC.

Focus on Western Countries: Incidence and Mortality Rates in the US and Europe

In the US, the Surveillance, Epidemiology and End Results (SEER) program collects incidence and survival data from cancer registries estimated to cover ~28% of the US population. In 2014, 33,190 new cases and 23,000 deaths are estimated to occur due to liver and biliary ducts cancer [7]. Analysis of data from the SEER registries showed that the incidence of HCC tripled in the US between 1975 and 2005, in particular among Hispanics, blacks and white middle-aged men [8]. The high prevalence of HCV infection among "baby-boomers," i.e., people born between 1945 and 1965, has been suggested to explain a substantial proportion of the increase in HCC rates in the US. Liver cancer incidence has been elevated historically among Asians/Pacific Islanders in comparison with other racial groups, because of the high prevalence of chronic HBV infection among older adults born outside the US [2]. The most recent data showed that HCC incidence was highest among Asians/Pacific Islanders (11.7/100,000) and lowest among white persons (4.2/100,000). Intermediate incidence rates were reported among Hispanics (9.5/100,000) and black people (7.5/100,000) [9]. However, after decades of increasing HCC incidence rates, during 2007-2010 the trend was no longer statistically significant, partly because of the reduction in HCC incidence rates among men aged 35-49 years and Asians/Pacific Islanders [9].

For this ethnic group, several factors are likely to have a role, including the implementation of HBV vaccination programs, the impact of antiviral therapy on HBV progression as well as changes in immigration patterns.

Overall liver cancer mortality rates increased during 2000-2010, driven by increasing mortality trends among whites, blacks and Hispanics (2.1%, 2.4% and 1.3% per year respectively). On the other hand, mortality rates significantly declined among Asians/Pacific Islanders (-1.6% per year) and among men aged 35-49 years in all ethnic groups [9]. Declining liver cancer mortality rates among young adults may suggest a possible decline in the overall US liver cancer mortality. This is what is happening in Japan, where liver cancer mortality peaked a generation earlier than in the US and a decrease in mortality due to liver cancer began around 1985, first in the sentinel group of 40-year old subjects [10, 11].

Reduced exposure to traditional risk factors for HCV such as injection drug use and contaminated blood product transfusion in the post-Second World War may have contributed to the declining trend.

The European Network of Cancer Registries provides estimates of cancer burden at the European and European Union (EU) member state level. According to the most recently available data, an estimated 63,420 liver (liver and intrahepatic bile ducts) cancer cases occurred in Europe in 2012 (ASR 6.2 per 100,000) [12, 13].

For the 27 countries of the EU (EU-27), 51,319 liver cancer cases were estimated to occur in 2012 (ASR 7 per 100,000). As expected, the incidence rate was higher in men than in women (ASR 10 vs. 3.3 respectively). The highest incidence rates were estimated in Moldova (ASR 12 per 100,000), Italy (ASR 10.5 per 100,000), France (ASR 9.5 per 100,000), Luxembourg (ASR 10.4 per 100,000) and Spain (ASR 8.6 per 100,000); on the other hand, the Netherlands (ASR 3.3 per 100,000), Iceland (ASR 3.4 per 100,000) and Norway (ASR 4.1 per 100,000) were the countries with the lowest estimated incidence rates. The male-to-female ratio was between two and four in most countries, with the greatest gender disparity in Portugal (4.8), France (4.6) and Switzerland (4.2) and the lowest in Bosnia and Herzegovina (1.5), Iceland (1.7), Albania (1.8) and Poland (1.8). Estimated mortality rates were very close to incidence rates, because of the poor survival rate associated with liver cancer. In 2012, there were an estimated 62,136 deaths due to liver cancer in Europe (ASR 5.9 per 100,000); the EU-27 accounted for an estimated 47,989 deaths (ASR 6.2 per 100,000). The highest mortality rates were estimated in Moldova (ASR 13.5 per 100,000), Romania (ASR 10.5 per 100,000) and Luxembourg (ASR 9.9 per 100,000) and the lowest in the Netherlands (ASR 2.8 per 100,000) and Norway (ASR 2.6 per 100,000) [12].

In some countries, the estimated mortality rates are higher than the incidence rates: an explanation is that the liver is the first site of metastasis for several malignancies and it may be problematic in cancer registries to distinguish accurately between primary and secondary liver cancer. A significant decline in male mortality from HCC has been reported over recent years in countries such as France and Italy, which had large upward trends until the mid-1990s, whereas slight upward trends were registered over the period 1980-2004 in Austria, Germany, Switzerland, and other Northern countries.

In women, a reduction in mortality has been observed in most European countries. The most favorable trends were reported among subjects aged 20-44 years for both males and females [14]. The changing prevalence of risk factors for HCC may have contributed to these trends: the decrease in southern European countries is thought to reflect screening of blood products for HCV and HBV, the reduction in alcohol consumption and smoking prevalence, as well as improved treatment for cirrhosis and/or liver cancer. In Southern Europe, HCV infection was highly prevalent among elderly people and this may explain the observed rise in liver cancer mortality up to the early 1990s and the subsequent decrease [14].

However, temporal trends in liver cancer incidence and mortality are often difficult to interpret because of the lack of standardized criteria across registries, along with changes in liver cancer coding procedures.

Moreover, few data on the prevalence and trends of hepatitis B and hepatitis C infection are available in several populations, limiting the possibility to adequately match trends in HCC incidence and mortality to underlying changes in risk-factor epidemiology.

The Epidemiology of Risk Factors for HCC

The overwhelming majority of HCC cases occur in patients with cirrhosis [2]. As a consequence, any cause of liver disease that may progress to cirrhosis should be considered a risk factor for HCC. Chronic viral hepatitis B and C account for more than 80% of cases worldwide. The epidemiology of HCC largely reflects the geographic distribution of HBV and HCV infection. In most high-risk countries of Africa and Asia, HBV infection and aflatoxins are the most important risk factors. In low-risk countries, HCV infection, alcohol abuse and metabolic syndrome have a major role. An exception is represented by Japan and Egypt, where the main risk factor for HCC is HCV infection [15].

HBV infection is the most common cause of HCC worldwide, accounting for 50-55% of cases. According to the World Health Organization (WHO), 350 million people around the world are estimated to be chronically infected by HBV [16]. In endemic areas, HBV is usually acquired by vertical and perinatal transmission; on the contrary, in low-prevalence regions HBV infection is usually acquired in adulthood through sexual and parenteral routes. The risk to develop chronic infection is significantly higher when infection is acquired during childhood (>90% vs. 5-10% of adults). The number of HCC cases attributed to HBV infection ranges from 70% in South Korea to 15% in Japan [17]; in Western countries, HBsAg seroprevalence among patients with HCC varies widely, being 3% in Sweden, 9% in the United States, 19% in Italy and 55% in Greece [15]. In a large study in Taiwan, Beasley et al. followed 22,707 male Chinese government employees for more than a decade, of whom 3,454 (15%) were HBsAg negative [18]. The age-adjusted annual incidence of HCC was 495 per 100,000 in HBsAg carriers compared with 5 per 100,000 in HBsAg-negative men. Chronic HBV infection was associated with a 98-fold higher relative risk (RR) for HCC. The lifetime risk of developing HCC is 15 to 20 times higher among HBV-infected subjects in comparison with the general population and is estimated to be 10% to 25% [19, 20, 21]. A systematic review of the natural history of chronic HBV infection in Asia reported the incidence rate of HCC to be 0.2 per 100 person-years in inactive carriers, 0.6 person-years for those with chronic HBV infection without cirrhosis, and 3.7 person-years for those with compensated cirrhosis [22]. In Western countries, there is a lack of high-quality studies: however, available data suggest that HCC incidence rate ranges from 0.02 per 100 person-years in inactive carriers to 2.2 per 100 person-years in subjects with compensated cirrhosis [2]. Though most HBV-infected individuals who develop HCC have cirrhosis, it is important to note that up to 30% of cases develop in noncirrhotic patients. On the contrary, almost all cases of HCV-related HCC occur in patients with cirrhosis. The fraction of HCC attributable to HCV is 30% and HCV appears to be the major risk factor for HCC in developed countries. According to the WHO, the global prevalence of HCV infection is estimated to be 3%, with more than 150 million chronic carriers at risk of developing liver cirrhosis and/or liver cancer [23]. Up to 85% of new cases may progress to chronic infection. Egypt has the highest rates of chronic HCV infection (approximately 20%), as a consequence of the past practice of intravenous therapy for schistosomiasis. Most European countries report a prevalence rate in the general population ranging between 0.003 and 4.5%, with high prevalence rates (>1.2%) in Southern and Eastern countries and low prevalence rates (≤0.1%) in Northern countries [24]. In the US, 1.3% of the population have antibodies to HCV [25]. 15-35% of subjects with chronic HCV develop cirrhosis in 25-30 years and the annual incidence of HCC among cirrhotic patients with HCV infection is 1 to 4% [26, 27]. The RR of developing HCC is 15- to 20-fold higher among HCV-infected subjects in comparison to uninfected ones; a meta-analysis of case-control studies showed that anti-HCV positive individuals had 17 times the risk of HCC when compared with anti-HCV-negative subjects [28]. Markers of HCV infection have been reported in 80-90% of HCC cases in Japan, 44-66% in Italy and 30-50% in the US [2, 29-31]. Two meta-analysis reported that HBV and HCV have an additive effect on the risk of developing HCC. Donato et al. found that the odds ratio (OR) for HCC was 165 in coinfected patients in comparison to an OR of 17 for HCV-infected subjects and an OR of 23 for HBV carriers [32]. A meta-analysis of 32 case-control studies carried out in China reported that the pooled OR for HCC was 14.1 for HBsAg-positive subjects, 4.6 for anti-HCV/HCV RNA positive individuals and 35.7 for coinfected ones [33].

However, an updated meta-analysis based on more recent studies (2000-2009) described opposing results: a subadditive effect of HBV and HCV coinfection was reported in recently published studies, cohort studies and studies conducted in HBV/HCV non-endemic areas. Conversely, an additive effect was reported in older studies, case-control studies and studies conducted in HCV endemic areas. From a pathogenetic point of view, the subadditive effect of HCV/HBV coinfection may be explained considering the reciprocal interference of one virus on the replication of the other [34].

Human immunodeficiency virus (HIV)-infected individuals have been suggested to have a 6-fold to 7-fold higher risk of developing HCC. The higher prevalence of chronic viral hepatitis among HIV-positive people is likely to have a significant impact, though HIV itself may promote fibrogenesis, accelerating the progression of HCV- and HBV-related liver disease to cirrhosis and HCC [35, 36].

In sub-Saharan Africa and Asia, dietary exposure to aflatoxins contributes to the development of HCC. Aflatoxins are carcinogens produced by Aspergillus species (A. *flavus* and A. *parasiticus*), infesting grain, peanuts, legumes, corn, particularly when they are stored in high-moisture conditions [37]. It is estimated that aflatoxins may play a causative role in 4.6-28.2% of all global HCC cases [38]. The risk of developing HCC in subjects exposed to aflatoxins and chronic HBV infection is markedly increased in comparison to those exposed to HBV or aflatoxins alone. In endemic regions, HBV is usually acquired early in life and exposure to aflatoxins begins even earlier, *in utero*. Aflatoxins and HBV have a synergistic impact on hepatocarcinogenesis: in a prospective cohort study carried out in China the risk of HCC was 4-fold greater among persons with increased levels of aflatoxin metabolites in urine, 7-fold greater among persons chronically infected with HBV and 60-fold greater among individuals with both risk factors [39].

According to the WHO report “European Status Report on Alcohol and Health 2010,” Europe is the region with the heaviest alcohol consumption in the world [40]. Chronic alcohol consumption is the leading cause of cirrhosis in Europe. Although there is weak evidence that ethanol is a carcinogen, its role in the development of cirrhosis is well-established. Considering that most cases of HCC occur in cirrhotic livers, it is not surprising to find that alcohol consumption may have a synergistic effect with both HBV and HCV on HCC risk. Moreover, heavy alcohol drinking has been associated with increased risk of developing HCC in the absence of viral infection: a meta-analysis of 20 studies, including 2294 patients with HCC, reported a direct relation between the risk of developing HCC and increasing alcohol intake.

The RR for HCC was 1.36 (95% confidence interval (CI) 1.23-1.51) for 50 g/day, and 1.86 (95% CI 1.53-2.27) for 100 g/day [41]. The impact of low or moderate alcohol intake on HCC risk remains unclear.

Nonalcoholic fatty liver disease (NAFLD) is the most common form of chronic liver disease in the US. NAFLD encompasses a clinicopathologic spectrum of disease ranging from hepatic steatosis to NASH, which can progress to cirrhosis and its complications, including hepatic failure and HCC [42]. In the US, NAFLD is estimated to affect 30% of the population and as high as 90% of the morbidly obese [43].

Similar rates have been reported in European countries [44-46]. One-third to one-half of patients with NASH have progressive fibrosis over 3 to 5 years and up to 20% may develop cirrhosis over 10 years [47]. Longitudinal studies have shown the prevalence of HCC to be 0%-0.5% in NAFLD and 0%-2.8% in NASH over time periods of up to 20 years [48-51]. Conversely, increased risk has been reported in the setting of NASH-cirrhosis, though the rates of HCC are lower when compared to cirrhosis due to chronic viral hepatitis [52-56].

Diabetes mellitus and obesity are implicated in the development of NAFLD but have also been independently associated with the risk of HCC. In a large cohort of veterans, El Serag et al. found that the incidence of HCC was significantly higher among patients with diabetes in comparison to those without diabetes (incidence rate 2.39 vs. 0.87 per 10,000 person-years). The risk remained higher even after excluding patients with underlying liver disease or other risk factors for HCC [57].

Several large population-based cohorts across Europe and the US have confirmed patients with diabetes to have a 1.86-fold to 4-fold higher risk of HCC [58-61]. Analogously, obesity has been associated with a 1.5-4 increased risk of HCC [62-65]. Obesity and diabetes have been suggested to have a synergistic effect: in a case-control study from Italy, the authors enrolled 185 patients with HCC and 404 hospital controls. They found that obesity and diabetes were associated with HCC risk (OR 1.9 and 3.7 respectively).

The association was still significant among subjects without chronic viral hepatitis (OR 3.5 for both obesity and diabetes) and a 10-fold increased risk was observed when these two conditions were combined [66].

Conclusion

HCC is a leading cause of cancer-related mortality worldwide. HBV infection still represents the major risk factor for HCC, although its impact is expected to decline in future generations because of vaccination programs. The incidence of HCV should also decline as a consequence of control measures, such as screening of blood and blood products, which have been routinely introduced in most developed countries in the early 1990s.

However, both vaccination for HBV infection and public health measures for HCV infection do not reduce the burden of patients living with chronic viral hepatitis at risk of developing HCC.

For those subjects, approaches to reduce HCC incidence rates include antiviral treatment, reduction of cofactors for liver disease progression, including alcohol, obesity and diabetes, and adequate surveillance of high-risk individuals.

References

[1] Ferlay, J., Soerjomataram, I., Ervik, M., Dikshit, R., Eser, S., Mathers, C., Rebelo, M., Parkin, D. M., Forman, D., Bray, F. GLOBOCAN 2012 v1.0, *Cancer Incidence and Mortality Worldwide: IARC CancerBase No. 11 [Internet]*. Lyon, France: International Agency for Research on Cancer; 2013. Available from: http://globocan.iarc.fr, accessed on 8/14/2014.

[2] El-Serag, H. B. Epidemiology of viral hepatitis and hepatocellular carcinoma. *Gastroenterology* 2012; 142(6): 1264-1273.

[3] Yuan, J. M., Ross, R. K., Stanczyk, F. Z., Govindarajan, S., Gao, Y. T., Henderson, B. E., Yu, M. C. A cohort study of serum testosterone and hepatocellular carcinoma in Shanghai, China. *Int. J. Cancer* 1995; 63(4): 491-493.

[4] Chiu, C. M., Yeh, S. H., Chen, P. J., Kuo, T. J., Chang, C. J., Chen, P. J., Yang, W. J., Chen, D. S. Hepatitis B virus X protein enhances androgen receptor responsive gene expression depending on androgen level. *Proc. Natl. Acad. Sci. US* 2007; 104(8): 2571-2578.

[5] Yeh, S. H., Chen, P. J. Gender disparity of hepatocellular carcinoma: the roles of sex hormones. *Oncology* 2010; 78(S1): 172-179.

[6] White, D. L., Tavakoli-Tabasi, S., Kuzniarek, J., Pascua, R., Ramsey, D. J., El-Serag, H. B. Higher serum testosterone is associated with increased risk of advanced hepatitis C-related liver disease in males. *Hepatology* 2012; 55(3): 759-768.

[7] SEER Cancer. *Surveillance Epidemiology and End Results*. Available from: http:// www.seer.cancer.gov/about, accessed on 8/14/2014.

[8] Altekruse, S. F., McGlynn, K. A., Reichman, M. E. Hepatocellular carcinoma incidence, mortality, and survival trends in the United States from 1975 to 2005. *J. Clin. Oncol.* 2009; 27(9): 1485-1491.

[9] Altekruse, S. F., Henley, S. J., Cucinelli, J. E., McGlynn, K. A. Changing Hepatocellular Carcinoma Incidence and Liver Cancer Mortality Rates in the United States. *Am. J. Gastroenterol.* 2014; 109(4): 542-553.

[10] Saika, K., Matsuda, T. Time trends in liver cancer mortality (1980-2008) in Japan, the US and Europe. *Jpn. J. Clin. Oncol.* 2012; 42(1): 84.

[11] Matsuda, T., Saika, K. Trends in liver cancer mortality rates in Japan, US, UK, France and Korea based on the WHO mortality database. *Jpn. J. Clin. Oncol.* 2012; 42(4): 360-361.

[12] Steliarova-Foucher, E., O'Callaghan, M., Ferlay, J., Masuyer, E., Forman, D., Comber, H., Bray, F. *European Cancer Observatory: Cancer Incidence, Mortality, Prevalence and Survival in Europe. Version 1.0* (September 2012) European Network of Cancer Registries, International Agency for Research on Cancer. Available from: http://eco.iarc .fr, accessed on 8/15/2014.

[13] Ferlay, J., Steliarova-Foucher, E., Lortet-Tieulent, J., Rosso, S., Coebergh, J. W., Comber, H., Forman, D., Bray, F. Cancer incidence and mortality patterns in Europe: estimates for 40 countries in 2012. *Eur. J. Cancer* 2013; 49(6): 1374-1403.

[14] Bosetti, C., Levi, F., Boffetta, P., Lucchini, F., Negri, E., La Vecchia, C. Trends in Mortality from Hepatocellular Carcinoma in Europe, 1980-2004. *Hepatology* 2008; 48 (1):137-145.

[15] Raza, S. A., Clifford, G. M., Franceschi, S. Worldwide variation in the relative importance of hepatitis B and hepatitis C viruses in hepatocellular carcinoma: a systematic review. *Br. J. Cancer* 2007; 96(7): 1127-1134.

[16] WHO. Hepatitis B 2014. *Fact sheet No. 204*. Available from: http://www.who.int/mediacentre/factsheets/fs204/en/, accessed on 9/13/14.

[17] Kim, S. R., Kudo, M., Hino, O., Han, K. H., Chung, Y. H., Lee, H. S.; Organizing Committee of Japan-Korea Liver Symposium. Epidemiology of hepatocellular carcinoma in Japan and Korea. *Oncology* 2008; 75(S1): 13-16.

[18] Beasley, R. P. Hepatitis B virus. The major etiology of hepatocellular carcinoma. *Cancer* 1988; 61(10): 1942-1956.

[19] Shi, J., Zhu, L., Liu, S., Xie, W. F. A meta-analysis of case-control studies on the combined effect of hepatitis B and C virus infections in causing hepatocellular carcinoma in China. *Br. J. Cancer* 2005; 92(3): 607-612.

[20] Donato, F., Boffetta, P., Puoti, M. A meta-analysis of epidemiological studies on the combined effect of hepatitis B and C virus infections in causing hepatocellular carcinoma. *Int. J. Cancer* 1998; 75(3): 347-354.

[21] Seeger, C., Mason, W. S. Hepatitis B virus biology. *Microbiol. Mol. Biol. Rev.* 2000; 64 (1): 51-68.

[22] Fattovich, G., Bortolotti, F., Donato, F. Natural history of chronic hepatitis B: special emphasis on disease progression and prognostic factors. *J. Hepatol.* 2008; 48(2): 335-352.

[23] WHO. Hepatitis C 2014. *Fact sheet No. 164*. Available from: http://www.who.int/mediacentre/factsheets/fs164/en/, accessed on 9/13/14.

[24] Muhlberger, N., Schwarzer, R., Lettmeier, B., Sroczynski, G., Zeuzem, S., Siebert, U. HCV -related burden of disease in Europe: a systematic assessment of incidence, prevalence, morbidity, and mortality. *BMC Public Health* 2009; 9: 34.

[25] Ditah, I., Ditah, F., Devaki, P., Ewelukwa, O., Ditah, C., Njei, B., Luma, H. N., Charlton, M. The changing epidemiology of hepatitis C virus infection in the United States: National Health and Nutrition Examination Survey 2001 through 2010. *J. Hepatol.* 2014; 60(4): 691-698.

[26] Freeman, A. J., Dore, G. J., Law, M. G., Thorpe, M., Von Overbeck, J., Lloyd, A. R., Marinos, G., Kaldor, J. M. Estimating progression to cirrhosis in chronic hepatitis C virus infection. *Hepatology* 2001; 34(4 Pt 1): 809-816.

[27] Fattovich, G., Giustina, G., Degos, F., Tremolada, F., Diodati, G., Almasio, P., Nevens, F., Solinas, A., Mura, D., Brouwer, J. T., Thomas, H., Njapoum, C., Casarin, C., Bonetti, P., Fuschi, P., Basho, J., Tocco, A., Bhalla, A., Galassini, R., Noventa, F., Schalm, S. W., Realdi, G. Morbidity and mortality in compensated cirrhosis type C: a retrospective follow-up study of 384 patients. *Gastroenterology* 1997; 112(2): 463-472.

[28] Donato, F., Tagger, A., Gelatti, U., Parrinello, G., Boffetta, P., Albertini, A., Decarli, A., Trevisi, P., Ribero, M. L., Martelli, C., Porru, S., Nardi, G. Alcohol and hepatocellular carcinoma: the effect of lifetime intake and hepatitis virus infections in men and women. *Am. J. Epidemiol.* 2002; 155(4): 323-331.

[29] Fasani, P., Sangiovanni, A., De Fazio, C., Borzio, M., Bruno, S., Ronchi, G., Del Ninno, E., Colombo, M. High prevalence of multinodular hepatocellular carcinoma in patients with cirrhosis attributable to multiple risk factors. *Hepatology* 1999; 29(6): 1704-1707.

[30] Stroffolini, T., Andreone, P., Andriulli, A., Ascione, A., Craxì, A., Chiaramonte, M., Galante, D., Manghisi, O. G., Mazzanti, R., Medaglia, C., Pilleri, G., Rapaccini, G. L., Albanese, M., Taliani, G., Tosti, M. E., Villa, E., Gasbarrini, G. Gross pathologic types of hepatocellular carcinoma in Italy. *Oncology* 1999; 56(3): 189-192.

[31] Yoshizawa, H. Hepatocellular carcinoma associated with hepatitis C virus infection in Japan: projection to other countries in the foreseeable future. *Oncology* 2002; 62(S1): 8-17.

[32] Donato, F., Boffetta, P., Puoti, M. A meta-analysis of epidemiological studies on the combined effect of hepatitis B and C virus infections in causing hepatocellular carcinoma. *Int. J. Cancer* 1998; 75(3): 347-354.

[33] Shi, J., Zhu, L., Liu, S., Xie, W. F. A meta-analysis of case-control studies on the combined effect of hepatitis B and C virus infections in causing hepatocellular carcinoma in China. *Br. J. Cancer* 2005; 92(3): 607-612.

[34] Cho, L. Y., Yang, J. J., Ko, K. P., Park, B., Shin, A., Lim, M. K., Oh, J. K., Park, S., Kim, Y. J., Shin, H. R., Yoo, K. Y., Park, S. K. Coinfection of hepatitis B and C viruses and risk of hepatocellular carcinoma: systematic review and meta-analysis. *Int. J. Cancer* 2011; 128(1): 176-184.

[35] Pinzone, M. R., Fiorica, F., Di Rosa, M., Malaguarnera, G., Malaguarnera, L., Cacopardo, B., Zanghì, G., Nunnari, G. Non-AIDS-defining cancers among HIV-infected people. *Eur. Rev. Med. Pharmacol. Sci.* 2012; 16(10): 1377-1388.

[36] Nunnari, G., Berretta, M., Pinzone, M. R., Di Rosa, M., Berretta, S., Cunsolo, G., Malaguarnera, M., Cosentino, S., De Paoli, P., Schnell, J. M., Cacopardo, B. Hepatocellular carcinoma in HIV positive patients. *Eur. Rev. Med. Pharmacol. Sci.* 2012; 16(9): 1257-1270.

[37] IARC. In: *Working Group on the Evaluation of Carcinogenic Risks to Humans, International Agency for Research on Cancer. Some traditional herbal medicines, some mycotoxins, naphthalene and styrene*, vol. 2010. Lyon (France): International Agency for Research on Cancer; 2002.

[38] Liu, Y., Wu, F. Global burden of aflatoxin-induced hepatocellular carcinoma: a risk assessment. *Environ. Health Perspect.* 2010; 118(6): 818-824.

[39] Qian, G. S., Ross, R. K., Yu, M. C., Yuan, J. M., Gao, Y. T., Henderson, B. E., Wogan, G. N., Groopman, J. D. A follow-up study of urinary markers of aflatoxin exposure and liver cancer risk in Shanghai, People's Republic of China. *Cancer Epidemiol. Biomarkers Prev.* 1994; 3(1): 3-10.

[40] WHO. *European Status Report on Alcohol and Health: World Health Organization.* Regional Office for Europe; 2010.

[41] Bagnardi, V., Blangiardo, M., La Vecchia, C., Corrao, G. A meta-analysis of alcohol drinking and cancer risk. *Br. J. Cancer* 2001; 85(11): 1700-1705.

[42] Ong, J. P., Younossi, Z. M. Epidemiology and natural history of NAFLD and NASH. *Clin. Liver Dis.* 2007; 11(1): 1-16, vii.

[43] Torres, D. M., Harrison, S. A. Diagnosis and therapy of nonalcoholic steatohepatitis. *Gastroenterology* 2008; 134(6): 1682-1698.

[44] Bedogni, G., Miglioli, L., Masutti, F., Castiglione, A., Croce, L. S., Tiribelli, C., Bellentani, S. Incidence and natural course of fatty liver in the general population: the Dionysos study. *Hepatology* 2007; 46(5): 1387-1391.

[45] Haring, R., Wallaschofski, H., Nauck, M., Dorr, M., Baumeister, S. E., Volzke, H. Ultrasonographic hepatic steatosis increases prediction of mortality risk from elevated serum gamma-glutamyl transpeptidase levels. *Hepatology* 2009; 50(5): 1403-1411.

[46] Castellares, C., Barreiro, P., Martin-Carbonero, L., Labarga, P., Vispo, M. E., Casado, R., Galindo, L., García-Gascó, P., García-Samaniego, J., Soriano, V. Liver cirrhosis in HIV-infected patients: prevalence, aetiology and clinical outcome. *J. Viral Hepat.* 2008; 15(3): 165-172.

[47] Farrell, G. C., Larter, C. Z. Nonalcoholic Fatty Liver Disease: From Steatosis to Cirrhosis. *Hepatology* 2006; 43(2 S1): S99-S112.

[48] Adams, L. A., Lymp, J. F., St Sauver, J., Sanderson, S. O., Lindor, K. D., Feldstein, A., Angulo, P. The natural history of nonalcoholic fatty liver disease: a population-based cohort study. *Gastroenterology* 2005; 129(1): 113-121.

[49] Ekstedt, M., Franzen, L. E., Mathiesen, U. L., Thorelius, L., Holmqvist, M., Bodemar, G., Kechagias, S. Long-term follow-up of patients with NAFLD and elevated liver enzymes. *Hepatology* 2006; 44(4): 865-873.

[50] Ong, J. P., Pitts, A., Younossi, Z. M. Increased overall mortality and liver-related mortality in non-alcoholic fatty liver disease. *J. Hepatol.* 2008; 49(4): 608-612.

[51] Rafiq, N., Bai, C., Fang, Y., Srishord, M., McCullough, A., Gramlich, T., Younossi, Z. M. Long-term follow-up of patients with nonalcoholic fatty liver. *Clin. Gastroenterol. Hepatol.* 2009; 7(2): 234-238.

[52] Ratziu, V., Bonyhay, L., Di Martino, V., Charlotte, F., Cavallaro, L., Sayegh-Tainturier, M. H., Giral, P., Grimaldi, A., Opolon, P., Poynard, T. Survival, liver failure, and hepatocellular carcinoma in obesity-related cryptogenic cirrhosis. *Hepatology* 2002; 35 (6): 1485-1493.

[53] Sanyal, A. J., Banas, C., Sargeant, C., Luketic, V. A., Sterling, R. K., Stravitz, R. T., Shiffman, M. L., Heuman, D., Coterrell, A., Fisher, R. A., Contos, M. J., Mills, A. S. Similarities and differences in outcomes of cirrhosis due to nonalcoholic steatohepatitis and hepatitis C. *Hepatology* 2006; 43(4): 682-689.

[54] Yatsuji, S., Hashimoto, E., Tobari, M., Taniai, M., Tokushige, K., Shiratori, K. Clinical features and outcomes of cirrhosis due to non-alcoholic steatohepatitis compared with cirrhosis caused by chronic hepatitis C. *J. Gastroenterol. Hepatol.* 2009; 24(2): 248-254.

[55] Ascha, M. S., Hanouneh, I. A., Lopez, R., Tamimi, T. A., Feldstein, A. F., Zein, N. N. The incidence and risk factors of hepatocellular carcinoma in patients with nonalcoholic steatohepatitis. *Hepatology* 2010; 51(6): 1972-1978.

[56] Bhala, N., Angulo, P., van der Poorten, D., Lee, E., Hui, J. M., Saracco, G., Adams, L. A., Charatcharoenwitthaya, P., Topping, J. H., Bugianesi, E., Day, C. P., George, J. The natural history of nonalcoholic fatty liver disease with advanced fibrosis or cirrhosis: an international collaborative study. *Hepatology* 2011; 54(4): 1208-1216.

[57] El-Serag, H. B., Tran, T., Everhart, J. E. Diabetes increases the risk of chronic liver disease and hepatocellular carcinoma. *Gastroenterology* 2004; 126(2): 460-468.

[58] Adami, H. O., Chow, W. H., Nyren, O., Berne, C., Linet, M. S., Ekbom, A., Wolk, A., McLaughlin, J. K., Fraumeni, J. F. Jr. Excess risk of primary liver cancer in patients with diabetes mellitus. *J. Natl. Cancer Inst.* 1996; 88(20): 1472-1477.

[59] Wideroff, L., Gridley, G., Mellemkjaer, L., Chow, W. H., Linet, M., Keehn, S., Borch-Johnsen, K., Olsen, J. H. Cancer incidence in a population based cohort of patients

hospitalized with diabetes mellitus in Denmark. *J. Natl. Cancer Inst.* 1997; 89(18): 1360-1365.

[60] Lagiou, P., Kuper, H., Stuver, S. O., Tzonou, A., Trichopoulos, D., Adami, H. O. Role of diabetes mellitus in the etiology of hepatocellular carcinoma. *J. Natl. Cancer Inst.* 2000; 92(13): 1096-1099.

[61] Davila, J. A., Morgan, R. O., Shaib, Y., McGlynn, K. A., El-Serag, H. B. Diabetes increases the risk of hepatocellular carcinoma in the United States: a population based case control study. *Gut* 2005; 54(4): 533-539.

[62] Wolk, A., Gridley, G., Svensson, M., Nyren, O., McLaughlin, J. K., Fraumeni, J. F., Adam, H. O. A prospective study of obesity and cancer risk (Sweden). *Cancer Causes Control* 2001; 12(1): 13-21.

[63] Calle, E. E., Rodriguez, C., Walker-Thurmond, K., Thun, M. J. Overweight, obesity, and mortality from cancer in a prospectively studied cohort of US adults. *N. Engl. J. Med.* 2003; 348(17): 1625-1638.

[64] Moller, H., Mellemgaard, A., Lindvig, K., Olsen, J. H. Obesity and cancer risk: a Danish record-linkage study. *Eur. J. Cancer* 1994; 30A(3): 344-350.

[65] Oh, S. W., Yoon, Y. S., Shin, S. A. Effects of excess weight on cancer incidences depending on cancer sites and histologic findings among men: Korea National Health Insurance Corporation Study. *J. Clin. Oncol.* 2005; 23(21): 4742-4754.

[66] Polesel, J., Zucchetto, A., Montella, M., Dal Maso, L., Crispo, A., La Vecchia, C., Serraino, D., Franceschi, S., Talamini, R. The impact of obesity and diabetes mellitus on the risk of hepatocellular carcinoma. *Ann. Oncol.* 2009; 20(2): 353-358.

In: Hepatocellular Carcinoma in the 3rd Millennium
Editors: M. Berretta and B. Cacopardo
ISBN: 978-1-63484-025-5

Chapter 2

Risk Factors for Hepatocellular Carcinoma

Marilia Rita Pinzone, Giuseppe Nunnari and Bruno Cacopardo*

Department of Clinical and Experimental Medicine,
Division of Infectious Diseases, University of Catania, Catania, Italy

Abstract

Hepatocellular carcinoma (HCC) is the second most common cause of death from cancer worldwide. The vast majority of cases occur in the setting of cirrhosis, usually due to hepatitis B virus (HBV) and hepatitis C virus (HCV) infection. In developed countries, chronic alcohol abuse is a significant risk factor for advanced liver disease and HCC; in addition, in Western countries obesity and diabetes are growing epidemics, which significantly contribute to the development of non-alcoholic fatty liver disease (NAFLD). NAFLD is an emerging risk factor for cirrhosis and HCC. Metabolic liver diseases, in particular hereditary hemochromatosis, account for a small number of liver cancers. In several regions of the world, including sub-Saharan Africa, Eastern Asia and parts of South America, aflatoxin exposure in food is a significant risk factor for HCC.

Unlike other cancers, risk factors for HCC can usually be identified at an individual level; moreover, the majority of risk factors are preventable. Vaccination against HBV is the most efficient primary prevention measure available in high-incidence countries, whereas antiviral treatment for HBV and HCV may reduce liver disease progression and the risk of HCC. Lifestyle modification, including weight loss and promotion of physical exercise, may have a significant impact in the management of NAFLD and its complications, including HCC.

* Corresponding author: Bruno Cacopardo, Department of Clinical and Experimental Medicine, Division of Infectious Diseases, ARNAS Garibaldi Nesima, University of Catania, via Palermo 636, 95125 Catania, Italy. Tel: +39095 7598650, fax: +39 095 7598666, e-mail: cacopardobruno@inwind.it.

INTRODUCTION

Hepatocellular carcinoma (HCC) is the second most common cause of death from cancer worldwide, responsible for ~750,000 deaths annually [1]. The vast majority of cases occur in the setting of cirrhosis, usually due to hepatitis B virus (HBV) and hepatitis C virus infection (HCV) [2]. In developed countries, chronic alcohol abuse is a significant risk factor for cirrhosis and HCC; in addition, in Western countries obesity and diabetes are growing epidemics, which significantly contribute to the development of non-alcoholic fatty liver disease (NAFLD). NAFLD is an emerging risk factor for the development of cirrhosis and HCC. Metabolic liver diseases, in particular hereditary hemochromatosis, account for a small number of liver cancers. In several regions, including sub-Saharan Africa, Eastern Asia and parts of South America, aflatoxin exposure in food is a significant risk factor for HCC [2].

In this chapter, we describe the main risk factors for HCC, with a focus on chronic viral hepatitis, alcohol abuse and NAFLD.

CHRONIC VIRAL HEPATITIS

Hepatitis B: HBV infection is the most common cause of HCC worldwide [2]. HBV is a DNA virus belonging to the *Hepadnaviridae* family. HBV transmission may occur by exposure to contaminated blood, as well as through sexual and other parenteral routes. In endemic countries, infection is usually acquired by vertical and perinatal transmission. The risk of developing a chronic infection is significantly higher among newborns and children (up to 80-90% of cases) in comparison to adults. The fraction of HCC attributable to HBV varies from less than 20% in the United States to 65% in China and Far East [3].

Most of HCC cases arise in the setting of cirrhosis. However, chronic HBV infection is a risk factor for HCC *per se*, even in the absence of cirrhosis. Multiple mechanisms contribute to the development of HCC, including liver chronic inflammation, induction of oxidative stress and direct viral effects. The direct role of HBV in carcinogenesis is primarily related to its capability to integrate in the host genome, causing insertional mutagenesis of cancer-related genes and increased chromosomal instability [4]. In fact, HBV DNA persists in infected hepatocytes both as episomal nuclear cccDNA and integrated DNA [5]. Viral insertions in "hot spots" may lead to the oncogenic transformation of infected cells. HBV preferentially integrates in genomic regions encoding for cell regulatory genes involved in survival, proliferation and apoptosis. In a recent study, HBV integration was described in more than 80% of HBV-associated HCC and was significantly more frequent in HCC tissues in comparison to the surrounding normal tissues [6]. Around 40% of HBV breakpoints within the HBV genome were located within a 1,800-bp region where the viral enhancer, X gene and core gene were located. The authors also identified some recurrent HBV integration events located in three cancer-related genes, namely telomerase reverse transcriptase (TERT), MLL4 and CCNE1. HBV integration in these regions was associated with up-regulated gene expression in tumoral tissue in comparison with normal one [6]. Some viral proteins, especially the HBx transactivator, are important cofactors in the oncogenetic process. The integrated HBx gene product may contribute directly to chromosomal instability and interfere with the mitotic phase, by interacting with a component of the mitotic checkpoint complex

(BubR1) [7]. Moreover, HBx has been reported to inhibit pituitary tumor-transforming gene 1 (PTTG1) ubiquitination, which in turn impairs its degradation by the proteasome, leading to accumulation of PTTG1, a protein implicated in inhibition of sister chromatid separation during mitosis [8].

The HBx protein has been shown to promote cell proliferation: it is able to trans-activate several cellular promoters and enhancers containing binding sites of nuclear transcription factors involved in cell growth, including the activator protein 1 (AP-1), AP-2, cAMP response element-binding (CREB) protein, TATA box-binding protein (TBP) and CCAAT enhancer-binding protein (c-EBP) [9, 10]. Moreover, it may activate the nuclear factor kappa-B (NF-kB) and STAT-3 pathways, the Ras-Raf-MAPK pathway, the PI3K-Akt pathway and the Src-dependent pathway [11-15].

HBx has also been associated with deregulated cell proliferation: in fact, it is able to inhibit the tumor suppressor retinoblastoma (pRb) signaling, which led to an increase in E2F1 activity and a subsequent continuous growth of HBV-infected cells [16]. HBx also modulates the DNA-binding specificity of the p53 tumor suppressor, altering the expression of its target genes. Of interest, p53 has been shown to repress HBV transcription and HBx may act as a co-repressor of the p53 promoter [17]. Along with pre-S2, HBx may up-regulate the expression and activity of hTERT, a crucial step in tumorigenesis [18, 19]. HBx may also modulate hypoxia-induced angiogenesis in HCC. In fact, it has been associated with increased expression of several factors involved in angiogenesis, such as inducible nitric oxide synthase (iNOS), hypoxia-inducible factor-1alpha (HIF-1α), angiopoietin-2 (Ang2) and vascular endothelial growth factor (VEGF) [20-23]. HBx is also able to promote the metastatic phenotype of tumoral cells, by modulate the expression and activation of matrix metalloproteinases (MMPs) [24-26]. HBx may be responsible for epigenetic changes, including hypermethylation or hypomethylation of tumor suppressor and tumor promoting genes respectively. In addition, HBx may alter the expression of certain microRNAs implicated in tumorigenesis [27].

Several virus-related and host-related factors may increase the risk of developing HCC among subjects with chronic HBV infection. Male gender and increasing age have been associated with greater risk of HCC [2]. Co-infection with Hepatitis D virus (HDV) is considered a risk factor: although HDV has not been directly associated with hepatocarcinogenesis, it probably boosts HCC development by increasing the severity of liver disease. As described elsewhere in this book, co-infection with HCV and/or HIV is also considered a risk factor for HCC. Analogously, alcohol abuse, smoking and dietary exposure to aflatoxins may contribute to HCC development [2].

Several genetic association studies have assessed the susceptible genetic variants for HBV-related HCC. These studies have been mainly conducted on Asian populations and should be validated in populations with different ethnicity to be applicable in clinical practice. The loss of heterozygosity on the KIF1B locus has been identified as a susceptibility marker for HCC in patients with chronic HBV as well as variations at chromosome 8p12. Some retrospective case-control studies have used a candidate gene approach to identify genes associated with HCC in patients with HBV. Some genes, such as cytotoxic T-lymphocyte antigen 4 gene, the promoter region of the MCM7 gene and enhancer II (EnhII), basal core promoter (BCP), and pre-core regions of HBV genes have been associated with HCC development [28-32]. However, these studies have been conducted on selected patients and selected samples (surgical resected HCC), limiting the general applicability of these findings.

Both HBV DNA serum levels and HBV genotype may affect the risk of developing HCC. In Asian studies, genotype C has been associated with more severe liver disease and higher risk of HCC when compared with genotype B. In Western Europe and North America genotype D has been associated with higher incidence of HCC in comparison with genotype A. Other studies have associated genotype B with the development of HCC in young subjects without cirrhosis [33, 34].

Patients with higher levels of HBV replication, as documented by high serum levels of HBV DNA and/or HbeAg positivity, have increased risk of HCC. In a cohort of 11,893 men in Taiwan, the incidence of HCC was significantly higher among HBsAg-positive and HbeAg-positive patients (1169 per 100,000 person-year) in comparison to those who were only HBsAg-positive (324 per 100,000 person-years) and those who were HBsAg-negative (39 per 100,000 person-years) [35]. In a community-based prospective study in Taiwan, the REVEAL-HBV study, the incidence of cirrhosis and HCC was significantly correlated with the levels of HBV DNA, even after adjusting for other factors, including age, sex, smoking, alcohol drinking and HbeAg status [36]. HBV inactive carriers had a 5-fold higher risk of developing HCC in comparison to HbsAg-negative controls [37]. High HBV DNA serum levels have been also associated with a worse prognosis of HBV-related HCC, including reduced hepatic functional reserve, which limits in turn the therapeutic options for HCC, as well as higher rates of recurrence after treatment [38].

Antiviral therapy has an important role in the management of patients with HBV-related HCC. However, the reduction in the rates of progression to cirrhosis and in the risk of hepatic decompensation associated with anti-HBV therapy may not necessarily translate in a parallel decline in the incidence of HCC. Since HBV viral load directly correlates with HCC risk, it may be hypothesized that control of HBV replication with antiviral treatment will also lower the risk of HCC, especially with the newer agents, which have an improved efficacy and resistance profile. Nevertheless, the prolonged survival of patients with chronic HBV infection may paradoxically lead to an increase in the incidence of HCC. Moreover, there is a paucity of data on the impact of antiviral therapy on HCC risk and they generally come from nonrandomized, short-term studies. Several meta-analysis have evaluated the role of Interferon (IFN)-α treatment on HCC risk with mixed results [39-42]. As for nucleoside analogs (NAs), in a meta-analysis published in 2008, the risk of developing HCC after treatment with NAs (lamivudine and adefovir) was reduced by 78% (relative risk (RR) 0.22, 95% confidence interval (CI) 0.10-0.50). Subgroup analysis showed a significant benefit for HBeAg-positive patients (RR 0.21, 95% CI 0.10-0.44), patients with early cirrhosis (RR 0.17, 95% CI 0.04-0.79) and non-cirrhotic subjects (RR 0.21, 95% CI 0.10-0.47) [40]. Sabbat et al. evaluated the impact of lamivudine on HCC risk in a cohort of 631 patients with cirrhosis or advanced fibrosis, who were randomized to receive lamivudine or placebo for a maximum of five years. The study was terminated early because of the benefits associated with lamivudine. In fact, lamivudine was shown to reduce the risk of hepatic decompensation as well as the risk of developing HCC. 3.9% of patients in the lamivudine group developed HCC in comparison to 7.4% in the placebo arm (hazard ratio (HR) 0.49, 95% CI 0.25-0.99, $p = 0.047$) [43]. Few studies have evaluated the risk of developing HCC among patients receiving high genetic barrier NAs, such as entecavir and tenofovir. The cumulative incidence of HCC was significantly lower among patients receiving entecavir in comparison to untreated controls after 5 years of follow up in a retrospective study in Japan (3.7 vs. 13.7%, $p < 0.001$). Entecavir reduced HCC risk by 63% (HR 0.37, 95% CI 0.15-0.91). However, the benefit of entecavir administration on HCC risk was significant only in cirrhotic patients (7 vs 39%, $p < 0.001$) but not in non-cirrhotic ones (2.5 vs 3.6%, $p = 0.44$) [44]. In another study [45], the authors used a prediction model to compare the incidence of HCC in 641 patients treated for 6 years with tenofovir with the predicted HCC rate estimated by the REACH-B risk calculator. The authors found that tenofovir significantly reduced HCC incidence compared to the predicted HCC risk. These findings suggest that treatment with high genetic barrier NAs is associated with reduced risk of HCC, especially in patients with cirrhosis. However, studies with longer follow up and enrolling patients with less advanced liver disease are required to assess the benefits of the latest NAs on HCC risk.

In the last three decades, vaccination against HBV has led to a significant decrease in the rates of new cases of hepatitis B worldwide. In 1984, Taiwan was the first country to start a program of universal vaccination of newborns, with a significant impact on the rate of HBsAg carriers among children, which declined from 9.8% in 1984 to 0.7% in 1999. In parallel, HCC incidence decreased from 0.70 per 100,000 children to 0.36 [46]. However, vaccine does not prevent HCC development among patients who already have chronic HBV. For these subjects, adequate surveillance/screening programs remain essential to early diagnose HCC.

Hepatitis C: HCV is responsible for around 20% of HCC cases worldwide. HCV is a single-stranded RNA virus of the *Flaviviridae* family. Approximately 50-80% of infected subjects progress to chronic infection, 20% of whom develop cirrhosis in 20-30 years. Once cirrhosis is established, HCC develops at an annual rate of 1-4%. An important difference with HBV is that HCV-related HCC usually occurs in the setting of cirrhosis [2]. Moreover, HCV does not integrate in the host genome. As a consequence, insertional mutagenesis is not a pathogenetic mechanism contributing to liver carcinogenesis. On the contrary, HCV-induced inflammation and immune responses are thought to play a key role in HCC development and progression [47].

Chronic HCV infection is characterized by liver lymphocyte infiltrates: T lymphocytes and natural killer cells sense HCV RNA motifs through RIG-I and TLR-3, leading to activation of the NF-κB pathway and generation of IFN and other pro-inflammatory cytokines. Furthermore, the viral polymerase nonstructural protein 5B (NS5B) may directly activate the inflammatory cascade through NF-κB, up-regulating the secretion of interleukin (IL)-6 and type I IFN [48].

Patients with chronic HCV infection show increased oxidative stress: several HCV proteins, such as NS3, NS5A and core protein have been found to induce endoplasmic reticulum stress and the production of reactive oxygen species (ROS). ROS are involved in the modulation of cell cycle, cell metabolism and cell death; moreover, ROS induce oxidative DNA damage, which represents a key step in cell transformation [49, 50].

Deregulation of cell cycle has been described in HCV infection. HCV core protein and NS5A have been reported to promote cell proliferation by interfering with several cellular targets, including pRb, p53 and c-myc [51-55]. Moreover, HCV has been suggested to block apoptosis: HCV NS5A may block the activation of caspase-3 and inhibit proteolytic cleavage of the death substrate poly (ADP-ribose) polymerase in tumor necrosis factor-alpha (TNF α)-induced cells [56]. It may also interact with PI3K, promoting the PI3K-AKT cell survival pathway, and impair the interaction between the mammalian target of rapamycin (mTOR) and FKBP38, inhibiting apoptosis through the mTOR pathway [57, 58]. HCV core protein has been found to inhibit caspase-8 activation by maintaining the expression of the cellular FADD-like IL-1 converting enzyme (c-FLIP), an endogenous caspase-8 inhibitor [59].

Furthermore, HCV core protein may inhibit p53 activity as well as deoxycholic acid-mediated apoptosis by increasing Bcl-x protein and decreasing Bax protein [54, 60].

HCV core protein is able to trigger hepatic angiogenesis, by stimulating the production of TGF-β2 and VEGF proteins by many pathways, including ERK and protein kinase C (PKC) [61]. Furthermore, it has been reported to favor the loss of epithelial homeostasis and the acquisition of a migratory mesenchymal phenotype, by shutting down TGF-β-dependent tumor suppressive activity in a JNK/ pSmad3L pathway-dependent manner [62, 63].

In a recent meta-analysis, HCV genotype 1b has been associated with increased risk of HCC in comparison with other genotypes (RR 1.78, CI 1.36-2.32) [64]. Of interest, the risk was higher in the early stages of liver disease (RR 2.46, CI 1.69-3.59) when compared with cirrhotic patients (RR 1.60, CI 1.07-2.39). Specific conformational features of the secondary structure of the N-terminus of the NS3 protein, characterizing certain strains of HCV 1b, have been suggested to contribute to the higher risk of HCC associated with this genotype [65].

As for host-related factors, older age, male sex, co-infection with HIV or HBV, diabetes, obesity and alcohol abuse are considered risk factors for HCC [2, 66, 67]. Modality of HCV acquisition seems to be an independent predictor of the incidence of cirrhosis and HCC: the highest pooled incidence rates for cirrhosis and HCC have been observed among subjects with transfusion-associated HCV (14 and 1 per 1000 person-years respectively), whereas lower pooled incidence has been reported among intravenous drug users (5 and 0 per 1000 person-years respectively) [68]. Among patients with HCV-related cirrhosis, lower platelet count, higher bilirubin and higher α-fetoprotein levels have been associated with increased risk of HCC [69-72].

Antiviral treatment may lead to the eradication of HCV infection. Patients achieving sustained virological response (SVR) have a significantly lower risk of developing HCC in comparison to untreated ones. In a meta-analysis of 14 studies reporting HCC rates after treatment with IFN in patients with HCV-related cirrhosis, the authors found a significantly lower incidence among treated patients (risk difference (RD) -12.8% (CI -8.3 to -17.2%, $p < 0.0001$). Of interest, HCC rates were lower not only in sustained responders vs. untreated patients (RD -19.1%, 95% CI -13.1 to 25.2%, $p < 0.00001$), but also in non-responders vs. untreated patients (RD -11.8%, 95% CI -6.4 to -19.1%, $p < 0.0001$) [39]. In a more recent meta-analysis of 20 studies comparing untreated patients with those receiving IFN alone or with ribavirin, the authors reported that antiviral therapy was associated with a significant reduction in the risk of HCC (RR 0.43, CI 0.33-0.56, $p < 0.00001$). Again, the most favorable results were observed among sustained responders (RR 0.35, CI 0.26-0.46, $p < 0.00001$) and in patients treated with ribavirin-based regimens (RR 0.25, CI 0.14-0.46) [73].

The HALT-C trial examined the effect of maintenance treatment with IFN in patients with advanced disease who had failed to achieve SVR with standard therapy. Maintenance therapy did not prevent complications of HCV cirrhosis, including HCC [74]. The aforementioned meta-analysis of Sood et al. confirmed no benefits of maintenance IFN in non-responders in terms of HCC risk reduction (RR 0.58, CI 0.33-1.03) [73]. However, a slightly lower risk of HCC seems to occur among patients who experienced a significant decline in HCV RNA during standard therapy but later broke through or relapsed [75].

The landscape of HCV treatment is rapidly changing, with the introduction of more effective drugs specifically targeting the viral replication cycle [76]. Future studies are needed to evaluate the long-term benefits of these direct-acting antiviral drugs, including HCC risk reduction.

ALCOHOL

Alcohol is the main cause of advanced liver disease in Western countries. Alcohol has been recently classified by the International Agency for Research on Cancer as "carcinogenic to humans," because it has been causally related to the occurrence of several malignant tumors, including cancer of the oral cavity, pharynx, larynx, esophagus, breast, colon and liver [77]. In the setting of liver cancer, several studies have shown an independent role of alcohol in the induction of both cirrhosis and HCC [78, 79].

A recent meta-analysis reported the relative risk of developing HCC was 1.86 (CI 1.53-2.27) for 100 g of alcohol intake per day. Of interest, the risk was still significantly higher for lower alcohol intake (RR 1.17 for 25 g/day and 1.36 for 50 g/day) and was higher among women in comparison to men (RR 9.15 vs. 1.62 for 100 g/day) [80].

Alcohol-related carcinogenesis is complex and related not only with alcohol metabolism in hepatocytes but also with the activation of other liver-resident populations, such as Kupffer cells (KCs) and hepatic stellate cells (HSCs).

Alcohol is metabolized by several pathways, the most common one involving alcohol dehydrogenase (ADH) and aldehyde dehydrogenase (ALDH) [81]. The majority of alcohol is absorbed in the duodenum and small intestine and transformed into acetaldehyde by ADH located in the cytoplasm of hepatocytes. Acetaldehyde is oxidized to acetate by the mitochondrial form of ALDH.

Acetate is then incorporated to form acetyl-coenzyme A and oxidized in the Krebs cycle. The cytochrome P450 2E1 (CYP2E1) of microsomal ethanol oxidizing system also breaks down alcohol to acetaldehyde. However, in moderate alcohol consumers CYP2E1 metabolizes only small amounts of alcohol; chronic alcohol abuse is associated with a marked induction of CYP2E1, leading to increased hepatic acetaldehyde production [81]. CYP2E1-dependent alcohol metabolism is responsible for increased hepatic oxidative stress and production of ROS. ROS can form DNA and protein adducts and react with cell membrane lipids, causing the formation of biologically reactive aldehyde molecules. In chronic alcohol abuse, CYP2E1 may also increase the conversion of several pro-carcinogens (including nitrosamines and azo-compounds) to carcinogen derivatives [81]. Moreover, alcohol abuse is associated with altered balance of bacterial flora, increased gut permeability and microbial translocation [82]. The increased hepatic levels of microbial products, especially lipopolysaccharide, are responsible for the activation of KCs, which in turn release several pro-inflammatory cytokines, such as TNF-α, interleukins and prostaglandins [83-85]. This pro-inflammatory milieu may favor in turn the trans-differentiation of HSCs to a myofibroblastic state, characterized by increased collagen synthesis and deposition [86, 87]. This mechanism leads to progressive fibrosis and finally liver cirrhosis. Previous studies have shown increased number of KCs and HSCs in HCC, which seems to be related to the chemokine CCL2 signaling. In fact, CCR-2 deficient mice, who do not express the receptor for CCL2, have a lower number and size of tumoral foci. Attraction of HSCs to the tumor has an important impact on angiogenesis, as HSCs may increase neo-vascularization by increasing the production of MMP-2 [88].

Alcohol acts synergistically with preexisting chronic liver diseases, such as viral hepatitis and fatty liver disease, further increasing the risk of HCC. Cirrhotic patients with HCV infection and heavy alcohol intake had a significantly higher risk of HCC than those with cirrhosis due to alcohol alone (HR 11.2, CI 2.3-55) [89]. HCC development seems to be accelerated and associated with reduced tumor-free survival among subjects with alcoholic and HCV-related cirrhosis [90]. Alcohol abuse and diabetes have been reported to have a synergistic effect on the risk of HCC. In a case-control study conducted from 1984 to 2002 and involving 295 HCC cases and 435 matched controls, heavy alcohol consumption was associated with a 2-fold to 3-fold increase in HCC risk after adjustment for HCV and HBV status. The risk of developing HCC synergistically increased among subjects with heavy alcohol consumption and diabetes (OR 4.2, 95% CI 2.6-5.8), as well as heavy alcohol consumption and viral hepatitis (OR 5.5, 95% CI 3.9-7) [91]. Obese alcohol users were reported to have a significantly higher risk of HCC in the REVEAL-HBV study, a cohort study of 2,260 Taiwanese men with chronic HBV infection [92]. Analogously, Beaugrand et al. found that overweight and diabetes were independently associated with the risk of HCC in a French cohort of patients with HCV- or alcohol-related cirrhosis [93].

The role of alcohol and smoking as cofactors in the development of HCC has been difficult to establish, because the two risk factors coexist in the majority of patients. However, some studies have shown a synergistic effect, especially in patients with chronic viral hepatitis [94, 95]. From a pathogenetic point of view, it has been postulated that carcinogenic compounds in cigarette smoke may have an increased effect in the context of alcohol-induced liver damage; moreover, CYP2E1 induction due to alcohol may enhance the carcinogenetic potential of tobacco compounds [96].

Alcohol and aflatoxin B1 have been reported to have a synergistic impact on the risk of developing HCC [97]. Aflatoxin B1 is metabolized by CYP2E1. As alcohol induces CYP2E1, it may potentiate the carcinogenetic effect of aflatoxin B1 and increase HCC risk.

Non-Alcoholic Fatty Liver Disease

NAFLD encompasses a histological spectrum ranging from liver steatosis to non-alcoholic steatohepatitis (NASH), which is characterized by steatosis and necroinflammation. NASH may progress to cirrhosis and its complications, including HCC [98].

NAFLD is emerging as the most common cause of liver disease in developed countries and its prevalence is expected to increase with the epidemics of diabetes and obesity. In fact, obesity and diabetes, as well as insulin resistance and hyperlipidemia, are risk factors for the development of NAFLD [98]. Several studies carried out in Europe reported NAFLD prevalence rates of 26-33% in the general population [99-101]. A large proportion of cryptogenetic cirrhosis is probably related with NASH. Although HCC usually develops in individuals with NASH-associated cirrhosis, few cases of HCC in non-cirrhotic patients with NASH have been described [102]. Longitudinal studies reported the prevalence of HCC in NAFLD to be 0%-0.5% and the prevalence of HCC in NASH to be 0%-2.8% over time periods of up to 19.5 years [103-106]. From a pathogenetic point of view, several mechanisms occurring in NASH may contribute to hepatocarcinogenesis. Insulin resistance leads to increased release of free fatty acids from adipocytes and increased circulating levels of proinflammatory cytokines, such as IL-6, leptin, resistin and TNF-α [107]. Moreover, hyperinsulinemia is responsible for upregulation of insulin-like growth factor-1(IGF-1), which inhibits apoptosis and stimulates liver cell proliferation [108, 109].

NASH is characterized by decreased circulating levels of adiponectin, a hormone with anti-inflammatory properties secreted by adipocytes. Interestingly, adiponectin has been reported to inhibit angiogenesis by modulating apoptosis [110, 111]. As a consequence, it may be hypothesized that low levels of adiponectin may promote uninhibited cell growth and contribute to liver inflammation.

NASH has also been associated with oxidative stress and increased production of ROS. In fact, in obese mice with fatty hepatocytes, ROS production is increased and related with the activation of several pro-oncogenic pathways [112]. Trans-4-hydroxy-2-nonenal, a product of lipid peroxidation, has been associated with mutations of the p53 tumor suppressor gene, which represent a common finding in a wide range of malignancies, including HCC [113]. The c-Jun amino-terminal kinase 1 (JNK1) is a ubiquitous mitogen-activated protein kinase, whose levels are elevated in obese patients [114]. Several factors, including ROS, free fatty acids and TNF-α, are able to activate JNK. JNK activation is responsible for the phosphorylation of insulin receptor substrate-1, which has been implicated not only in the induction of insulin resistance but also in liver inflammation and apoptosis [114, 115]. In NAFLD, JNK activity seems related to the levels of liver histologic activity: patients with NASH have increased levels of phosphorylated JNK in comparison to those with steatosis [115]. Moreover, mouse models have demonstrated that JNK1 promotes the development of steatohepatitis [116], whereas the absence of JNK1 has a protective effect against the development of insulin resistance, liver steatosis and inflammation [117]. These findings suggest that JNK inhibitors may potentially have a role in the treatment of NASH. JNK is over-activated in more than 50% of human HCC samples; the sustained over-activation of JNK, especially JNK1, leads to an aberrant increase in the expression of several genes involved in hepatocyte proliferation [118-120]. ROS have been reported to potentiate JNK, by inactivating JNK phosphatases and boosting JNK activity [121].

The use of statins has been associated with decreased risk of HCC in patients with diabetes [122]. Of interest, atorvastatin has been found to decrease JNK expression in patients with abdominal aortic aneurysms [123]. It may be hypothesized that statins could have a role in the prevention and treatment of NASH as well as NASH-related HCC. However, further studies are needed to establish the best therapeutic approach to this disease.

Other Risk Factors

Few cases of HCC are a consequence of inherited metabolic liver diseases, including α1-antitrypsin deficiency, hereditary hemochromatosis (HH) and Wilson's disease.

Patients with HH have been reported to have an increased risk of HCC in comparison with the general population. The relative risk of developing HCC ranges from 20 in population-based cohort studies [124] to 200 in studies with a high prevalence of cirrhotic patients with HH [125]. HCC develops in 8-10% of subjects with HH and is responsible for approximately 45% of deaths in this subset of patients. HH seems to be an independent risk factor for the development of HCC, regardless of any other underlying liver disease [126].

α1-antitrypsin deficiency is associated with the development of cirrhosis and HCC. In a cross-sectional study, no difference in HCC prevalence was reported between patients with cirrhosis due to α1-antitrypsin deficiency and those with cirrhosis of other causes.

However, the majority of patients with α1-antitrypsin deficiency who developed HCC were infected with HBV and/or HCV, whereas none of the patients with α1-antitrypsin deficiency but without signs of chronic liver disease had HCC [127]. These data suggest that chronic viral infections are likely to play a more important role than α1-antitrypsin deficiency in the development of cirrhosis and HCC.

Similarly, available data suggest that in the absence of HCV or HBV infection, HCC is a rare complication in patients with Wilson's disease, as well as those with primary sclerosing cholangitis, autoimmune hepatitis and primary biliary cirrhosis [128].

Conclusion

Unlike other malignancies, HCC is potentially a preventable cancer: in fact, the underlying cause can usually be identified at an individual level and in the majority of cases risk factors for liver disease are largely amenable to primary prevention.

Vaccination against HBV represents a paradigmatic example, as it has been associated with a significant reduction in the incidence of HBV-related HCC.

The growing epidemics of obesity and diabetes are expected to increase the incidence of HCC due to NAFLD. As a consequence, lifestyle modification programs are fundamental to reduce the prevalence of several risk factors for HCC, including heavy alcohol consumption, smoking and obesity.

References

[1] Ferlay, J., Soerjomataram, I., Ervik, M., Dikshit, R., Eser, S., Mathers, C., Rebelo, M., Parkin, D. M., Forman, D., Bray, F. GLOBOCAN 2012 v1.0, *Cancer Incidence and Mortality Worldwide: IARC CancerBase No. 11 [Internet]*. Lyon, France: International Agency for Research on Cancer; 2013. Available from: http://globocan.iarc.fr, accessed on 8/14/2014.

[2] El-Serag, H. B. Epidemiology of viral hepatitis and hepatocellular carcinoma. *Gastroenterology* 2012; 142(6): 1264-1273.

[3] WHO. Hepatitis B 2014. *Fact sheet No. 204*. Available from: http://www.who.int/mediacentre/factsheets/fs204/en/, accessed on 9/13/14.

[4] Feitelson, M. A., Lee, J. Hepatitis B virus integration, fragile sites, and hepatocarcinogenesis. *Cancer Lett*. 2007; 252(2): 157-170.

[5] Levrero, M., Pollicino, T., Petersen, J., Belloni, L., Raimondo, G., Dandri, M. Control of cccDNA function in hepatitis B virus infection. *J. Hepatol*. 2009; 51(3): 581-592.

[6] Sung, W.-K., Zheng, H., Li, S., Chen, R., Liu, X., Li, Y. et al. Genome-wide survey of recurrent HBV integration in hepatocellular carcinoma. *Nat. Genet*. 2012; 44(7): 765-769.

[7] Kim, S., Park, S. Y., Yong, H., Famulski, J. K., Chae, S., Lee, J. H., Kang, C. M., Saya, H., Chan, G. K., Cho, H. HBV X protein targets hBubR1, which induces dysregulation of the mitotic checkpoint. *Oncogene* 2008; 27(24): 3457-3464.

[8] Molina-Jimenez, F., Benedicto, I., Murata, M., Martín-Vílchez, S., Seki, T., Antonio Pintor-Toro, J., Tortolero, M., Moreno-Otero, R., Okazaki, K., Koike, K., Barbero, J. L., Matsuzaki, K., Majano, P. L., López-Cabrera, M. Expression of pituitary tumor transforming gene 1 (PTTG1)/securin in hepatitis B virus (HBV)-associated liver diseases: evidence for an HBV X protein-mediated inhibition of PTTG1 ubiquitination and degradation. *Hepatology* 2010; 51(3): 777-787.

[9] Cougot, D., Neuveut, C., Buendia, M. A. HBV induced carcinogenesis. *J. Clin. Virol.* 2005; 34(S1): S75-78.

[10] Brechot, C., Kremsdorf, D., Soussan, P., Pineau, P., Dejean, A., Paterlini-Brechot, P., Tiollais, P. Hepatitis B virus (HBV)-related hepatocellular carcinoma (HCC): Molecular mechanisms and novel paradigms. *Pathol. Biol.* (Paris) 2010; 58(4): 278-287.

[11] Bouchard, M., Giannakopoulos, S., Wang, E. H., Tanese, N., Schneider, R. J. Hepatitis B virus HBx protein activation of cyclin A-cyclin-dependent kinase 2 complexes and G1 transit via a Src kinase pathway. *J. Virol.* 2001; 75(9): 4247-4257.

[12] Klein, N. P., Schneider, R. J. Activation of Src family kinases by hepatitis B virus HBx protein and coupled signaling to Ras. *Mol. Cell. Biol.* 1997; 17(11): 6427-6436.

[13] Shan, C., Xu, F., Zhang, S., You, J., You, X., Qiu, L., Zheng, J., Ye, L., Zhang, X. Hepatitis B virus X protein promotes liver cell proliferation via a positive cascade loop involving arachidonic acid metabolism and p-ERK1/2. *Cell Res.* 2010; 20(5): 563-575.

[14] Wang, H. D., Trivedi, A., Johnson, D. L. Regulation of RNA polymerase I-dependent promoters by the hepatitis B virus X protein via activated Ras and TATA binding protein. *Mol. Cell. Biol.* 1998; 18(12): 7086-7094.

[15] Yun, C., Cho, H., Kim, S. J., Lee, J. H., Park, S. Y., Chan, G. K., Cho, H. Mitotic aberration coupled with centrosome amplification is induced by hepatitis B virus X oncoprotein via the Ras-mitogen-activated protein/extracellular signal-regulated kinase-mitogen activated protein pathway. *Mol. Cancer Res.* 2004; 2(3): 159-169.

[16] Choi, B. H., Choi, M., Jeon, H. Y., Rho, H. M. Hepatitis B viral X protein overcomes inhibition of E2F1 activity by pRb on the human Rb gene promoter. *DNA Cell. Biol.* 2001; 20(2): 75-80.

[17] Lee, S. G., Rho, H. M. Transcriptional repression of the human p53 gene by hepatitis B viral X protein. *Oncogene* 2000; 19(3): 468-471.

[18] Zhang, X., Dong, N., Zhang, H., You, J., Wang, H., Ye, L. Effects of hepatitis B virus X protein on human telomerase reverse transcriptase expression and activity in hepatoma cells. *J. Lab. Clin. Med.* 2005; 145(2): 98-104.

[19] Liu, H., Luan, F., Ju, Y., Shen, H., Gao, L., Wang, X., Liu, S., Zhang, L., Sun, W., Ma, C. In vitro transfection of the hepatitis B virus PreS2 gene into the human hepatocarcinoma cell line HepG2 induces upregulation of human telomerase reverse transcriptase. *Biochem. Biophys. Res. Commun.* 2007; 355(2): 379-384.

[20] Majano, P. L., Garcia-Monzon, C., Lopez-Cabrera, M., Lara-Pezzi, E., Fernández-Ruiz, E., García-Iglesias, C., Borque, M. J., Moreno-Otero, R. Inducible nitric oxide synthase expression in chronic viral hepatitis. Evidence for a virus-induced gene upregulation. *J. Clin. Invest.* 1998; 101(7): 1343-1352.

[21] Moon, E. J., Jeong, C. H., Jeong, J. W., Kim, K. R., Yu, D. Y., Murakami, S., Kim, C. W., Kim, K. W. Hepatitis B virus X protein induces angiogenesis by stabilizing hypoxia-inducible factor-1alpha. *FASEB J.* 2004; 18(2): 382-384.

[22] Lee, S. W., Lee, Y. M., Bae, S. K., Murakami, S., Yun, Y., Kim, K. W. Human hepatitis B virus X protein is a possible mediator of hypoxia-induced angiogenesis in hepatocarcinogenesis. *Biochem. Biophys. Res. Commun.* 2000; 268(2): 456-461.
[23] Yang, J. C., Teng, C. F., Wu, H. C., Tsai, H. W., Chuang, H. C., Tsai, T. F., Hsu, Y. H., Huang, W., Wu, L. W., Su, I. J. Enhanced expression of vascular endothelial growth factor-A in ground glass hepatocytes and its implication in hepatitis B virus hepatocarcinogenesis. *Hepatology* 2009; 49(6): 1962-1971.
[24] Chung, T. W., Lee, Y. C., Kim, C. H. Hepatitis B viral HBx induces matrix metalloproteinase-9 gene expression through activation of ERK and PI-3K/AKT pathways: involvement of invasive potential. *FASEB J.* 2004; 18(10): 1123-1125.
[25] Liu, L. P., Liang, H. F., Chen, X. P., Zhang, W. G., Yang, S. L., Xu, T., Ren, L. The role of NF-kappaB in Hepatitis b virus X protein-mediated upregulation of VEGF and MMPs. *Cancer Invest.* 2010; 28(5): 443-451.
[26] Yu, F. L., Liu, H. J., Lee, J. W., Liao, M. H., Shih, W. L. Hepatitis B virus X protein promotes cell migration by inducing matrix metalloproteinase-3. *J. Hepatol.* 2005; 42 (4): 520-527.
[27] Tian, Y., Yang, W., Song, J., Wu, Y., Ni, B. Hepatitis B virus X protein-induced aberrant epigenetic modifications contributing to human hepatocellular carcinoma pathogenesis. *Mol. Cell. Biol.* 2013; 33(15): 2810-2816.
[28] Zhang, H., Zhai, Y., Hu, Z. et al. Genome-wide association study identifies 1p36.22 as a new susceptibility locus for hepatocellular carcinoma in chronic hepatitis B virus carriers. *Nat. Genet.* 2010; 42(9): 755-758.
[29] Chan, L. K., Ko, F. C., Sze, K. M., Ng, I. O., Yam, J. W. Nuclear-targeted deleted in liver cancer 1 (DLC1) is less efficient in exerting its tumor suppressive activity both in vitro and in vivo. *PLoS One* 2011; 6(9): e25547.
[30] Gu, X., Qi, P., Zhou, F., Ji, Q., Wang, H., Dou, T., Zhao, Y., Gao, C. 149G > A polymorphism in the cytotoxic T-lymphocyte antigen-4 gene increases susceptibility to hepatitis B-related hepatocellular carcinoma in a male Chinese population. *Hum. Immunol.* 2010; 71(1): 83-87.
[31] Chou, Y. C., Yu, M. W., Wu, C. F., Yang, S. Y., Lin, C. L., Liu, C. J., Shih, W. L., Chen, P. J., Liaw, Y. F., Chen, C. J. Temporal relationship between hepatitis B virus enhancer II/basal core promoter sequence variation and risk of hepatocellular carcinoma. *Gut* 2008; 57(1): 91-97.
[32] Liu, Y., Zhang, Y., Wen, J., Liu, L., Zhai, X., Liu, J., Pan, S., Chen, J., Shen, H., Hu, Z. A genetic variant in the promoter region of miR-106b-25 cluster and risk of HBV infection and hepatocellular carcinoma. *PLoS One* 2012; 7(2): e32230.
[33] Chan, H. L., Tse, C. H., Mo, F., Koh, J., Wong, V. W., Wong, G. L., Lam Chan, S., Yeo, W., Sung, J. J., Mok, T. S. High viral load and hepatitis B virus subgenotype are associated with increased risk of hepatocellular carcinoma. *J. Clin. Oncol.* 2008; 26(2): 177-182.
[34] Ni, Y. H., Chang, M. H., Wang, K. J., Hsu, H. Y., Chen, H. L., Kao, J. H., Yeh, S. H., Jeng, Y. M., Tsai, K. S., Chen, D. S. Clinical relevance of hepatitis B virus genotype in children with chronic infection and hepatocellular carcinoma. *Gastroenterology* 2004; 127(6): 1733-1738.
[35] Yang, H. I., Lu, S. N., Liaw, Y. F., You, S. L., Sun, C. A., Wang, L. Y., Hsiao, C. K., Chen, P. J., Chen, D. S., Chen, C. J.; Taiwan Community-Based Cancer Screening

Project Group. Hepatitis B e antigen and the risk of hepatocellular carcinoma. *N. Engl. J. Med.* 2002; 347(3): 168-174.

[36] Chen, C. J., Yang, H. I., Iloeje, U. H. Hepatitis B virus DNA levels and outcomes in chronic hepatitis B. *Hepatology* 2009; 49(5S): S72-84.

[37] Chen, J. D., Yang, H. I., Iloeje, U. H., You, S. L., Lu, S. N., Wang, L. Y., Su, J., Sun, C. A., Liaw, Y. F., Chen, C. J.; Risk Evaluation of Viral Load Elevation and Associated Liver Disease/Cancer in HBV (REVEAL-HBV) Study Group. Carriers of inactive hepatitis B virus are still at risk for hepatocellular carcinoma and liver-related death. *Gastroenterology* 2010; 138(5): 1747-1754.

[38] Yu, S. J., Kim, Y. J. Hepatitis B viral load affects prognosis of hepatocellular carcinoma. *World J. Gastroenterol.* 2014; 20(34): 12039-12044.

[39] Cammà, C., Giunta, M., Andreone, P., Craxì, A. Interferon and prevention of hepatocellular carcinoma in viral cirrhosis: an evidence-based approach. *J. Hepatol.* 2001; 34(4): 593-602.

[40] Sung, J. J., Tsoi, K. K., Wong, V. W., Li, K. C., Chan, H. L. Meta-analysis: treatment of hepatitis B infection reduces risk of hepatocellular carcinoma. *Aliment. Pharmacol. Ther.* 2008; 28(9): 1067-1077.

[41] Yang, Y. F., Zhao, W., Zhong, Y. D., Xia, H. M., Shen, L., Zhang, N. Interferon therapy in chronic hepatitis B reduces progression to cirrhosis and hepatocellular carcinoma: a meta-analysis. *J. Viral Hepat.* 2009; 16(4): 265-271.

[42] Miyake, Y., Kobashi, H., Yamamoto, K. Meta-analysis: the effect of interferon on development of hepatocellular carcinoma in patients with chronic hepatitis B virus infection. *J. Gastroenterol.* 2009; 44(5): 470-475.

[43] Liaw, Y. F., Sung, J. J., Chow, W. C., Farrell, G., Lee, C. Z., Yuen, H., Tanwandee, T., Tao, Q. M., Shue, K., Keene, O. N., Dixon, J. S., Gray, D. F., Sabbat, J.; Cirrhosis Asian Lamivudine Multicentre Study Group. Lamivudine for patients with chronic hepatitis B and advanced liver disease. *N. Engl. J. Med.* 2004; 351(15): 1521-1531.

[44] Hosaka, T., Suzuki, F., Kobayashi, M., Seko, Y., Kawamura, Y., Sezaki, H., Akuta, N., Suzuki, Y., Saitoh, S., Arase, Y., Ikeda, K., Kobayashi, M., Kumada, H. Long-term entecavir treatment reduces hepatocellular carcinoma incidence in patients with hepatitis B virus infection. *Hepatology* 2013; 58(1): 98-107.

[45] Kim, W. R., Berg, T., Loomba, R., Aguilar Schall, R., Dinh, P., Yee, L. J., Martins, E. B., Flaherty, J. F., Gurel, S., Buti, M., Marcellin, P. Long Term Tenofovir Disoproxil Fumarate (TDF) Therapy and the Risk of Hepatocellular Carcinoma. *J. Hepatol.* 2013; 58: S19.

[46] Chang, M. H., Chen, C. J., Lai, M. S., Hsu, H. M., Wu, T. C., Kong, M. S., Liang, D. C., Shau, W. Y., Chen, D. S. Universal hepatitis B vaccination in Taiwan and the incidence of hepatocellular carcinoma in children. Taiwan Childhood Hepatoma Study Group. *N. Engl. J. Med.* 1997; 336(26): 1855-1859.

[47] Castello, G., Scala, S., Palmieri, G., Curley, S. A., Izzo, F. HCV-related hepatocellular carcinoma: From chronic inflammation to cancer. *Clin. Immunol.* 2010; 134(3): 237-250.

[48] Yu, G. Y., He, G., Li, C. Y., Tang, M., Grivennikov, S., Tsai, W. T., Wu, M. S., Hsu, C. W., Tsai, Y., Wang, L. H., Karin, M. Hepatic expression of HCV RNA-dependent RNA polymerase triggers innate immune signaling and cytokine production. *Mol. Cell* 2012; 48(2): 313-321.

[49] Okuda, M., Li, K., Beard, M. R., Showalter, L. A., Scholle, F., Lemon, S. M., Weinman, S. A. Mitochondrial injury, oxidative stress, and antioxidant gene expression are induced by hepatitis C virus core protein. *Gastroenterology* 2002; 122(2): 366-375.

[50] Korenaga, M., Wang, T., Li, Y., Showalter, L. A., Chan, T., Sun, J., Weinman, S. A. Hepatitis C virus core protein inhibits mitochondrial electron transport and increases reactive oxygen species (ROS) production. *J. Biol. Chem.* 2005; 280(45): 37481-37488.

[51] Munakata, T., Nakamura, M., Liang, Y., Li, K., Lemon, S. M. Down-regulation of the retinoblastoma tumor suppressor by the hepatitis C virus NS5B RNA-dependent RNA polymerase. *Proc. Natl. Acad. Sci. US* 2005; 102(50): 18159-18164.

[52] Munakata, T., Liang, Y., Kim, S., McGivern, D. R., Huibregtse, J., Nomoto, A., Lemon, S. M. Hepatitis C virus induces E6AP-dependent degradation of the retinoblastoma protein. *PLoS Pathog.* 2007; 3(9): 1335-1347.

[53] Hassan, M., Ghozlan, H., Abdel-Kader, O. Activation of RB/E2F signaling pathway is required for the modulation of hepatitis C virus core protein-induced cell growth in liver and non-liver cells. *Cell Signal.* 2004; 16(12): 1375-1385.

[54] Ray, R. B., Steele, R., Meyer, K., Ray, R. Transcriptional repression of p53 promoter by hepatitis C virus core protein. *J. Biol. Chem.* 1997; 272(17): 10983-10986.

[55] Honda, M., Kaneko, S., Shimazaki, T., Matsushita, E., Kobayashi, K., Ping, L. H., Zhang, H. C., Lemon, S. M. Hepatitis C virus core protein induces apoptosis and impairs cell-cycle regulation in stably transformed Chinese hamster ovary cells. *Hepatology* 2000; 31(6): 1351-1359.

[56] Ghosh, A. K., Majumder, M., Steele, R., Meyer, K., Ray, R., Ray, R. B. Hepatitis C virus NS5A protein protects against TNF-alpha mediated apoptotic cell death. *Virus Res.* 2000; 67(2): 173-178.

[57] He, Y., Nakao, H., Tan, S. L., Polyak, S. J., Neddermann, P., Vijaysri, S., Jacobs, B. L., Katze, M. G. Subversion of cell signaling pathways by hepatitis C virus nonstructural 5A protein via interaction with Grb2 and P85 phosphatidylinositol 3-kinase. *J. Virol.* 2002; 76(18): 9207-9217.

[58] Peng, L., Liang, D., Tong, W., Li, J., Yuan, Z. Hepatitis C Virus NS5A activates the mammalian target of rapamycin (mTOR) pathway, contributing to cell survival by disrupting the interaction between FK506-binding protein 38 (FKBP38) and mTOR. *J. Biol. Chem.* 2010; 285(27): 20870-20881.

[59] Saito, K., Meyer, K., Warner, R., Basu, A., Ray, R. B., Ray, R. Hepatitis C virus core protein inhibits tumor necrosis factor alpha-mediated apoptosis by a protective effect involving cellular FLICE inhibitory protein. *J. Virol.* 2006; 80(9): 4372-4379.

[60] Hara, Y., Hino, K., Okuda, M., Furutani, T., Hidaka, I., Yamaguchi, Y., Korenaga, M., Li, K., Weinman, S. A., Lemon, S. M., Okita, K. Hepatitis C virus core protein inhibits deoxycholic acid-mediated apoptosis despite generating mitochondrial reactive oxygen species. *J. Gastroenterol.* 2006; 41(3): 257-268.

[61] Hassan, M., Selimovic, D., Ghozlan, H., Abdel-kader, O. Hepatitis C virus core protein triggers hepatic angiogenesis by a mechanism including multiple pathways. *Hepatology* 2009; 49(5): 1469-1482.

[62] Matsuzaki, K., Murata, M., Yoshida, K., Sekimoto, G., Uemura, Y., Sakaida, N., Kaibori, M., Kamiyama, Y., Nishizawa, M., Fujisawa, J., Okazaki, K., Seki, T. Chronic inflammation associated with hepatitis C virus infection perturbs hepatic transforming

growth factor beta signaling, promoting cirrhosis and hepatocellular carcinoma. *Hepatology* 2007; 46(1): 48-57.

[63] Battaglia, S., Benzoubir, N., Nobilet, S., Charneau, P., Samuel, D., Zignego, A. L., Atfi, A., Bréchot, C., Bourgeade, M. F. Liver cancer-derived hepatitis C virus core proteins shift TGF-beta responses from tumor suppression to epithelial mesenchymal transition. *PLoS One* 2009; 4(2): e4355.

[64] Raimondi, S., Bruno, S., Mondelli, M. U., Maisonneuve, P. Hepatitis C virus genotype 1b as a risk factor for hepatocellular carcinoma development: a meta-analysis. *J. Hepatol.* 2009; 50(6): 1142-1154.

[65] Nishise, Y., Saito, T., Sugahara, K., Ito, J. I., Saito, K., Togashi, H., Nagano-Fujii, M., Hotta, H., Kawata, S. Risk of hepatocellular carcinoma and secondary structure of hepatitis C virus (HCV) NS3 protein aminoterminus, in patients infected with HCV subtype 1b. *J. Infect. Dis.* 2007; 196(7): 1006-1009.

[66] Pinzone, M. R., Fiorica, F., Di Rosa, M., Malaguarnera, G., Malaguarnera, L., Cacopardo, B., Zanghì, G., Nunnari, G. Non-AIDS-defining cancers among HIV-infected people. *Eur. Rev. Med. Pharmacol. Sci.* 2012; 16(10): 1377-1388.

[67] Nunnari, G., Berretta, M., Pinzone, M. R., Di Rosa, M., Berretta, S., Cunsolo, G., Malaguarnera, M., Cosentino, S., De Paoli, P., Schnell, J. M., Cacopardo, B. Hepatocellular carcinoma in HIV positive patients. *Eur. Rev. Med. Pharmacol. Sci.* 2012; 16(9): 1257-1270.

[68] El-Serag, H. B. Hepatocellular carcinoma and hepatitis C in the United States. *Hepatology* 2002; 36(5 S1): S74-83.

[69] Fattovich, G., Pantalena, M., Zagni, I., Realdi, G., Schalm, S. W., Christensen, E.; European Concerted Action on Viral Hepatitis (EUROHEP). Effect of hepatitis B and C virus infections on the natural history of compensated cirrhosis: A cohort study of 297 patients. *Am. J. Gastroenterol.* 2002; 97(11): 2886-2895.

[70] Degos, F., Christidis, C., Ganne-Carrie, N., Farmachidi, J. P., Degott, C., Guettier, C., Trinchet, J. C., Beaugrand, M., Chevret, S. Hepatitis C virus related cirrhosis: Time to occurrence of hepatocellular carcinoma and death. *Gut* 2000; 47(1): 131-136.

[71] Fattovich, G., Schalm, S. W. Hepatitis C and cirrhosis. In: Liang, T. J., Hoofnagle, J. H., eds. *Hepatitis C*. San Diego: Academic Press, 2000: 241-263.

[72] Taura, N., Fukuda, S., Ichikawa, T., Miyaaki, H., Shibata, H., Honda, T., Yamaguchi, T., Kubota, Y., Uchida, S., Kamo, Y., Yoshimura, E., Isomoto, H., Matsumoto, T., Takeshima, F., Tsutsumi, T., Tsuruta, S., Nakao, K. Relationship of α-fetoprotein levels and development of hepatocellular carcinoma in hepatitis C patients with liver cirrhosis. *Exp. Ther. Med.* 2012; 4(6): 972-976.

[73] Singal, A. K., Singh, A., Jaganmohan, S., Guturu, P., Mummadi, R., Kuo, Y. F., Sood, G. K. Antiviral therapy reduces risk of hepatocellular carcinoma in patients with hepatitis C virus-related cirrhosis. *Clin. Gastroenterol. Hepatol.* 2010; 8(2): 192-199.

[74] Lee, W. M., Dienstag, J. L., Lindsay, K. L., Lok, A. S., Bonkovsky, H. L., Shiffman, M. L., Everson, G. T., Di Bisceglie, A. M., Morgan, T. R., Ghany, M. G., Morishima, C., Wright, E. C., Everhart, J. E.; HALT-C Trial Group. Evolution of the HALT-C Trial: pegylated interferon as maintenance therapy for chronic hepatitis C in previous interferon nonresponders. *Control Clin. Trials* 2004; 25(5): 472-492.

[75] Shiffman, M. L., Morishima, C., Dienstag, J. L., Lindsay, K. L., Hoefs, J. C., Lee, W. M., Wright, E. C., Naishadham, D., Everson, G. T., Lok, A. S., Di Bisceglie, A. M.,

Bonkovsky, H. L., Ghany, M. G.; HALT-C Trial Group. Effect of HCV RNA suppression during peginterferon alfa-2a maintenance therapy on clinical outcomes in the HALT-C trial. *Gastroenterology* 2009; 137(6): 1986-1994.

[76] Kim, D. Y., Ahn, S. H., Han, K. H. Emerging Therapies for Hepatitis C. *Gut Liver* 2014; 8(5): 471-479.

[77] Alcoholic beverage consumption and ethyl caramate (urethane). *IARC monographs on the evaluation of carcinogenic risks to humans 96*. Lyon: International Agency for Research on Cancer.

[78] Corrao, G., Aricò, S. Independent and combined action of hepatitis C virus infection and alcohol consumption on the risk of symptomatic liver cirrhosis. *Hepatology* 1998; 27(4): 914-919.

[79] Donato, F., Tagger, A., Gelatti, U., Parrinello, G., Boffetta, P., Albertini, A., Decarli, A., Travisi, P., Ribero, M. L., Martelli, C., Porru, S., Nardi, G. Alcohol and hepatocellular carcinoma: the effect of lifetime intake and hepatitis virus infections in men and women. *Am. J. Epidemiol.* 2002; 155(4): 323-331.

[80] Bagnardi, V., Blangiardo, M., La Vecchia, C., Corrao, G. A meta-analysis of alcohol drinking and cancer risk. *Br. J. Cancer* 2001; 85(11): 1700-1705.

[81] Grewal, P., Viswanathen, V. A. Liver Cancer and Alcohol. *Clin. Liver Dis.* 2012; 16(4): 839-850.

[82] Pinzone, M. R., Celesia, B. M., Di Rosa, M., Cacopardo, B., Nunnari, G. Microbial translocation in chronic liver diseases. *Int. J. Microbiol.* 2012; 2012: 694629.

[83] Roberts, R. A., Ganey, P. E., Ju, C., Kamendulis, L. M., Rusyn, I., Klaunig, J. E. Role of the Kupffer cell in mediating hepatic toxicity and carcinogenesis. *Toxicol. Sci.* 2007; 96(1): 2-15.

[84] Thurman, R. G. II. Alcoholic liver injury involves activation of Kupffer cells by endotoxin. *Am. J. Physiol.* 1998; 275(4 Pt 1): G605-G611.

[85] Thakur, V., McMullen, M. R., Pritchard, M. T., Nagy, L. E. Regulation of macrophage activation in alcoholic liver disease. *J. Gastroenterol. Hepatol.* 2007; 22(S1): S53-56.

[86] Friedman, S. L. Hepatic stellate cells: protean, multifunctional, and enigmatic cells of the liver. *Physiol. Rev.* 2008; 88(1): 125-172.

[87] Sato, M., Suzuki, S., Senoo, H. Hepatic stellate cells: unique characteristics in cell biology and phenotype. *Cell Struct. Funct.* 2003; 28(2): 105-112.

[88] Yang, X., Lu, P., Ishida, Y., Kuziel, W. A., Fujii, C., Mukaida, N. Attenuated liver tumor formation in the absence of CCR2 with a concomitant reduction in the accumulation of hepatic stellate cells, macrophages and neovascularization. *Int. J. Cancer* 2006; 118(2): 335-345.

[89] Berman, K., Tandra, S., Vuppalanchi, R., Ghabril, M., Sandrasegaran, K., Nguyen, J., Caffrey, H., Liangpunsakul, S., Lumeng, L., Kwo, P., Chalasani, N. Hepatic and extrahepatic cancer in cirrhosis: a longitudinal cohort study. *Am. J. Gastroenterol.* 2011; 106(5): 899-906.

[90] Miyakawa, H., Sato, C., Tazawa, J., Izumi, N., Hattori, K., Ebata, A., Maeda, M., Ikeda, T., Hirata, R., Mae, S. A prospective study on hepatocellular carcinoma in liver cirrhosis respective roles of alcohol and hepatitis C virus infection. *Alcohol Alcohol.* Suppl. 1994; 29(1): 75-79.

[91] Yuan, J. M., Govindarajan, S., Arakawa, K., Yu, M. C. Synergism of alcohol, diabetes, and viral hepatitis on the risk of hepatocellular carcinoma in blacks and whites in the US. *Cancer* 2004; 101(5): 1009-1017.

[92] Loomba, R., Yang, H. I., Su, J., Brenner, D., Iloeje, U., Chen, C. J. Obesity and alcohol synergize to increase the risk of incident hepatocellular carcinoma in men. *Clin. Gastroenterol. Hepatol.* 2010; 8(10): 891-898.

[93] N'Kontchou, G., Paries, J., Htar, M. T., Ganne-Carrie, N., Costentin, L., Grando-Lemaire, V., Trinchet, J. C., Beaugrand, M. Risk factors for hepatocellular carcinoma in patients with alcoholic or viral C cirrhosis. *Clin. Gastroenterol. Hepatol.* 2006; 4(8): 1062-1068.

[94] Kuper, H., Tzonou, A., Kaklamani, E., Hsieh, C. C., Lagiou, P., Adami, H. O., Trichopoulos, D., Stuver, S. O. Tobacco smoking, alcohol consumption and their interaction in the causation of hepatocellular carcinoma. *Int. J. Cancer* 2000; 85(4): 498-502.

[95] Marrero, J. A., Fontana, R. J., Fu, S., Conjeevaram, H. S., Su, G. L., Lok, A. S. Alcohol, tobacco and obesity are synergistic risk factors for hepatocellular carcinoma. *J. Hepatol.* 2005; 42(2): 218-224.

[96] Staretz, M. E., Murphy, S. E., Patten, C. J., Nunes, M. G., Koehl, W., Amin, S., Koenig, L. A., Guengerich, F. P., Hecht, S. S. Comparative metabolism of the tobacco-related carcinogens benzo[a]pyrene, 4-(methylnitrosamino)-1-(3-pyridyl)-1-butanone,4-(methylnitrosamino)-1-(3-pyridyl)-1-butanol, and N'- nitrosonornicotine in human hepatic microsomes. *Drug Metab. Dispos.* 1997; 25(2): 154-162.

[97] Bulatao-Jayme, J., Almero, E. M., Castro, C. A., Jardeleza, M. T., Salamat, L. A. A case-control dietary study of primary liver cancer risk from aflatoxin exposure. *Int. J. Epidemiol.* 1982; 11(2): 112-119.

[98] Starley, B. Q., Calcagno, C. J., Harrison, S. A. Nonalcoholic Fatty Liver Disease and Hepatocellular Carcinoma: A Weighty Connection. *Hepatology* 2010; 51(5): 1820-1832.

[99] Bedogni, G., Miglioli, L., Masutti, F., Castiglione, A., Croce, L. S., Tiribelli, C., Bellentani, S. Incidence and natural course of fatty liver in the general population: the Dionysos study. *Hepatology* 2007; 46(5): 1387-1391.

[100] Gastaldelli, A., Kozakova, M., Hojlund, K., Flyvbjerg, A., Favuzzi, A., Mitrakou, A., Balkau, B.; RISC Investigators. Fatty liver is associated with insulin resistance, risk of coronary heart disease, and early atherosclerosis in a large European population. *Hepatology* 2009; 49(5): 1537-1544.

[101] Haring, R., Wallaschofski, H., Nauck, M., Dorr, M., Baumeister, S. E., Volzke, H. Ultrasonographic hepatic steatosis increases prediction of mortality risk from elevated serum gamma-glutamyl transpeptidase levels. *Hepatology* 2009; 50(5): 1403-1411.

[102] Guzman, G., Brunt, E. M., Petrovic, L. M., Chejfec, G., Layden, T. J., Cotler, S. J. Does nonalcoholic fatty liver disease predispose patients to hepatocellular carcinoma in the absence of cirrhosis? *Arch. Pathol. Lab. Med.* 2008; 132(11): 1761-1766.

[103] Adams, L. A., Lymp, J. F., St Sauver, J., Sanderson, S. O., Lindor, K. D., Feldstein, A., Angulo, P. The natural history of nonalcoholic fatty liver disease: a population-based cohort study. *Gastroenterology* 2005; 129(1): 113-121.

[104] Ekstedt, M., Franzen, L. E., Mathiesen, U. L., Thorelius, L., Holmqvist, M., Bodemar, G., Kechagias, S. Long-term follow-up of patients with NAFLD and elevated liver enzymes. *Hepatology* 2006; 44(4): 865-873.

[105] Ong, J. P., Pitts, A., Younossi, Z. M. Increased overall mortality and liver-related mortality in non-alcoholic fatty liver disease. *J. Hepatol.* 2008; 49(4): 608-612.

[106] Rafiq, N., Bai, C., Fang, Y., Srishord, M., McCullough, A., Gramlich, T., Younossi, Z. M. Long-term follow-up of patients with nonalcoholic fatty liver. *Clin. Gastroenterol. Hepatol.* 2009; 7(2): 234-238.

[107] Bugianesi, E. Non-alcoholic steatohepatitis and cancer. *Clin. Liver Dis.* 2007; 11(1): 191-207, x-xi.

[108] Ish-Shalom, D., Christoffersen, C. T., Vorwerk, P., Sacerdoti-Sierra, N., Shymko, R. M., Naor, D., De Meyts, P. Mitogenic properties of insulin and insulin analogues mediated by the insulin receptor. *Diabetologia* 1997; 40(S2): S25-S31.

[109] Tanaka, S., Mohr, L., Schmidt, E. V., Suqimachi, K., Wands, J. R. Biological effects of human insulin receptor substrate-1 overexpression in hepatocytes. *Hepatology* 1997; 26 (3): 598-604.

[110] Ukkola, O., Santaniemi, M. Adiponectin: a link between excess adiposity and associated comorbidities? *J. Mol. Med.* 2002; 80(11): 696-702.

[111] Brakenhielm, E., Veitonmaki, N., Cao, R., Kihara, S., Matsuzawa, Y., Zhivotovsky, B., Funahashi, T., Cao, Y. Adiponectin-induced antiangiogenesis and antitumor activity involve caspase-mediated endothelial cell apoptosis. *Proc. Natl. Acad. Sci. US* 2004; 101(8): 2476-2481.

[112] Yang, S., Zhu, H., Li, Y., Lin, H., Gabrielson, K., Trush, M. A., Diehl, A. M. Mitochondrial adaptations to obesity-related oxidant stress. *Arch. Biochem. Biophys.* 2000; 378(2): 259-268.

[113] Hu, W., Feng, Z., Eveleigh, J., Iyer, G., Pan, J., Amin, S., Chung, F. L., Tang, M. S. The major lipid peroxidation product, trans-4-hydroxy-2-nonenal, preferentially forms DNA adducts at codon 249 of human p53 gene, a unique mutational hotspot in hepatocellular carcinoma. *Carcinogenesis* 2002; 23(11): 1781-1789.

[114] Hirosumi, J., Tuncman, G., Change, L., Gorgun, C. Z., Uysal, K. T., Maeda, K., Karin, M., Hotamisligil, G. S. A central role for JNK in obesity and insulin resistance. *Nature* 2002; 420(6913): 333-336.

[115] Puri, P., Mirshahi, F., Cheung, O., Natarajan, R., Maher, J. W., Kellum, J. M., Sanyal, A. J. Activation and dysregulation of the unfolded protein response in nonalcoholic fatty liver disease. *Gastroenterology* 2008; 134(2): 568-576.

[116] Schattenberg, J. M., Singh, R., Wang, Y., Lefkowitch, J. H., Rigoli, R. M., Scherer, P. E., Czaja, M. J. JNK1 but not JNK2 promotes the development of steatohepatitis in mice. *Hepatology* 2006; 43(1): 163-172.

[117] Singh, R., Wayn, Y., Xiang, Y., Tanaka, K. E., Gaarde, W. A., Czaja, M. J. Differential effects of JNK1 and JNK2 inhibition on murine steatohepatitis and insulin resistance. *Hepatology* 2009; 49(1): 87-96.

[118] Chang, Q., Zhang, Y., Beezhold, K. J., Bhatia, D., Zhao, H., Chen, J., Castranova, V., Shi, X., Chen, F. Sustained JNK1 activation is associated with altered histone H3 methylations in human liver cancer. *J. Hepatol.* 2009; 50(2): 323-333.

[119] Hui, L., Zatloukal, H., Scheuch, H., Stepniak, E., Wagner, E. F. Proliferation of human HCC cells and chemically induced mouse liver cancers requires JNK1-dependent p21 downregulation. *J. Clin. Invest.* 2008; 118(12): 3943-3953.
[120] Chen, F., Castanova, V. Beyond apoptosis of JNK1 in liver cancer. *Cell Cycle* 2009; 8 (8): 1145-1147.
[121] Rhee, S. G., Bae, Y. S., Lee, S. R., Kwon, J. Hydrogen peroxide: a key messenger that modulates protein phosphorylation through cysteine oxidation. *Sci. STKE* 2000; 2000 (53): pe1.
[122] El-Serag, H. B., Johnson, M. L., Hachem, C., Morgana, R. O. Statins are associated with a reduced risk of hepatocellular carcinoma in a large cohort of patients with diabetes. *Gastroenterology* 2009; 136(5): 1601-1608.
[123] Kajimoto, K., Miyauchi, K., Kasai, T., Shimada, K., Kojima, Y., Shimada, A., Niinami, H., Amano, A., Daida, H. Short-term 20-mg atorvastatin therapy reduces key inflammatory factors including c-Jun N-terminal kinase and dendritic cells and matrix metalloproteinase expression in human abdominal aortic aneurysmal wall. *Atherosclerosis* 2009; 206(2): 505-511.
[124] Elmberg, M., Hultcrantz, R., Ekbom, A., Brandt, L., Olsson, S., Olsson, R., Lindgren, S., Loof, L., Stal, P., Wallerstedt, S., Almer, S., Sandberg-Gertzen, H., Askling, J. Cancer risk in patients with hereditary hemochromatosis and in their first-degree relatives. *Gastroenterology* 2003; 125(6): 1733-1741.
[125] Niederau, C., Fischer, R., Sonnenberg, A., Stremmel, W., Trampisch, H. J., Strohmeyer, G. Survival and causes of death in cirrhotic and in noncirrhotic patients with primary hemochromatosis. *N. Engl. J. Med.* 1985; 313(20): 1256-1262.
[126] Fracanzani, A. L., Conte, D., Fraquelli, M., Taioli, E., Mattioli, M., Losco, A., Fargion, S. Increased cancer risk in a cohort of 230 patients with hereditary hemochromatosis in comparison to matched control patients with non-iron-related chronic liver disease. *Hepatology* 2001; 33(3): 647-651.
[127] Propst, T., Propst, A., Dietze, O., Judmaier, G., Braunsteiner, H., Vogel, W. Prevalence of hepatocellular carcinoma in alpha-1-antitrypsin deficiency. *J. Hepatol.* 1994; 21(6): 1006-1011.
[128] Fattovich, G., Stroffolini, T., Zagni, I., Donato, F. Hepatocellular Carcinoma in Cirrhosis: Incidence and Risk Factors. *Gastroenterology* 2004; 127(5 S1): S35-S50.

In: Hepatocellular Carcinoma in the 3rd Millennium
Editors: M. Berretta and B. Cacopardo
ISBN: 978-1-63484-025-5

Chapter 3

HEPATOCELLULAR CARCINOMA GENETIC LANDSCAPE

Michele Simbolo, Paola Capelli, Ivana Cataldo* and Aldo Scarpa
Department of Pathology and Diagnostics,
University and Hospital Trust of Verona, Verona, Italy

ABSTRACT

Liver cancer is the sixth most commonly diagnosed cancer worldwide and the third leading cause of cancer death. The number of cases has also been rapidly increasing in Western countries, and globally, more than 700,000 new patients are diagnosed annually. HCC arising from hepatocytes, represents the most common histological subtype of liver cancers, accounting for approximately 70–85% of all cases. Multiple etiological factors for HCC have been identified. The most important risk factor is infection with hepatitis viruses, mainly HBV and HCV. Alcohol-induced liver damage also ranks high, especially in Western countries. Virus infection or metabolic stress results in liver damage including fatty change, hepatitis, and cirrhosis, which set premalignant conditions for HCC. Chronic inflammation, virus infection, and liver regeneration in cirrhosis have been reported to induce genetic and epigenetic damage to the host genome. Most HCCs gradually develop from these premalignant stages by the accumulation of these alterations. Accordingly, highly damaged livers are extremely susceptible to multiple tumors. The next-generation sequencing (NGS) era enabled whole-genome or exome sequencing of the cancer genome within a reasonable time frame and cost. This approach is rapidly and exhaustively identify potential key genetic events, including potential molecular therapeutic targets, in HCC.

The current review summarizes the data about molecular pathogenesis and signal transduction pathways in hepatocellular carcinoma considering recent results in molecular research.

---

* Correspondence to: Prof. Aldo Scarpa, Department of Pathology and Diagnostics, University and Hospital Trust of Verona, Verona, Italy. Email:aldo.scarpa@univr.it

INTRODUCTION

Liver cancer is the sixth most commonly diagnosed cancer worldwide and the third leading cause of cancer death [1, 2]. Prevalence of this cancer is different among ethnic groups; HCC is more frequent in East Asian and African populations [3, 4]. The number of cases has also been rapidly increasing in Western countries, and globally, more than 700,000 new patients are diagnosed annually [3].

Hepatocellular carcinoma (HCC), arising from hepatocytes, represents the most common histological subtype of liver cancers, accounting for approximately 70–85% of all cases [5].

Multiple etiological factors for HCC have been identified [4]. The most important risk factor is infection with hepatitis viruses, mainly HBV and HCV. Alcohol-induced liver damage also ranks high, especially in Western countries. Recently, metabolic diseases such as obesity and diabetes mellitus have become well recognized risk factors for HCC [6]. Virus infection or metabolic stress results in liver damage including fatty change, hepatitis, and cirrhosis, which set premalignant conditions for HCC. Chronic inflammation, virus infection, and liver regeneration in cirrhosis have been reported to induce genetic and epigenetic damage to the host genome [7]. Most HCCs gradually develop from these premalignant stages by the accumulation of these alterations. Accordingly, highly damaged livers are extremely susceptible to multiple tumors.

Next-generation sequencing (NGS) technology enables whole-genome or exome sequencing of the cancer genome within a reasonable time frame and cost. This approach is rapidly and exhaustively identifying key genetic events, such as potential molecular therapeutic targets, in cancers, including HCC and biliary tract malignancies [8, 9, 10].

The current review summarizes the data about molecular pathogenesis and signal transduction pathways in hepatocellular carcinoma considering recent results in molecular research.

HISTOPATHOLOGICAL CARCINOGENESIS: AN OVERVIEW

Hepatocarcinogenesis is a slow process during which genomic changes progressively alter the hepatocellular phenotype to produce cellular intermediates that evolve into hepatocellular carcinoma (Figure 1) [7].

This neoplasm arises in normal livers, abnormal but non-cirrhotic livers and in cirrhotic livers as a result of different environmental risk factors [11, 12]. Each of these scenarios involves different genetic and epigenetic alterations, chromosomal aberrations, gene mutations resulting in altered molecular pathways. Hepatocellular carcinoma evolves in a period of around 30 years after chronic HBV or HCV infection is first diagnosed [13]. In this time frame the disease develops through three steps: preneoplastic, dysplastic and neoplastic [7].

Preneoplastic steps begin after establishment of chronic hepatitis caused by viral infection [14, 15] or aflatoxin B1exposure [16] or presence of cirrhotic status [17-21] leading to phenotypical alterations of hepatocytes.

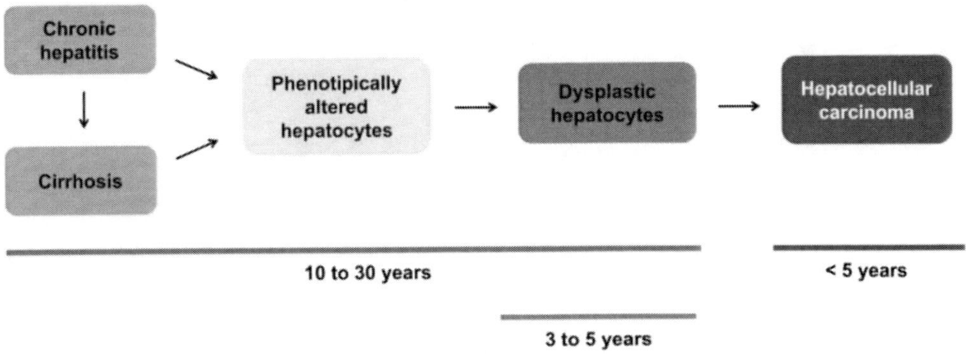

Figure 1. Chronologic sequence of cellular lesions culminating in the development of hepatocellular carcinoma in human.

Foci of phenotypically altered hepatocytes in chronic hepatitis and cirrhosis represent the first morphologically recognizable tissue lesions. The appearance of dysplastic cells characterizes the second phase that finally evolves in overt carcinoma. These morphological changes reflect the accumulation of genomic alterations in the transforming hepatocytes [7].

WNT PATHWAY

Wnt proteins are secreted extracellular auto-paracrine glycoproteins that interact with Frizzled receptors (FZD), a seven transmembrane domain protein, resembling the G-protein-coupled receptor (GPCR) family (Figure 2). They represent members of a highly conserved family that is involved in several processes including embryonic development, cell fate determination, proliferation, polarity, migration, and stem cell maintenance. In addition, Wnt/ß-catenin signaling has been found to play key roles in metabolic zonation of adult liver, regeneration [22]. The binding of Wnt to an FZD receptor can trigger the activation of at least three different pathways. The first is the Wnt/ß-catenin cascade, also called the Wnt-canonical pathway; the remaining two are the planar cell polarity (PCP) and the Wnt/calcium pathways, respectively. The two latter are ß-catenin independent and represent examples of the Wnt non-canonical cascades [23]. The activation of Wnt pathway induces regulation of expression of specific proto-oncogenes, including c-myc, cyclin D, and survivin.

The alterations in genes involved in this pathway is a feature of HCC. Unfortunately it constitutes the most undruggable pathway [24]. Recent exome studies confirmed *CTNNB1* the most frequent altered gene in HCC [25-27]. This gene encodes for ß-catenin that is the principal effector of the Wnt-canonical pathway, where it plays as transcriptional activator by binding TCF/LEF in nucleus and replacing the TLE-1 repressor, thus forming a transcriptional complex that activates the expression of its target genes [28].

AXIN1 and *APC* were affected by inactivating mutations in 15.2% and 1.6%, respectively [25, 26]. *AXIN1* encodes for a protein which composes a scaffold of proteins with APC, and two serine/threonine kinases: the glycogen synthase kinase 3b (GSK3b) and the casein kinase 1 (CK1). This targets ß-catenin for degradation in the absence of the canonical Wnt signaling [29].

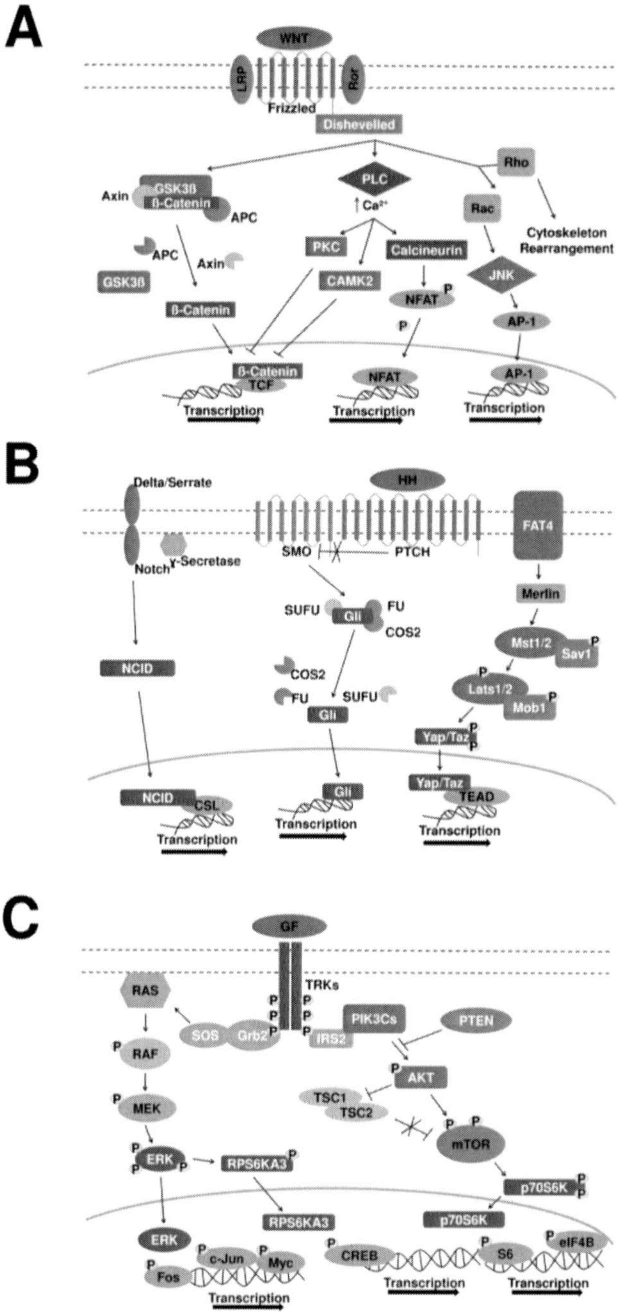

Figure 2. Significantly altered pathway in hepatocellular carcinoma: extracellular signaling *A*. Wnt pathway is the principal altered pathway in hepatocellular carcinoma. On the left, the Wnt canonical pathway which leads to the activation of β-catenin as transcriptional factor; in the middle the non canonical Wnt pathway known as WNT-Ca^{2+} is shown; on the right, the non canonical Wnt pathway known as Planar Cell Polarity (PCP) pathway which is involved in cytoskeleton rearrangement. *B*. Development and differentiation pathway. On the left side, Notch signaling is shown; in the middle the Hedgehog pathway and on the right side the Hippo pathway are represented. *C*. On the left the RAS/MEK pathway, on the right the PIK3/MTOR pathway. Although altered in a small proportion of cases, the PI3K signaling is one of the most targetable pathway in this tumor type.

This leads to a non-regulation of Wnt-canonical pathway and traslocation of ß-catenin in nucleus in the absence of Wnt signaling.

Other type of dysregulation of this pathway in HCC is the modulation of Wnt ligands or FZD receptor expression. As reported in many studies, they could account for Wnt/ß-catenin pathway activation without any mutation in *CTNNB1*, *APC*, or *AXIN* genes. Indeed, up-regulation of activators, such as ligands (Wnt1/3/4/5a/10b) or receptors/coreceptors (FZD3/6/7, Lrp6), and down-regulation of inhibitors (sFRP1/4/5, Wif1, Dkk3, Dkk4) have been reported in HCC and surrounding precancerous liver tissues, which emphasizes that their over and/or under-expression may be early molecular events during hepato-carcinogenesis [30-37].

DNA Integrity and Cell Cycle Control

The presence of *TP53* mutations in HCC dates back of more than 20 years [38, 39]. Recent exome studies confirmed that *TP53* mutations occur in more than 20% [25, 27] of cases, making this gene the second most altered in HCC. Copy number alterations (CNA) consisting in the loss of *TP53* locus at chromosome 17p13 is also frequent and often accompanies the mutation [40].

Mutations in the *IRF2* gene have been reported in 4.8% of wild type *TP53* HCCs [25]. In fact, IRF2 protein interacts with the p53 inhibitor MDM2, and acts as a transcriptional regulator through its DNA-binding activity and protein-protein interactions [41, 42].

MYC, *RB* and *BRCA2* genes that are involved in the DNA integrity and cell cycle control have been found altered in HCC. These genes are not altered by mutations but by copy number alterations (CNA) consisting in amplification of *MYC* and deletion of *RB* and *BRCA2* [43, 44, 45].

Moreover, the negative regulators of cell cycle progression p15/p16 (*CDKN2A/CDKN2B*) have also been reported as frequently deleted [25, 46] whereas *CCND1*, an oncogenic driver and positive regulator of cell cycle, has been found amplified [46]. *CDKN2A*, which encodes $p16^{INK4a}$ protein, has also been suggested to be silenced through CpG island hyper-methylation [47].

The *TERT* gene encodes a telomerase reverse transcriptase, the catalytic subunit of the telomerase enzyme, which maintains telomere length by the addition of the telomere repeat sequence at the end of each chromosome, and its expression plays an essential role in overriding cellular senescence. Dysregulation of telomerase expression in somatic cells is involved in carcinogenesis, and cancer cells frequently overexpress TERT [48]. Previous studies indicated that HBV integration occurs in genes encoding molecules that are important in the control of cell signaling and proliferation, including the *TERT* gene [49, 50]. In a genome sequencing study of 27 HCCs including 11 HBV-associated and 14 HCV-associated HCCs, HBV integration was detected within or upstream of the TERT gene in 4 of the 11 HBV-related HCCs, consistent with previous reports of recurrent HBV integration at the *TERT* gene locus [25]. In summary, more than 20% of HBV-associated HCCs have HBV virus DNA integrated into the *TERT* gene leading to its over-expression, thus enabling replicative immortality which is a hallmark of HCC.

Chromatin Remodeling

In the last years SWI/SNF chromatin remodeling pathway acquired a central role in tumorigenesis of different cancer type [51, 52]. Several exome sequencing studies on solid tumor identified the genes involved in this pathway as most frequent altered in cancer and HCC is no exception [25, 27, 53]. The combination of proteins encoded by these genes composes five possible complexes deputed to specific roles in cellular development and maintenance by modifying chromatin structure to enhance or silence transcriptional activity [54]. Interestingly, two of the most frequently altered genes, *ARID1A* and *ARID2*, are mutated in different proportions of HCCs according to their specific etiology. In fact, *ARID2* mutations are significantly enriched in HCV-associated HCC compared to HBV-associated HCC (14% vs. 2%, P value = 0.046) [27], and *ARID1A* mutation appears to be associated with alcohol intake (P value = 0.002) [25]. A recent study on 110 HBV-associated HCCs confirmed the presence of *ARID1A* mutations in 13% of cases, and suggested a crucial role of these anomalies in tumor metastasis [55].

Less frequent mutations of other SWI/SNF components, including *SMARCA2*, *SMARCA4*, and *SMARCB1*, the BAF subunit (*SMARCA1*), and the PBAF subunit (*PBRM1*), have been identified in HCC. The SMARC family includes a series of genes encoding the catalytic core of chromatin remodeling complex [56] whereas *PBRM1* has preferential binding to different acetylated lysine configurations of histone tails, indicating that it may contribute to the 'reading' of the histone code [57]. Recurrent mutations of histone methyltransferases, including *MLL* in 1.7% and *MLL3* in 4.2% of cases have also been identified [53]. Of particular interest is the report of a HBV integration site into the MLL4 methyltransferase gene in one tumor [58]. The transcriptional impact of HBV integration was evaluated with RNA sequencing which showed that integration of HBV DNA into the 3rd exon of *MLL4* resulted in a human-viral fusion transcript and a 20-fold increase of MLL4 transcription in comparison with the adjacent normal liver tissue [58].

Ras and Pi3k Signaling

Despite the rarity of *KRAS* mutations in HCC [59], a high prevalence of *KRAS* mutations has been detected in HCCs associated with high exposure of vinyl chloride [60]. Recurrent mutations in *RPS6KA3* have been found in 9.6% of cases. *RPS6KA3* is a gene located on chromosome X that encodes the ribosomal S6 protein kinase 2 (RSK2). RSK2 is a serine/threonine kinase of the Ras/MAPK signaling pathway that is directly phosphorylated and activated by extracellular-regulated kinases 1 and 2 (ERK1/2). RSK2 exerts feedback inhibition on the ERK1/2 pathway by phosphorylating and inhibiting the guanine nucleotide exchange factor SOS [61, 62]. These mutations may cause aberrant activation of the ERK pathway.

Dysregulation in components of mTOR pathway has been reported in a small proportion of cases. A targeted next generation sequencing study on 14 advanced/metastatic HCCs found aberrations leading to putative activation of the PI3K/AKT/mTOR pathway [63]. In a large cohort of 125 cases *PIK3CA* was altered in only 1.6% of cases, while *PTEN* and *PIK3CG* were altered in less than 1% of cases [25].

Oxidative Stress Response Pathway

NFE2L2 encodes a master transcription factor that is crucial for cellular redox homeostasis and oxidative stress response. Hotspot missense mutations in the DLG and ETGF motifs have been reported in lung cancers [67]. Recurrent *NFE2L2* hotspot mutations were identified in HCC (8/125, 6.4%) [25]. Further, inactivating mutations of *KEAP1*, a negative regulator of NFE2L2, have been reported in HCC [25, 68]. *NEF2L2* or *KEAP1* mutations coexisted with the deregulation of the WNT pathway by *CTNNB1* or *AXIN1* mutations [25], suggesting a potential synergistic association between the oxidative stress pathway and WNT signaling in HCC.

The Keap1-Nrf2 pathway is the major regulator of cytoprotective responses to endogenous and exogenous stresses caused by reactive oxygen species (ROS) and electrophiles [64]. The key signaling proteins within the pathway are the transcription factorNrf2 (nuclear factor erythroid 2-related factor 2 encoded by *NFE2L2* gene) that binds together with small Maf proteins to the antioxidant response element (ARE) in the regulatory regions of target genes, and Keap1 (Kelch ECH associating protein 1), a repressor protein that binds to Nrf2 and promotes its degradation by the ubiquitin proteasome pathway.

In basal conditions of the Nrf2-Keap1 signaling pathway, two Keap1 molecules bind to Nrf2 and Nrf2 is polyubiquitylated by the Cul3-based E3 ligase complex. This polyubiquitylation results in rapid Nrf2 degradation by the proteasome. A small proportion of Nrf2 escapes the inhibitory complex and accumulates in the nucleus to mediate basal ARE-dependent gene expression, thereby maintaining the cellular homeostasis. Under stress conditions, inducers modify the Keap1 cysteines leading to the inhibition of Nrf2 ubiquitylation via dissociation of the inhibitory complex [65, 66].

Differentiation and Development

Notch signaling pathway plays an important role in cell-cellcommunications and participates in the regulation of multiple cell differentiation processes during embryonic development and stem/progenitor cell staging [69, 70]. Two studies have demonstrated that NOTCH1 overexpression inhibits HCC cell growth by promoting cell cycle arrest and apoptosis [71, 72]. Despite this, there is evidence for an oncogenic role of Notch activation in hepatocarcinogenesis [73]. Also significant over-expression of NOTCH1 and NOTCH3 was detected by immunohistochemistry in 60 HCCs [74].

Hedgehog signaling pathway is required for embryogenesis and regulation of a variety of essential functions, from differentiation to regeneration, as well as in stem cell biology, through control of cellular proliferation, apoptosis, and migration. It is activated by the interaction of Hh ligands (i.e., sonic, Indian, and dessert hedgehog) with the transmembrane Smoothened (SMO) receptor, resulting in nuclear translocation of Gli and transcriptional activation of target genes among which *MYC* and *CYCLIN-D1*. Hh signaling targets include ß-catenin and different cyclins, along with Hh negative regulators such as PTCH and HHIP. In diseased livers, the Hh pathway promotes hepatic regeneration; however, excessive or continuous activation of Hh has been shown to halt successful regeneration and contribute to liver fibrosis [75]. In HCC, the initial findings demonstrated aberrant over-expression of GLI1 and SMO together with down-regulation of HHIP in a subset of HCCs [76].

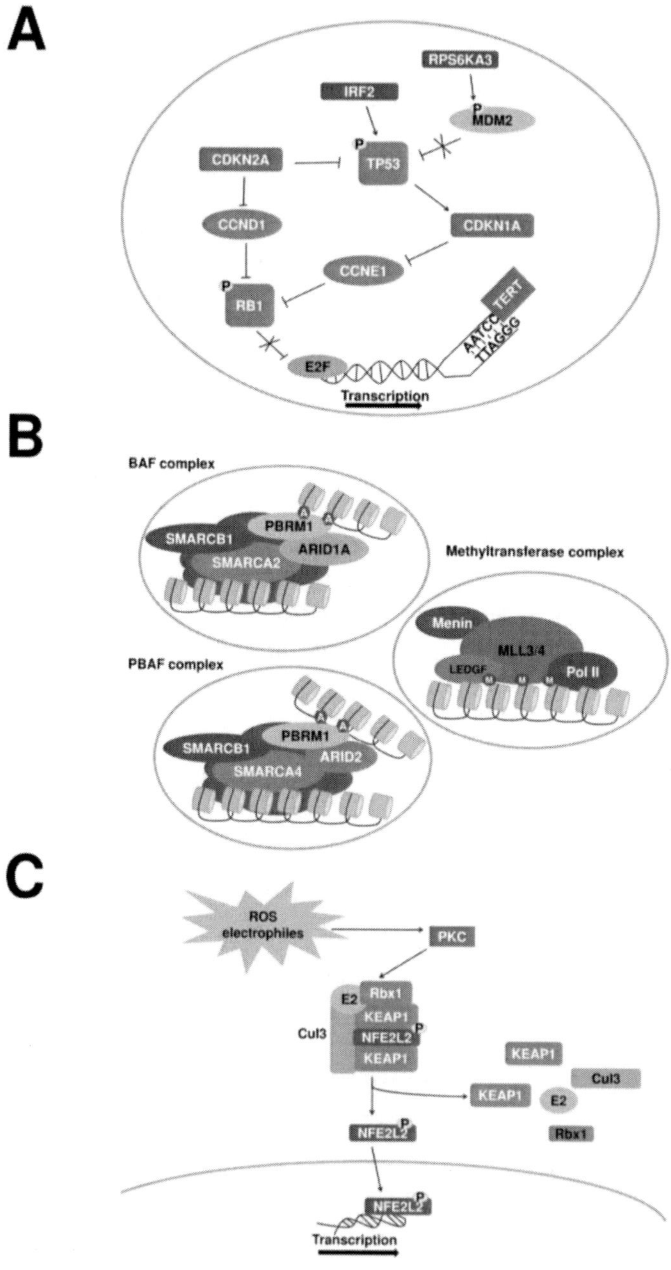

Figure 3. Significantly altered pathway in hepatocellular carcinoma: cytoplasmic and nucleus signaling. *A.* DNA integrity and cell cycle control include a series of genes frequently altered in hepatocellular carcinoma in particular *TP53* which is the second most altered gene in this tumor. *B.* Chromatin remodeler genes have been found altered in different tumor types. The genes involved in the BAF/PBAF complexes and Methyltransferase complex appear to be the most altered in hepatocellular carcinoma. *C.* Oxidative stress response pathway included a series of genes coding for proteins involved in the response to ROS and electrophiles stimuli.

The hippo pathway is an evolutionary conserved cascade that plays an essential role in the control of organ size and cell contact inhibition by regulating cell proliferation and apoptosis. Recent evidence has pointed towards an oncogenic role for this pathway in human cancer, including HCC [77]. While the key components and upstream regulators of the hippo pathway (e.g., FAT, NF2, and FDM6) are mostly considered to participate as tumor suppressors, downstream mediators such as TAZ, YAP, and TEADs are mostly involved in oncogenic events. Interestingly, approximately 30% of HCCs present with low levels of phospho-YAP and an inactive cleaved form of MST1 is present in the majority of these cases [78]. Moreover, a heterozygous deletion of YAP was able to suppress development of HCC caused by NF2 inactivation [79]. Altogether, these findings indicate that inhibition of YAP by MST1/2 can be considered as an important pathway for HCC suppression.

Conclusion

Characterization of the genetic alterations associated with HCC is an essential step to increase our knowledge of hepatocarcinogenesis. In recent years, remarkable progress has been made in elucidating the molecular pathology of hepatic tumors. With the new sequencing technologies, elucidation of the nature of the liver cancer genome has become possible. The emerging molecular characterization of HCC is of utmost importance and may open the door to novel innovative targeted therapies in HCC. Sequencing analysis has further helped identify the molecular complexity of multi-centric lesions and intratumoral heterogeneity. Detailed analysis of somatic mutation signatures and hepatitis related virus genome integration sites will clarify the molecular basis of liver carcinogenesis. Finally, comprehensive studies may find clinical application to identify markers useful for the early detection of tumors, the assessment of prognosis or to find new therapeutic targets.

References

[1] Center MM, Jemal A: International trends in liver cancer incidence rates. *Cancer Epidemiol. Biomarkers Prev.,* 20:2362-8, 2011.

[2] Jemal A, Bray F, Center MM, et al. Global cancer statistics. *CA Cancer J. Clin.,* 61:69-90, 2011.

[3] Yang JD, Roberts LR: Hepatocellular carcinoma: A global view. *Nat. Rev. Gastroenterol. Hepatol.,* 7:448-58, 2010.

[4] Altekruse SF, McGlynn KA, Reichman ME: Hepatocellular carcinoma incidence, mortality, and survival trends in the United States from 1975 to 2005. *J. Clin. Oncol.,* 27:1485-91, 2009.

[5] Perz JF, Armstrong GL, Farrington LA, et al. The contributions of hepatitis B virus and hepatitis C virus infections to cirrhosis and primary liver cancer worldwide. *J. Hepatol.,* 45:529-38, 2006.

[6] El-Serag HB: Epidemiology of viral hepatitis and hepatocellular carcinoma. *Gastroenterology,* 142:1264-1273 e1, 2012.

[7] Thorgeirsson SS, Grisham JW: Molecular pathogenesis of human hepatocellular carcinoma. *Nat. Genet.,* 31:339-46, 2002.
[8] Chin L, Andersen JN, Futreal PA: Cancer genomics: from discovery science to personalized medicine. *Nat. Med.,* 17:297-303, 2011.
[9] Tao Y, Ruan J, Yeh SH, et al. Rapid growth of a hepatocellular carcinoma and the driving mutations revealed by cell-population genetic analysis of whole-genome data. *Proc. Natl. Acad. Sci. USA,* 108:12042-7, 2011.
[10] Simbolo M, Fassan M, Ruzzenente A, et al. Multigene mutational profiling of cholangiocarcinomas identifies actionable molecular subgroups. *Oncotarget,* 5:2839-52, 2014.
[11] Llovet JM, Bruix J: Systematic review of randomized trials for unresectable hepatocellular carcinoma: Chemoembolization improves survival. *Hepatology,* 37:429-42, 2003.
[12] Llovet JM, Burroughs A, Bruix J: Hepatocellular carcinoma. *Lancet,* 362:1907-17, 2003.
[13] Tong MJ, el-Farra NS, Reikes AR, et al. Clinical outcomes after transfusion-associated hepatitis C. *N. Engl. J. Med.,* 332:1463-6, 1995.
[14] Takano S, Yokosuka O, Imazeki F, et al. Incidence of hepatocellular carcinoma in chronic hepatitis B and C: a prospective study of 251 patients. *Hepatology,* 21:650-5, 1995.
[15] Chu CM: Natural history of chronic hepatitis B virus infection in adults with emphasis on the occurrence of cirrhosis and hepatocellular carcinoma. *J. Gastroenterol. Hepatol.,* 15 Suppl:E25-30, 2000.
[16] Moudgil V, Redhu D, Dhanda S, et al. A review of molecular mechanisms in the development of hepatocellular carcinoma by aflatoxin and hepatitis B and C viruses. *J. Environ. Pathol. Toxicol. Oncol.,* 32:165-75, 2013.
[17] Oka H, Kurioka N, Kim K, et al. Prospective study of early detection of hepatocellular carcinoma in patients with cirrhosis. *Hepatology,* 12:680-7, 1990.
[18] Ikeda K, Saitoh S, Koida I, et al. A multivariate analysis of risk factors for hepatocellular carcinogenesis: a prospective observation of 795 patients with viral and alcoholic cirrhosis. *Hepatology,* 18:47-53, 1993.
[19] Kato Y, Nakata K, Omagari K, et al. Risk of hepatocellular carcinoma in patients with cirrhosis in Japan. Analysis of infectious hepatitis viruses. *Cancer,* 74:2234-8, 1994.
[20] del Olmo JA, Serra MA, Rodriguez F, et al. Incidence and risk factors for hepatocellular carcinoma in 967 patients with cirrhosis. *J. Cancer Res. Clin. Oncol.,* 124:560-4, 1998.
[21] Chiaramonte M, Stroffolini T, Vian A, et al. Rate of incidence of hepatocellular carcinoma in patients with compensated viral cirrhosis. *Cancer,* 85:2132-7, 1999.
[22] Gebhardt R, Hovhannisyan A: Organ patterning in the adult stage: the role of Wnt/beta-catenin signaling in liver zonation and beyond. *Dev. Dyn.,* 239:45-55, 2010.
[23] Huelsken J, Behrens J: The Wnt signalling pathway. *J. Cell Sci.,* 115: 3977-8, 2002.
[24] Moon RT, Kohn AD, De Ferrari GV, et al. WNT and beta-catenin signalling: diseases and therapies. *Nat. Rev. Genet.,* 5:691-701, 2004.
[25] Guichard C, Amaddeo G, Imbeaud S, et al. Integrated analysis of somatic mutations and focal copy-number changes identifies key genes and pathways in hepatocellular carcinoma. *Nat. Genet.,* 44:694-8, 2012.

[26] Totoki Y, Tatsuno K, Yamamoto S, et al. High-resolution characterization of a hepatocellular carcinoma genome. *Nat. Genet.,* 43:464-9, 2011.

[27] Li M, Zhao H, Zhang X, et al. Inactivating mutations of the chromatin remodeling gene ARID2 in hepatocellular carcinoma. *Nat. Genet.,* 43:828-9, 2011.

[28] Brantjes H, Roose J, van De Wetering M, et al. All Tcf HMG box transcription factors interact with Groucho-related co-repressors. *Nucleic Acids Res.,* 29:1410-9, 2001.

[29] MacDonald BT, Tamai K, He X: Wnt/beta-catenin signaling: components, mechanisms, and diseases. *Dev. Cell,* 17:9-26, 2009.

[30] Bengochea A, de Souza MM, Lefrancois L, et al. Common dysregulation of Wnt/Frizzled receptor elements in human hepatocellular carcinoma. *Br. J. Cancer,* 99:143-50, 2008.

[31] Kim M, Lee HC, Tsedensodnom O, et al. Functional interaction between Wnt3 and Frizzled-7 leads to activation of the Wnt/beta-catenin signaling pathway in hepatocellular carcinoma cells. *J. Hepatol.,* 48:780-91, 2008.

[32] Wei W, Chua MS, Grepper S, et al. Blockade of Wnt-1 signaling leads to anti-tumor effects in hepatocellular carcinoma cells. *Mol. Cancer,* 8:76, 2009.

[33] Tung EK, Wong BY, Yau TO, et al. Upregulation of the Wnt co-receptor LRP6 promotes hepatocarcinogenesis and enhances cell invasion. *PLoS One,* 7:e36565, 2012.

[34] Yoshikawa H, Matsubara K, Zhou X, et al. WNT10B functional dualism: beta-catenin/Tcf-dependent growth promotion or independent suppression with deregulated expression in cancer. *Mol. Biol. Cell,* 18:4292-303, 2007.

[35] Deng Y, Yu B, Cheng Q, et al. Epigenetic silencing of WIF-1 in hepatocellular carcinomas. *J. Cancer Res. Clin. Oncol.,* 136:1161-7, 2010.

[36] Ding Z, Qian YB, Zhu LX, et al. Promoter methylation and mRNA expression of DKK-3 and WIF-1 in hepatocellular carcinoma. *World J. Gastroenterol.,* 15:2595-601, 2009.

[37] Fatima S, Lee NP, Tsang FH, et al. Dickkopf 4 (DKK4) acts on Wnt/beta-catenin pathway by influencing beta-catenin in hepatocellular carcinoma. *Oncogene,* 31:4233-44, 2012.

[38] Oda T, Tsuda H, Scarpa A, et al. p53 gene mutation spectrum in hepatocellular carcinoma. *Cancer Res.,* 52:6358-64, 1992.

[39] Hsu IC, Metcalf RA, Sun T, et al. Mutational hotspot in the p53 gene in human hepatocellular carcinomas. *Nature,* 350:427-8, 1991.

[40] Wang G, Zhao Y, Liu X, et al. Allelic loss and gain, but not genomic instability, as the major somatic mutation in primary hepatocellular carcinoma. *Genes Chromosomes Cancer,* 31:221-7, 2001.

[41] Tamura T, Yanai H, Savitsky D, et al. The IRF family transcription factors in immunity and oncogenesis. *Annu. Rev. Immunol.,* 26:535-84, 2008.

[42] Pettersson S, Kelleher M, Pion E, et al. Role of Mdm2 acid domain interactions in recognition and ubiquitination of the transcription factor IRF-2. *Biochem. J.,* 418:575-85, 2009.

[43] Kusano N, Shiraishi K, Kubo K, et al. Genetic aberrations detected by comparative genomic hybridization in hepatocellular carcinomas: their relationship to clinicopathological features. *Hepatology,* 29:1858-62, 1999.

[44] Pedica F, Ruzzenente A, Bagante F, et al. A re-emerging marker for prognosis in hepatocellular carcinoma: the add-value of fishing c-myc gene for early relapse. *PLoS One,* 8:e68203, 2013.

[45] Knuutila S, Aalto Y, Autio K, et al. DNA copy number losses in human neoplasms. *Am. J. Pathol.,* 155:683-94, 1999.

[46] Wang K, Lim HY, Shi S, et al. Genomic landscape of copy number aberrations enables the identification of oncogenic drivers in hepatocellular carcinoma. *Hepatology,* 58:706-17, 2013.

[47] Matsuda Y, Ichida T, Matsuzawa J, et al. p16(INK4) is inactivated by extensive CpG methylation in human hepatocellular carcinoma. *Gastroenterology,* 116:394-400, 1999.

[48] Cao Y, Bryan TM, Reddel RR: Increased copy number of the TERT and TERC telomerase subunit genes in cancer cells. *Cancer Sci.,* 99:1092-9, 2008.

[49] Wang J, Chenivesse X, Henglein B, et al. Hepatitis B virus integration in a cyclin A gene in a hepatocellular carcinoma. *Nature,* 343:555-7, 1990.

[50] Paterlini-Brechot P, Saigo K, Murakami Y, et al. Hepatitis B virus-related insertional mutagenesis occurs frequently in human liver cancers and recurrently targets human telomerase gene. *Oncogene,* 22:3911-6, 2003.

[51] Oike T, Ogiwara H, Nakano T, et al. Inactivating mutations in SWI/SNF chromatin remodeling genes in human cancer. *Jpn. J. Clin. Oncol.,* 43:849-55, 2013.

[52] Masliah-Planchon J, Bieche I, Guinebretiere JM, et al. SWI/SNF Chromatin Remodeling and Human Malignancies. *Annu. Rev. Pathol.,* 2014.

[53] Fujimoto A, Totoki Y, Abe T, et al. Whole-genome sequencing of liver cancers identifies etiological influences on mutation patterns and recurrent mutations in chromatin regulators. *Nat. Genet.,* 44:760-4, 2012.

[54] Hohmann AF, Vakoc CR: A rationale to target the SWI/SNF complex for cancer therapy. *Trends Genet.,* 30:356-63, 2014.

[55] Huang J, Deng Q, Wang Q, et al. Exome sequencing of hepatitis B virus-associated hepatocellular carcinoma. *Nat. Genet.,* 44:1117-21, 2012.

[56] Wang X, Haswell JR, Roberts CW: Molecular pathways: SWI/SNF (BAF) complexes are frequently mutated in cancer--mechanisms and potential therapeutic insights. *Clin. Cancer Res.,* 20:21-7, 2014.

[57] Chandrasekaran R, Thompson M: Polybromo-1-bromodomains bind histone H3 at specific acetyl-lysine positions. *Biochem. Biophys. Res. Commun.,* 355:661-6, 2007.

[58] Jiang Z, Jhunjhunwala S, Liu J, et al. The effects of hepatitis B virus integration into the genomes of hepatocellular carcinoma patients. *Genome Res.,* 22:593-601, 2012.

[59] Tsuda H, Hirohashi S, Shimosato Y, et al. Low incidence of point mutation of c-Ki-ras and N-ras oncogenes in human hepatocellular carcinoma. *Jpn. J. Cancer Res.,* 80:196-9, 1989.

[60] Weihrauch M, Benick M, Lehner G, et al. High prevalence of K-ras-2 mutations in hepatocellular carcinomas in workers exposed to vinyl chloride. *Int. Arch. Occup. Environ Health,* 74:405-10, 2001.

[61] Douville E, Downward J: EGF induced SOS phosphorylation in PC12 cells involves P90 RSK-2. *Oncogene,* 15:373-83, 1997.

[62] Schneider A, Mehmood T, Pannetier S, et al. Altered ERK/MAPK signaling in the hippocampus of the mrsk2_KO mouse model of Coffin-Lowry syndrome. *J. Neurochem.,* 119:447-59, 2011.

[63] Janku F, Kaseb AO, Tsimberidou AM, et al. Identification of novel therapeutic targets in the PI3K/AKT/mTOR pathway in hepatocellular carcinoma using targeted next generation sequencing. *Oncotarget,* 5:3012-22, 2014.

[64] Kansanen E, Jyrkkanen HK, Levonen AL: Activation of stress signaling pathways by electrophilic oxidized and nitrated lipids. *Free Radic. Biol. Med.,* 52:973-82, 2012.

[65] Kansanen E, Kivela AM, Levonen AL: Regulation of Nrf2-dependent gene expression by 15-deoxy-Delta12,14-prostaglandin J2. *Free Radic. Biol. Med.,* 47:1310-7, 2009.

[66] Taguchi K, Motohashi H, Yamamoto M: Molecular mechanisms of the Keap1-Nrf2 pathway in stress response and cancer evolution. *Genes Cells,* 16:123-40, 2011.

[67] Shibata T, Ohta T, Tong KI, et al. Cancer related mutations in NRF2 impair its recognition by Keap1-Cul3 E3 ligase and promote malignancy. *Proc. Natl. Acad. Sci. USA,* 105:13568-73, 2008.

[68] Lee DF, Kuo HP, Liu M, et al. KEAP1 E3 ligase-mediated downregulation of NF-kappaB signaling by targeting IKKbeta. *Mol. Cell,* 36:131-40, 2009.

[69] Radtke F, Raj K: The role of Notch in tumorigenesis: oncogene or tumour suppressor? *Nat. Rev. Cancer,* 3:756-67, 2003.

[70] Zaret KS: Genetic programming of liver and pancreas progenitors: lessons for stem-cell differentiation. *Nat. Rev. Genet.,* 9:329-40, 2008.

[71] Qi R, An H, Yu Y, et al. Notch1 signaling inhibits growth of human hepatocellular carcinoma through induction of cell cycle arrest and apoptosis. *Cancer Res.,* 63:8323-9, 2003.

[72] Wang C, Qi R, Li N, et al. Notch1 signaling sensitizes tumor necrosis factor-related apoptosis-inducing ligand-induced apoptosis in human hepatocellular carcinoma cells by inhibiting Akt/Hdm2-mediated p53 degradation and up-regulating p53-dependent DR5 expression. *J. Biol. Chem.,* 284:16183-90, 2009.

[73] Villanueva A, Alsinet C, Yanger K, et al. Notch signaling is activated in human hepatocellular carcinoma and induces tumor formation in mice. *Gastroenterology,* 143:1660-1669 e7, 2012.

[74] Giovannini C, Gramantieri L, Chieco P, et al. Selective ablation of Notch3 in HCC enhances doxorubicin's death promoting effect by a p53 dependent mechanism. *J. Hepatol.,* 50:969-79, 2009.

[75] Omenetti A, Choi S, Michelotti G, et al. Hedgehog signaling in the liver. *J. Hepatol.,* 54:366-73, 2011.

[76] Patil MA, Zhang J, Ho C, et al. Hedgehog signaling in human hepatocellular carcinoma. *Cancer Biol. Ther.,* 5:111-7, 2006.

[77] Chan SW, Lim CJ, Chen L, et al. The Hippo pathway in biological control and cancer development. *J. Cell Physiol.,* 226:928-39, 2011.

[78] Zhou D, Conrad C, Xia F, et al. Mst1 and Mst2 maintain hepatocyte quiescence and suppress hepatocellular carcinoma development through inactivation of the Yap1 oncogene. *Cancer Cell,* 16:425-38, 2009.

[79] Zhang N, Bai H, David KK, et al. The Merlin/NF2 tumor suppressor functions through the YAP oncoprotein to regulate tissue homeostasis in mammals. *Dev. Cell,* 19:27-38, 2010.

In: Hepatocellular Carcinoma in the 3rd Millennium
Editors: M. Berretta and B. Cacopardo
ISBN: 978-1-63484-025-5

Chapter 4

NON-INVASIVE DIAGNOSIS OF HEPATOCELLULAR CARCINOMA

M. D'Onofrio*, E. Demozzi, R. De Robertis, S. Crosara and R. Pozzi Mucelli
Department of Radiology, G.B. Rossi Hospital –
University of Verona, Italy

INTRODUCTION

Hepatocellular carcinoma (HCC), the most common primary malignancy of the liver, represents 1 of the leading causes of cancer deaths in the world [1].

The main risk factor for HCC is the presence of chronic liver disease, particularly when the disease has already resulted in liver cirrhosis. The constant process of destruction and repair within the parenchyma that is associated with cirrhosis increases hepatocyte metabolism and amplifies the risk of mutations in a multistep progression from hyper-plastic nodule to early HCC and finally to moderately/poorly differentiated HCC. Hepatitis B and C viruses (HBV and HCV) are known to have oncogenic potential, and the risk of HCC in HBV and HCV carriers is increased independently of the presence of cirrhosis [2, 3].

The diagnosis of a hepatocellular carcinoma (HCC) strongly relies on imaging. Ultrasonography (US) plays a crucial role in surveillance, due to wide availability, relative inexpensiveness, and biological safety. According to the American Association for the Study of the Liver Diseases (AASLD) 2011 guidelines, US is recommended for surveillance of patients at risk of developing HCC; [4] namely, US should be performed every 6 months in patients with chronic B hepatitis and cirrhotic patients, regardless of the cause. However, literature data indicate highly variable sensitivity rates for the US detection of HCC, ranging from 33% to 96% [5]. Each suspected HCC discovered at US in a patient under surveillance must be therefore confirmed with multiphasic dynamic imaging [6]. CT and MRI must be used for the non-invasive diagnosis of HCC in patients under surveillance; according to the

* Correspondence to: Prof. Mirko D'Onofrio, Department of Radiology, G.B. Rossi Hospital – University of Verona. E-mail: mirko.donofrio@univr.it

AASLD 2011 guidelines [7] and to the European Association for the Study of the Liver (EASL) and the European Organization for Research and Treatment of Cancer (EORTC) [8], hyper-vascularity during hepatic arterial phase and wash-out on either portal venous or delayed phase are hallmark imaging features for the diagnosis of HCC. When present in patients under US surveillance, these features are sufficient for a non-invasive diagnosis [9, 10].

HEPATOCARCINOGENESIS

HCC develops through a multistep carcinogenesis starting from regenerative nodules, to low-/high-grade dysplastic nodules (LG- and HG-DN), early HCC, and finally into an overt HCC. Changes in blood supply, cellular content, microscopic architecture (cellular density, cords number) and biliary impairment take place during hepatocarcinogenesis [11]. This multistep carcinogenesis has the pathological meaning of a progressive de-differentiation of phenotypically abnormal lesions. Precursors of HCC have therefore specific and different pathological features: regenerative nodules are composed of normal hepatic parenchyma surrounded by a fibrous stroma: they present as innumerable, well-defined rounded regions of cirrhotic parenchyma surrounded by scar tissue, typically measuring 1–15 mm. These nodules lack clonal features and their cells are phenotypically normal so they usually are considered benign, even if dysplastic. Dysplastic nodules differ both macroscopically (size, color and consistency) and microscopically from regenerative nodules and background parenchyma and are classified as low grade or high grade, depending on the degree of cytologic and architectural atypia. Histologically, LG-DN do not show cytologic atypia neither expansive sub nodules nor architectural alterations. In HG-DN cells show cellular atypia, although not sufficient to establish a diagnosis of HCC, and may exhibit clone-like features. Early HCCs are analogous to "carcinoma in situ" or "micro invasive carcinoma" of other organs. Macroscopically they rarely exceed 2 cm and present as vaguely nodular lesions with indistinct margins, without a capsule. Progressed HCCs smaller than 2 cm are usually well-defined nodules; unlike early HCCs, small and progressed HCCs present an expansive growth with possible invasion of the adjacent parenchyma and structures. They are typically surrounded by a capsule and contain internal fibrous septa. HCCs exceeding 2 cm in diameter are known as "large HCCs." "Mosaic" architecture, defined as the presence of multiple internal tumor nodules separated by fibrous septa and areas of hemorrhage, necrosis, and fatty changes, is typical. Angiogenesis progresses along with hepatocarcinogenesis. Angiogenesis is histologically characterized by the onset of unpaired (or "non-triadal") arteries and sinusoidal capillarization [12, 13]. Unpaired arteries are isolated vessels not accompanied by bile ducts and/or portal veins. These arteries are absent in regenerative nodules; sometimes they are present in small number in LG-DN, while are present with increasing size and number in HG-DN, early HCCs and progressed HCCs [14]. The relative reduction of portal vessels causes a gradual reduction of portal blood flow to the nodules, which is accompanied to a compensatory increase of the arterial flow, due to the development of unpaired arteries [12, 13]. Venous drainage also evolves during hepatocarcinogenesis, shifting from hepatic veins (regenerative and dysplastic nodules, early HCCs) to sinusoids (progressed HCCs without fibrous capsules) to portal veins (progressed HCCs with fibrous capsules)

[15, 16]. During early phases of hepatocarcinogenesis there is an equilibrium between the arterial flow and the preservation of a portal flow, while in latter phases portal blood flow declines until it becomes absent, while arterial flow increases. As a consequence, LG-DN usually have a balanced vascular supply, similar to that of regenerative nodules and therefore will be isoenhancing at imaging as compared to the background liver, while HG-DN and early HCCs tend to a diminished arterial and portal flow, hence they can show hypo-enhancement. Moderately differentiated and progressed HCCs usually have elevated arterial flow with reduced or absent portal venous flow: this is the pathologic base that explains the typical contrastographic wash-in and wash-out. Progressed HCCs may also be associated with a peripheral enhancement during late arterial or early portal venous phases; this is probably caused by the passage of contrast medium from tumor through draining sinusoids and portal venules into surrounding sinusoids.

Early HCCs, being drained by hepatic veins, are not associated with this peripheral enhancement. Moreover, progressed HCCs tend to invade draining sinusoids and portal venules, leading to intra-hepatic metastatic spread: these metastases often manifest as satellite nodules located within the parenchyma that receives the venous drainage from the primary tumor. During the early stages of hepatocarcinogenesis hepatocytes may accumulate fat, therefore LG-DN, HG-DN, and early HCCs may show higher fat deposition than background liver [17]. The probability of intra-nodular lipid storage increases from LG-DNs to early HCCs: 40% of these latter present a diffuse fat storage. The peak frequency of diffuse steatosis is in 1.5 cm early HCCs and declines with increasing tumor size and grade [18]. Therefore, in a patient with cirrhosis or chronic hepatitis B, a fatty lesion is very likely to be a dysplastic nodule or an early HCC. Iron may accumulate in LG-DNs and some HG-DNs of patients without a systemic iron overload [19]. These iron-rich nodules are commonly described as "siderotic nodules." With further de-differentiation, hepatocytes may become "resistant" to iron accumulation, therefore most HG-DNs, early HCCs and progressed HCCs are iron free; even high-grade DNs and HCC sub nodules developing from otherwise siderotic precursors may not show iron deposition [20]. A siderotic nodule in a patient with cirrhosis or chronic B hepatitis is very likely to be a dysplastic nodule rather than an HCC. The development of an iron-free sub nodule within a siderotic nodule, however, suggests the incidental development of an HCC.

Organic anionic transporting polypeptides (OATP) are a family of proteins expressed in hepatocytes along the sinusoidal membrane, involved in bile transportation [21]. One of these transporters, OATP 8, is thought to play a crucial role for the uptake of two gadolinium-chelates contrast agents, gadoxetate disodium (Gd-EOB-DTPA) and gadobenate dimeglumine (Gd-BOPTA), by hepatocytes.

Literature data suggest that the expression of these transporters tends to decrease during hepatocarcinogenesis: expression levels are therefore higher in regenerative nodule and LG-DNs and lower in most HG-DNs, early HCCs and progressed HCCs [22]. Therefore, nodules with OATP-8 under-expression will appear hypointense as compared to the background liver during the hepato-biliary phase of MRI.

ULTRASONOGRAPHY

US plays a key role in the diagnosis of HCC. Surveillance programs aim is the early detection of HCCs in high-risk patients and are based on US examinations performed at variable (6-12 months) time intervals [23]. The 2011 AASLD guidelines recommend that surveillance of high-risk patients for HCC should be based only on US at 6-month intervals [24], because alpha-fetoprotein (AFP) determination lacks sensitivity and specificity for an effective surveillance.

Screening for HCC is most important in high-risk groups such as patients with cirrhosis, independently from the cause (viral, alcoholic, primary biliary cirrhosis, genetic hemochromatosis, alpha 1-antitrypsin deficiency), or hepatitis virus B carriers even without cirrhosis; [15, 25] surveillance is deemed of "uncertain benefit" for non-cirrhotic non-alcoholic fatty liver disease (NAFLD) patients [24]. According to the 2011 AASLD guidelines [24], the diagnostic algorithm for HCC starts from suspect nodules found during US surveillance. Lesions smaller than 1 cm, which include most regenerative nodules, require strict US follow-up (every 3 months) until dimensional increase is found. Lesions larger than 1 cm require further evaluation with multiphase contrast-enhanced examinations (four-phase CT or MRI).

At US, HCC usually presents as a well-defined nodule with heterogeneous echogenicity or a "mosaic pattern"; a hypoechoic rim could be present. However, small HCCs among many regenerative nodules could be missed at US, because they frequently have poor defined margins [26]. In addition, small HCCs may be undistinguishable from hemangiomas [27], particularly within a steatosis liver. Eco-Doppler techniques allow the study of pathological vessels traveling through lesions, providing both a qualitative and a quantitative evaluation of blood flow.

At eco-color-Doppler examination, HCC appears as a highly vascularized nodule. Two patterns of vascularization were historically described for HCC: the "basket pattern," which present a thin web of vascular signals that embraces the nodule as a basket, and the "vessel-within-the-tumor-pattern," in which vessels travels into the tumor.

CONTRAST-ENHANCED ULTRASONOGRAPHY (CEUS)

The introduction of CEUS has led to great improvements in the diagnostic capabilities of US [28]. CEUS is the only imaging method that allows a continuous real-time evaluation of contrast medium distribution within lesions. Harmonic, microbubble-specific imaging with a low acoustic US pressure (mechanical index <0,2) is required for CEUS. All background signals are filtered and deleted from CEUS-specific software, therefore enhancement is related only to the harmonic responses of the contrast medium. The dynamic evaluation of contrast medium distribution during different enhancement phases (arterial, portal/venous and late phases) begins immediately after microbubbles injection [29]. At CEUS, HCC is typically hypervascular with slow and mild wash-out (Figure 1).

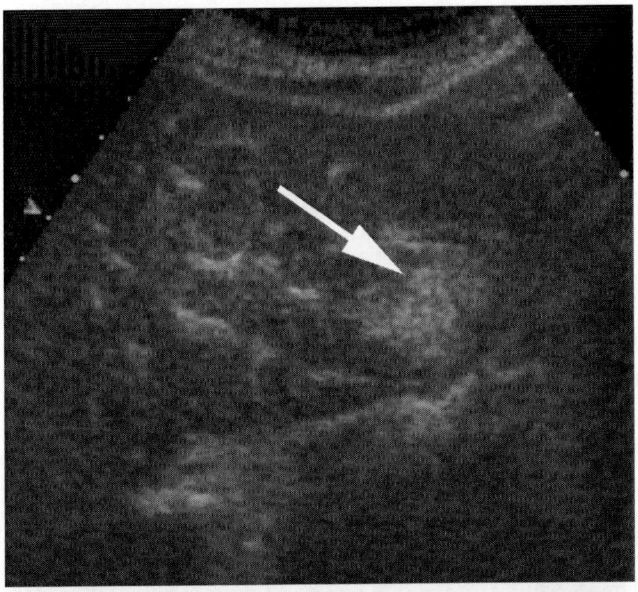

a

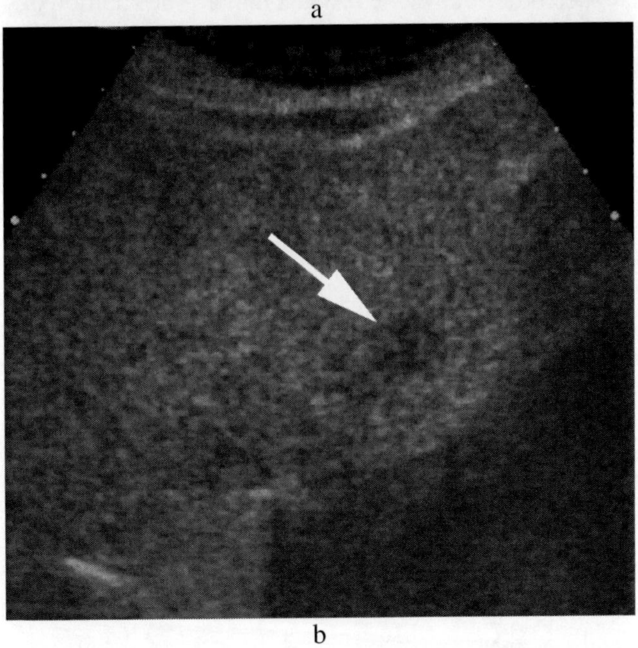

b

Figure 1a,b. HCC of the left liver lobe hypervascular at contrast-enhanced ultrasound appearing hyperechoic (arrow in a) in the early dynamic phase with clear wash-out resulting in hypoechoic aspect (arrow in b) in the late phases.

As above reported, the 2011 AASLD guidelines stated that the diagnosis of HCC in patient under US surveillance can be obtained with either contrast-enhanced CT or MRI; in the previous guidelines of the same Society, the non-invasive diagnosis of HCC was obtainable thanks to the concordance of two dynamic imaging methods, including CEUS [4]. CEUS was then removed from the more recent guidelines owing to the possibility of false positives: intra-hepatic cholangiocarcinoma may in fact present the same enhancement pattern of HCC, and cirrhosis is a well known risk factor for both diseases. Second-generation contrast agents as Sonazoid (Perfluorobutane, Daiichi-Sankyo, Tokyo, Japan) enable both the evaluation of perfusion and of Kupffer's cells presence during the delayed phase, because these microbubbles remains stable for at least to 3 hours after injection and are phagocytized by Kupffer's cells [30]. During this phase, liver parenchyma shows persistent homogenous enhancement, while lesions that contain few or no Kupffer's cells, as HCCs, can be recognized as perfusion defects. Dual-phase CEUS with Sonazoid could therefore greatly improve the diagnostic accuracy of CEUS for HCC detection [31].

Moreover, CEUS prior to biopsy procedures can increase the diagnostic yield by 10% especially in large tumors with necrotic areas. CEUS can localize the site for biopsy much more accurately than conventional US and color-Doppler imaging by demonstrating vascularized regions that have to be targeted and regions of necrosis, which should be avoided [32].

Unenhanced US is commonly used to guide procedures and loco-regional therapies such as ablation, whatever the modality used, and transarterial chemo/radioembolization. It is easy to use and widely available but, even when combined with Doppler, it does not provide useful information on the extent of the ablated neoplastic tissue. Assessment of tissue perfusion is crucial to differentiate necrotic from viable residual tumor. The addition of CEUS can provide important information also in this field [32].

Computed Tomography (CT)

CT is commonly used for the diagnosis and the staging of HCC. The standard protocol for liver examination relies on a multiphase dynamic acquisition: unenhanced, late arterial, portal, and delayed phases. Typically, iodine contrast agents are administered intravenously at a flow rate of at least 3-3,5 mL/s, followed by a saline flush. The contrast agent dose is usually tailored on body weight (1,5 mL/Kg of body weight, assuming a iodine concentration of 370 mg/mL). Liver CT needs a precise synchronization of post-injection scan delay; test bolus or bolus tracking techniques can be helpful. Fixed time delays should not be used. As previously stated, hyper-enhancement during arterial phase and washout during portal or delayed phases are pathognomonic of HCCs (Figure 2) in patients under surveillance [33].

The arterial phase for the CT evaluation of the liver coincides with a late arterial phase, about 15 seconds after the aortic threshold enhancement (200 Hounsfield Units). The portal/venous phase, characterized by a high degree of enhancement of liver parenchyma, along with hepatic and portal veins enhancement, is acquired 60-80 seconds after contrast medium injection. The delayed phase is acquired 3-5 minutes after contrast medium injection. Most regenerative nodules are undetectable or barely visible at un-enhanced CT, being small and isodense; large dysplastic nodules may instead appear hyperdense. HCCs appear iso- or hypo-attenuating at pre-contrast CT, and rarely hyperdense owing to the reduction of liver density caused by steatosis or to the increase of intra-tumoral metallic ions (iron, copper). HCC could also present an inhomogeneous density, with necrotic hypodense areas or hyperdense areas, related to hemorrhagic foci or calcifications; these features are quite rare, but more frequent in big size tumors, which could therefore present a typical "mosaic pattern" [34, 35]. After contrast medium injection, most regenerative nodules enhance to the same degree as the adjacent liver parenchyma or slightly less.

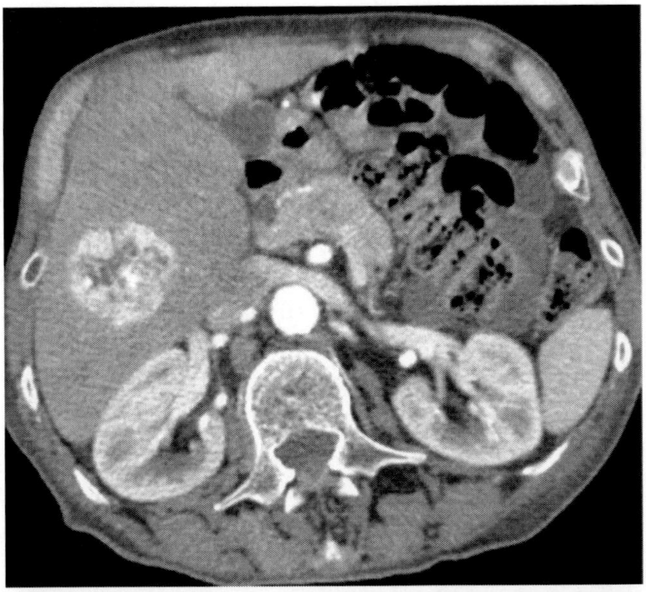

a

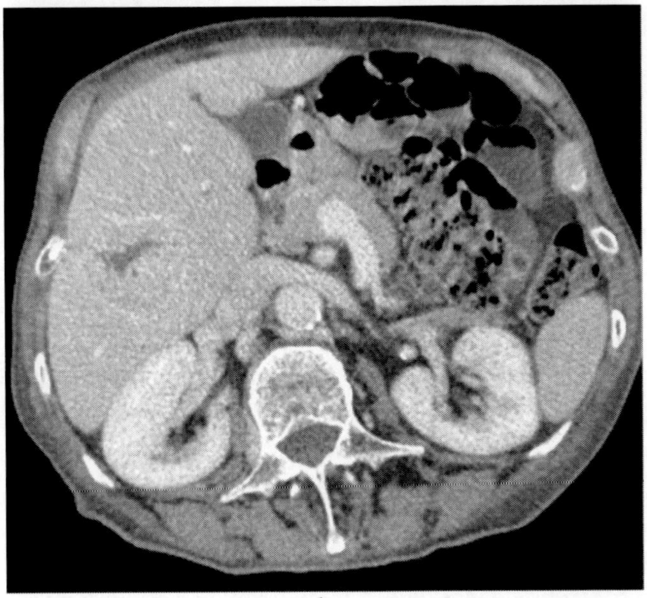

b

Figure 2a,b. HCC of the right liver lobe hypervascular at dynamic MDCT appearing inhomogeneously hyperdense in the late arterial phase with wash-out resulting slightly hypodense in the late phases.

Most dysplastic nodules are iso- or hypodense during arterial, portal and delayed phases; large dysplastic nodules may also appear isodense after contrast medium injection. HCC is typically hyperdense during arterial phase (wash-in); an inhomogenous enhancement can be present, with viable neoplastic tissue being hypervascular as compared to other portions of the tumor.

Sometimes satellite nodules can be identified. A small percentage (about 10%) of HCCs are hypovascular during the arterial phase; these are generally well-differentiated HCCs [36, 37]. During portal phase, HCC becomes inhomogenously hypodense because of the lack of portal perfusion (wash-out). The portal and delayed phases may also be helpful to measure the real size of the nodule, to depict hypovascular nodules (including early HCCs) [38] and to identify vascular thrombosis. In encapsulated HCCs, contrast medium out-flow is directed toward portal branches because of high interstitial intra-tumoral pressure, while non-encapsulated tumors drain directly into hepatic veins [39].

Encapsulated HCCs frequently appear hypodense during portal and delayed phases; tumor conspicuity during these phases can be increased by a slight enhancement of the highly fibrotic parenchyma typical of cirrhosis. CT is a good technique also for the evaluation of vascular involvement, which is quite frequent in HCCs [40]. In particular, portal branches invasion can be present in 30-70% of cases: a significant correlation between tumor size and portal invasion has been reported, and literature data reports a worse prognosis in these cases. Portal vein invasion is better detected on post-contrast images [41, 42].

Magnetic Resonance Imaging (MRI)

MRI has a very high diagnostic value for the detection and the characterization of HCCs [43-46], particularly for small lesions: the sensitivity for all sizes, <2 cm, and >2 cm HCCs has reported to be 96,9%, 92,3% and 100% for MRI and 87,5%, 92,3% and 84,2% for CT, respectively [45]. Moreover, MRI is biologically safe [47]. Liver MRI protocols are based on pre-contrast T1-weighted gradient recalled echo (GRE) in/out phase and fat-suppressed, T2-weighted turbo spin echo (TSE) with and without fat-suppression and half-Fourier acquisition single shot turbo spin echo (HASTE), and diffusion-weighted (DWI) with acquisition of at least three b-values (for example, 50, 400, and 800 s/mm^2) sequences. The dynamic study is based on 3D T1-weighted GRE fat suppressed sequences (for example, volume interpolated breath hold examination – VIBE sequences) before and after (arterial, portal, and delayed phases) gadolinium-chelates administration. As previously stated, Gd-EOB-DTPA and Gd-BOPTA have a selective uptake by hepatocytes and biliary excretion. In particular, Gd-EOB-DTPA has 50% uptake through an active transport mechanism. Biliary excretion manifests as an increased signal intensity of the hepatic parenchyma on T1-weighted images that peaks at approximately 20 minutes post injection. Regenerative nodules are isointense on T1- and T2-weighted images as compared to the background hepatic parenchyma. High T1 signal may be observed in some regenerative nodules due to lipid, protein, metals and/or metal-binding proteins. When iron is present in regenerative nodules, susceptibility effects can result in decreased signal intensity on both T1- and T2-weighted images. A reliable finding of regenerative nodules is the absence of enhancement in the arterial phase (no wash-in) [48]. Dysplastic nodules typically show T2 isointensity and variable signal intensity on T1-weighted images, like regenerative nodules. Most LG- and HG-DN are isoattenuating or isointense to the liver during the late hepatic arterial phase of MRI (no wash-in); some HG-DN have elevated arterial supply due to neo-arterialization and enhance more than liver in the late hepatic arterial phase (wash-in) and therefore they could be mistaken for progressed HCC. Dysplastic nodules, however, do not show washout during portal phase, because the portal supply remains comparable to that of the adjacent liver. The analysis of portal venous and delayed phase images is therefore fundamental to evaluate arterial-phase hyperenhancing nodules. Some HG-DNs contain one or more well-differentiated or moderately differentiated HCC sub nodules ("nodule-in-nodule" configuration); these are more appropriately categorized as "HCC arising in high-grade dysplastic nodule" [49]. Diffusion-weight imaging (DWI) is an MRI technique that depicts the diffusion of water molecules; restriction of their diffusion is present in densely cellular lesions, or when the normal functionality of cellular membranes, causing alteration in water molecules diffusion, is impaired. DWI has an improved sensitivity for HCC detection, which is particularly applicable to well-differentiated HCC with atypical features. On DWI, HCCs show high signal intensity with increasing b-values and corresponding low signal in the apparent diffusion coefficient (ADC) maps as compared to the surrounding liver parenchyma. HCCs show variable signal intensity on T1-weighted images, ranging from hypo- to hyper-intensity. Intra-tumoral lipids can be detected with dual echo T1-weighted GRE images (in/out phase sequences): signal intensity drops in out-phase images compared with in-phase images. The presence of lipids can be helpful to characterize lesions with an atypical appearance [50]. The appearance of HCC on T2-weighted images is also variable. Most commonly, HCC appears isointense; a high T2 signal can be useful to differentiate HCC from dysplastic nodule. In the "nodule-in-nodule" configuration, a slightly high signal may be observed, representing the focus of HCC within the hypointense dysplastic nodule; DWI can present restricted diffusion in the HCC spot [51]. The hallmark diagnostic features of HCC are arterial phase enhancement followed by portal venous or delayed phase washout [52-57], which are related both to neo-arterialization and loss of portal vessels. The combination of arterial wash-in and portal/delayed washout is highly specific for HCC in patients with cirrhosis: [52, 55-57] this enhancement pattern has approximately 100% specificity for HCCs >20 mm and approximately 90% for 10-19 mm HCCs [55, 56, 58, 59]. Additionally the washout rate is very important: an early washout seems predictive of a higher tumor grade [60, 61] and a higher probability of micro-vascular invasion [57] and therefore poor prognosis. A tumor capsule is a frequent pathologic feature of progressed HCC but not of early HCC, dysplastic nodules or cirrhotic nodules [58, 59]. The capsule corresponds to compressed adjacent liver parenchyma with nonspecific inflammatory cells; [53] as a consequence, the capsule is hyper intense during portal phase. Extra-capsular extension with presence of satellite nodules is frequently observed in large progressed HCCs [62]. These satellite nodules represent intra-hepatic metastases, generally within the venous drainage area around the main lesion [63] and present a high risk of recurrence and a lower survival after transplantation, resection or local ablation [64]. DWI can helps in the detection of very small satellite nodules. As above mentioned, Gd-BOPTA and Gd-EOB-DTPA are carried by OATP receptors into hepatocytes and then excreted into bile canaliculi via a multidrug resistance-associated protein (cMOAT) [65]. The accumulation of gadolinium into the liver parenchyma leads to a slight enhancement during the delayed hepato-biliary phase, typically acquired 60–120 minutes after Gd-BOPTA administration and 20 minutes with Gd-EOB [66]. Hepatocyte-specific contrast media permit therefore the assessment of both tumor vascularity and hepatocellular function [67]. Since OATP expression declines during hepatocarcinogenesis, most early HCCs and some HG-DNs are hypointense during hepato-biliary phase [68]. On the contrary, most regenerative nodules and LG-DNs, some HG-DNs and a minority of HCCs are isointense or hyperintense during this phase due to a preserved expression of OATP [69]. Nodules in cirrhotic liver that are hypointense during hepatobiliary phase are therefore likely to be malignant or premalignant [70], even in the absence of arterial phase enhancement or venous phase wash-out. Hepato-biliary phase of hepatospecific contrast media has therefore a great value for the diagnosis of HCCs [71], being 11% more sensitive for the diagnosis of HG-DN/early HCC than dynamic MRI; however, given that the distinction between early HCCs from dysplastic nodules can be challenging using conventional sequences alone [72, 73], liver-specific MR contrast agents play also an important role for the early diagnosis of HCC [74, 75]. Although most HCCs are hypointense in the hepatobiliary phase, about 5%–12% are hyperintense [76-78], owing to an over-expression of OATP [76, 79]. Compared with hepatobiliary phase hypointense HCCs, HCCs with isointensity or hyperintensity in the hepatobiliary phase are biologically more indolent, with lower grade [78], less frequent vascular invasion [78, 80, 81], and longer recurrence-free survival after resection [78, 81, 82]. Given that all lesions that do not contain hepatocytes (cysts, hemangiomas, metastases, and cholangiocarcinomas) will appear hypointense during hepatobiliary phase, hepatobiliary phase must be always evaluated in conjunction with other dynamic phases and sequences to differentiate HCC from other entities.

Conclusion

The identification, characterization, diagnosis, staging, and management of HCC in patients under surveillance are based on imaging. The surveillance of high-risk populations must be based on 6-months trans-abdominal US. The hallmark diagnostic features of HCC at CT or MRI are arterial phase wash-in followed by portal/delayed phase washout. Typical imaging features can be absent in precursors or atypical HCCs, which can therefore be missed: the addition of new techniques as hepato-specific contrast agents and DWI can therefore improve the non-invasive diagnostic capabilities of imaging. MRI should be therefore chosen for the lesion characterization in patients with a suspect HCC identified at US, given that a multi-parametric evaluation could provide more information regarding the real extent of the disease. Nevertheless, CEUS and CT are helpful and should be chosen for the re-evaluation of patients who underwent loco-regional therapies such as radiofrequency ablation or trans-arterial chemoembolization or chemotherapy.

References

[1] Siegel R, Naishadham D, Jemal A. Cancer statistics, 2013. *CA Cancer J Clin.* 2013;63:11-30.

[2] Yang HI, Sherman M, Su J, Chen PJ, Liaw YF, Iloeje UH, Chen CJ. Nomograms for risk of hepatocellular carcinoma in patients with chronic hepatitis B virus infection. *J Clin Oncol.* 2010;28:2437–2444.

[3] Lok AS, Seeff LB, Morgan TR, di Bisceglie AM, Sterling RK, Curto TM, Everson GT, Lindsay KL, Lee WM, Bonkovsky HL, et al. Incidence of hepatocellular carcinoma and associated risk factors in hepatitis C-related advanced liver disease. *Gastroenterology.* 2009;136:138–148.

[4] Bruix J, Sherman M, Llovet JM, Beaugrand M, Lencioni R, Burroughs AK, et al. EASL Panel of Experts on HC. Clinical management of hepatocellular carcinoma.

Conclusions of yhe Barcelona-2000 EASL conference. European Association for the Study of the Liver. *J Hepatol* 2001;35:421-430.

[5] Digumarthy SR, Sahani DV, Saini S. MRI in detection of hepatocellular carcinoma (HCC). *Cancer Imaging* 2005; 5:20-24.

[6] Jeong Min Lee, Jeong-Hee Yoon, and Kyung Won Kimb. Diagnosis of Hepatocellular Carcinoma: Newer Radiological Tools. *Seminars in Oncology,* Vol 39, No 4, August 2012, p 399-409.

[7] Bruix J, Sherman M. American Association for the Study of Liver Diseases. Management of hepatocellular carcinoma: an update. *Hepatology* 2011;53:1020-1022.

[8] EASL-EORTC clinical practice guidelines: management of hepatocellular carcinoma. *J Hepatol* 2012;56:908-943.

[9] Forner A, Vilana R, Ayuso C, et al. Diagnosis of hepatic nodules 20 mm or smaller in cirrhosis: prospective validation of the noninvasive diagnostic criteria for hepatocellular carcinoma. *Hepatology* 2008;47:97-104.

[10] Bolondi L, Gaiani S, Celli N, et al. Characterization of small nodules in cirrhosis by assessment of vascularity: the problem of hypovascular hepatocellular carcinoma. *Hepatology* 2005;42:27-34.

[11] Kudo M. Multistep human hepatocarcinogenesis: correlation of imaging with pathology. *J Gastroenterol* 2009;44(Suppl 19):112-118.

[12] Palmer WC, Patel T. Are common factors involved in the pathogenesis of primary liver cancers? A meta-analysis of risk factors for intrahepatic cholangiocarcinoma. *J Hepatol* 2012;57:69-76.

[13] Coleman WB. Mechanisms of human hepatocarcinogenesis. Curr Mol Med 2003;3:573-588

[14] Kitao A, Matsui O, Yoneda N, et al. The uptake transporter OATP8 expression decreses during multistep hepatocarcinogenesis: correlation with gadoxetic acid enhanced MR imaging. *Eur Radiol* 2011;21(10):2056-2066.

[15] Ueda K, Matsui O, Kawamori Y, et al. Hypervascular hepatocellular carcinoma: evaluation of hemodynamics with dynamic CT during hepatic arteriography. *Radiology* 1998;206(1):161-166.

[16] Kitao A, Zen Y, Matsui O, Gabata T, Nakanuma Y. Hepatocarcinogenesis: multistep changes of drainage vessels at CT during arterial portography and hepatic arteriography-radiologic-pathologic correlation. *Radiology* 2009;52:605-614.

[17] Takayama T, Makuuchi M, Hirohashi S, et al. Malignant transformation of adenomatous hyperplasia to hepatocellular carcinoma. *Lancet* 1990;336(8724):1150-1153.

[18] Kutami R, Nakashima Y, Nakashima O, Shiota K, Kojiro M. Pathomorphologic study on the mechanism of fatty change in small hepatocellular carcinoma of humans. *J Hepatol* 2000;33:282-289.

[19] International Consensus Group for Hepatocellular Neoplasia. Pathologic diagnosis of early hepatocellular carcinoma: a report of the international consensus group for hepatocellular neoplasia. *Hepatology* 2009;49:658-664.

[20] Terada T, Kadoya M, Nakanuma Y, Matsui O. Iron-accumulating adenomatous hyperplastic nodule with malignant foci in the cirrhotic liver. Histopathologic, quantitative iron, and magnetic resonance imaging in vitro studies. *Cancer* 1990;65:1994-2000.

[21] Nassif A, Jia J, Keiser M, et al. Visualization of hepatic uptake transporter function in healthy subjects by using gadoxetic acid enhanced MR imaging. *Radiology* 2012; 264(3):741-750.

[22] Choi JY, Lee JM, Sirlin CB. CT and MRI imaging and staging of Hepatocellular carcinoma: Part I. Development, growth and spread: key pathologic and imaging aspects. *Radiology* 2014; 272:635-654.

[23] Bolondi L. Screening for hepatocellular carcinoma in cirrhosis. *J Hepatol* 2003;39:1076-1084.

[24] Bruix J, Sherman M. Management of hepatocellular carcinoma: an update. *Hepatology* 2011;53:1020-2.

[25] Evans AA, Chen G, Ross EA, Shen FM, Lin WY, London WT. Eight-year follow-up of the 90,000-person Haimen City cohort: I. Hepatocellular carcinoma mortality, risk factors, and gender differences. *Cancer Epidemiol Biomarkers Prev* 2002;11:369-376.

[26] Lee JY, Choi BI, Han JK, Lee JM, Kim SH. State-of-the-art ultrasonography of hepatocellular carcinoma. *Eur J Radiol.* 2006;58:177-85.

[27] Caturelli E, Pompili M, Bartolucci F, Siena DA, Sperandeo M, Andriulli A et al. Hemangioma-like lesions in chronic liver disease: diagnostic evaluation in patients. *Radiology* 2001;220:337-342.

[28] Claudon M, Cosgrove D, Albrecht T, Bolondi L, Bosio M, Calliada F, Correas JM, Darge K, Dietrich C, D'Onofrio M, Evans DH, Filice C, Greiner L, Jäger K, Jong N, Leen E, Lencioni R, Lindsell D, Martegani A, Meairs S, Nolsøe C, Piscaglia F, Ricci P, Seidel G, Skjoldbye B, Solbiati L, Thorelius L, Tranquart F, Weskott HP, Whittingham T. Guidelines and good clinical practice recommendations for contrast enhanced ultrasound (CEUS) - update 2008. *Ultraschall Med* 2008;29:28-44.

[29] D'Onofrio M, Mansueto G, Falconi M, Procacci C. Neuroendocrine pancreatic tumor: value of contrast enhanced ultrasonography. *Abdom Imaging* 2004;29:246-258.

[30] Inoue T, Kudo M, Maenishi O, et al. Value of liver parenchymal phase contrast-enhanced sonography to diagnose premalignant and borderline lesions and overt hepatocellular carcinoma. *AJR Am J Roentgenol.* 2009;192:698-705.

[31] Moriyasu F, Itoh K. Efficacy of perflubutane microbubble-enhanced ultrasound in the characterization and detection of focal liver lesions: phase 3 multicenter clinical trial. *AJR AM J Roentgenol.* 2009;193:86-95.

[32] Claudon M, Dietrich CF, Choi BI, Cosgrove DO, Kudo M, Nolsøe CP, Piscaglia F, Wilson SR, Barr RG, Chammas MC, Chaubal NG, Chen MH, Clevert DA, Correas JM, Ding H, Forsberg F, Fowlkes JB, Gibson RN, Goldberg BB, Lassau N, Leen EL, Mattrey RF, Moriyasu F, Solbiati L, Weskott HP, Xu HX.; Guidelines and good clinical practice recommendations for contrast enhanced ultrasound (CEUS) in the liver--update 2012: a WFUMB-EFSUMB initiative in cooperation with representatives of AFSUMB, AIUM, ASUM, FLAUS and ICUS. *Ultraschall Med.* 2013 Feb;34(1):11-29.

[33] Ayyappan AP, Jhaveri KS. CT and MRI of hepatocellular carcinoma: an update. *Expert Rev Anticancer Ther.* 2010;10:507-19.

[34] Jeong YY, Yim NY, Kang HK. Hepatocellular carcinoma in the cirrhotic liver with helical CT and MRI: imaging spectrum and pittfalls of cirrhosis-related nodules. *Am J Roentgenol* 2005;185:1024-1032.

[35] Baron RL, Brancatelli G. Computed tomographic imaging of hepatocellular carcinoma. *Gastroenterology* 2004;127:133-143.

[36] Atasoy C, Akyar S. Multidetector CT: contribution in liver imaging. *Eur J Radiol* 2004;52:2-17.

[37] Li CS, Chen RC, Tu HY. Imaging well-differentiated hepatocellular carcinoma with dynamic triple-phase helical computed tomography. *Br J Radiol* 2006;79:659-665.

[38] Takayasu K, Furukawa H, Wakao F, et al. CT diagnosis of early hepatocellular carcinoma: sensitivity, findings, and CT-pathologic correlation. *AJR Am J Roentgenol* 1995;164:885-890.

[39] Tanaka T, Yamanaka N, Oriyama T et al. Factors regulating tumor pressure in hepatocellular carcinoma and implications for tumor spread. *Hepatology* 1997;26:283-287.

[40] Nakao N, Miura K, Takayasu Y et al. CT angiography in hepatocellular carcinoma. *J Comput Assist Tomogr* 1983;7:780-787.

[41] Mathieu D, Grenier P, Larde D, Vasile N. Portal vein involvement in hepatocellular carcinoma. Dynamic CT feautures. *Radiology* 1984;152:127-132.

[42] Karahan OI, Yikilmaz A, Isisn S, Orhan S. Characterization of hepatocellular carcinomas with triphasic CT and correlation with histopathologuc findings. *Acta Radiol* 2003;44:566-571.

[43] Pitton MB, Kloeckner R, Herber S, Otto G, Kreitner KF, Dueber C. MRI versus 64-row MDCT for diagnosis of hepatocellular carcinoma. *World J Gastroenterol* 2009; 15:6044-6051.

[44] Purysko AS, Remer EM, Coppa CP, Leão Filho HM, Thupili CR, Veniero JC. LIRADS: a case-based review of the new categorization of liver findings in patients with end-stage liver disease. *Radiographics* 2012; 32:1977-1995.

[45] Tada T, Kumada T, Toyoda H, Ito T, Sone Y, Okuda S, Ogawa S, Igura T, Imai Y. Diagnostic accuracy for macroscopic classification of nodular hepatocellular carcinoma: comparison of gadolinium ethoxybenzyl diethylenetriamine pentaacetic acid-enhanced magnetic resonance imaging and angiography-assisted computed tomography. *J Gastroenterol* 2014 [Epub ahead of print] DOI 10.1007/s00535-014-0947-x.

[46] Khalili K, Kim TK, Jang HJ, et al. Optimization of imaging diagnosis of 1-2 cm hepatocellular carcinoma: an analysis of diagnostic performance and resource utilization. *J Hepatol* 2011; 54:723-728.

[47] Catalano OA, Choy G, Zhu A, Hahn PF, Sahani DV. Differentiation of malignant thrombus from bland thrombus of the portal vein in patients with hepatocellular carcinoma: application of diffusion-weighted MR imaging. *Radiology* 2010; 254:154-162.

[48] Willatt JM, Hussain HK, Adusumilli S, Marrero JA. MR Imaging of hepatocellular carcinoma in the cirrhotic liver: challenges and controversies. *Radiology* 2008;247:311-330.

[49] Roskams T, Kojiro M. Pathology of early hepatocellular carcinoma: conventional and molecular diagnosis. *Semin Liver Dis* 2010;30:17-25.

[50] Stevens WR, Gulino SP, Batts KP, Stephens DH, Johnson CD. Mosaic pattern of hepatocellular carcinoma: histologic basis for a characteristic CT appearance. *J ComputAssist Tomogr* 1996;20(3):337-342.

[51] Hina Arif-Tiwari, Bobby Kalb, Surya Chundru, Puneet Sharma, James Costello, Rainner W. Guessner,Diego R. Martin. MRI of hepatocellular carcinoma: an update of current practices. *Diagn Interv Radiol* 2014; 20:209-221.
[52] Forner A, Vilana R, Ayuso C, et al. Diagnosis of hepatic nodules 20 mm or smaller in cirrhosis: Prospective validation of the noninvasive diagnostic criteria for hepatocellular carcinoma. *Hepatology* 2008;47(1):97-104.
[53] American College of Radiology. Liver Imaging Reporting and Data System version 2013.1. http://www.acr.org/Quality-Safety/Resources/LIRADS/. Accessed July 19, 2013.
[54] Pomfret EA, Washburn K, Wald C, et al. Report of a national conference on liver allocation in patients with hepatocellular carcinoma in the United States. *Liver Transpl* 2010;16(3):262-278.
[55] Kim TK, Lee KH, Jang HJ, et al. Analysis of gadobenate dimeglumine-enhanced MRfindings for characterizing small (1-2-cm) hepatic nodules in patients at high risk for hepatocellular carcinoma. *Radiology* 2011;259(3):730-738.
[56] Marrero JA, Hussain HK, Nghiem HV, Umar R, Fontana RJ, Lok AS. Improving the prediction of hepatocellular carcinoma in cirrhotic patients with an arterially-enhancing liver mass. *Liver Transpl* 2005;11(3):281-289.
[57] Rimola J, Forner A, Tremosini S, et al. Noninvasive diagnosis of hepatocellular carcinoma >2 cm in cirrhosis. Diagnostic accuracy assessing fat, capsule and signal intensity at dynamic MRI. *J Hepatol* 2012;56(6):1317-1323.
[58] Khan AS, Hussain HK, Johnson TD, Weadock WJ, Pelletier SJ, Marrero JA. Value of delayed hypointensity and delayed enhancing rim in magnetic resonance imaging diagnosis of small hepatocellular carcinoma in the cirrhotic liver. *J Magn ResonImaging* 2010;32(2):360-366.
[59] Lim JH, Choi D, Park CK, Lee WJ, Lim HK. Encapsulated hepatocellular carcinoma: CT-pathologic correlations. *Eur Radiol* 2006;16(10):2326-2333.
[60] Enomoto S, Tamai H, Shingaki N, et al. Assessment of hepatocellular carcinomas using conventional magnetic resonance imaging correlated with histological differentiation and a serum marker of poor prognosis. *Hepatol Int* 2011;5(2):730-737.
[61] Okamoto D, Yoshimitsu K, Nishie A, et al. Enhancement pattern analysis of hypervascular hepatocellular carcinoma on dynamic MR imaging with histopathological correlation: validity of portal phase imaging for predicting tumor grade. *Eur J Radiol* 2012;81(6):1116-1121.
[62] Kojiro M. Histopathology of liver cancers. *Best Pract Res Clin Gastroenterol* 2005;19(1):39-62.
[63] Sakamoto M, Hirohashi S, Tsuda H, Shimosato Y, Makuuchi M, Hosoda Y. Multicentric independent development of hepatocellular carcinoma revealed by analysis of hepatitis B virus integration pattern. *Am J Surg Pathol* 1989;13(12):1064-1067.
[64] Kim SH, Choi SB, Lee JG, et al. Prognostic factors and 10-year survival in patients with hepatocellular carcinoma after curative hepatectomy. *J Gastrointest Surg* 2011;15(4):598-607.
[65] Narita M, Hatano E, Arizono S, et al. Expression of OATP1B3 determines uptake of Gd-EOB-DTPA in hepatocellular carcinoma. *J Gastroenterol* 009;44:793-798.
[66] Frydrychowicz A, Lubner MG, Brown JJ, et al. Hepatobiliary MR imaging with gadolinium-based contrast agents. *J Magn Reson Imaging* 2012;35:492-51.

[67] Choi JY, Lee JM, Sirlin CB. CT and MR imaging diagnosis and staging of Hepatocellular carcinoma. Part II. Extracellular agents, hepatobiliary agents and ancillary imaging features. *Radiology* 2014;273:30-50.

[68] Sano K, Ichikawa T, Motosugi U, et al. Imaging study of early hepatocellular carcinoma: usefulness of gadoxetic acid-enhanced MR imaging. *Radiology* 2011;261(3):834-844.

[69] Kudo M. Multistep human hepatocarcinogenesis: correlation of imaging with pathology. *J Gastroenterol* 2009;44(Suppl 19):112-118.

[70] Golfieri R, Grazioli L, Orlando E, et al. Which is the best MRI marker of malignancy for atypical cirrhotic nodules: hypointensity in hepatobiliary phase alone or combined with other features? Classification after Gd-EOB-DTPA administration. *J Magn Reson Imaging* 2012;36(3):648-657.

[71] Forner A, Vilana R, Ayuso C, et al. Diagnosis of hepatic nodules 20 mm or smaller in cirrhosis: prospective validation of the noninvasive diagnostic criteria for hepatocellular carcinoma. *Hepatology* 2008;47:97-104.

[72] Takayasu K, Muramatsu Y, Furukawa H, et al. Early hepatocellular carcinoma: appearance at CT during arterial portography and CT arteriography with pathologic correlation. *Radiology* 1995;194:101-105.

[73] Hayashi M, Matsui O, Ueda K, et al. Correlation between the blood supply and grade of malignancy of hepatocellular nodules associated with liver cirrhosis: evaluation by CT during intraarterial injection of contrast medium. *AJR Am J Roentgenol* 1999; 172:969-976.

[74] Bashir MR, Gupta RT, Davenport MS, et al. Hepatocellular carcinoma in a North American population: does hepatobiliary MR imaging with Gd-EOB-DTPA improve sensitivity and confidence for diagnosis? *J Magn Reson Imaging* 2013;37:398-406.

[75] Haradome H, Grazioli L, Tinti R, et al. Additional value of gadoxetic acid-DTPA-enhanced hepatobiliary phase MR imaging in the diagnosis of early-stage hepatocellular carcinoma: comparison with dynamic triple-phase multidetector CT imaging. *J Magn Reson Imaging* 2011;34:69-78.

[76] Narita M, Hatano E, Arizono S, et al. Expression of OATP1B3 determines uptake of Gd-EOB-DTPA in hepatocellular carcinoma. *J Gastroenterol* 2009;44(7):793-798.

[77] Suh YJ, Kim MJ, Choi JY, Park YN, Park MS, Kim KW. Differentiation of hepatic hyperintense lesions seen on gadoxetic acidenhanced hepatobiliary phase MRI. *AJR Am J Roentgenol* 2011;197:44-52.

[78] Kitao A, Matsui O, Yoneda N, et al. Hypervascular hepatocellular carcinoma: correlation between biologic features and signal intensity on gadoxetic acid-enhanced MR images. *Radiology* 2012;265(3):780-789.

[79] Kitao A, Zen Y, Matsui O, et al. Hepatocellular carcinoma: signal intensity at gadoxetic acid-enhanced MR Imaging-correlation with molecular transporters and histopathologic features. *Radiology* 2010;256(3):817–826.

[80] Kim JY, Kim MJ, Kim KA, Jeong HT, Park YN. Hyperintense HCC on hepatobiliary phase images of gadoxetic acid-enhanced MRI: correlation with clinical and pathological features. *Eur J Radiol* 2012;81(12): 3877-3882.

[81] Vasuri F, Golfieri R, Fiorentino M, et al. OATP 1B1/1B3 expression in hepatocellular carcinomas treated with orthotopic liver transplantation. *Virchows Arch* 2011;459(2):141-146.

[82] Choi JW, Lee JM, Kim SJ, et al. Hepatocellular carcinoma: imaging patterns on gadoxetic acid-enhanced MR Images and their value as an imaging biomarker. *Radiology* 2013;267(3):776-786.

In: Hepatocellular Carcinoma in the 3rd Millennium
Editors: M. Berretta and B. Cacopardo
ISBN: 978-1-63484-025-5

Chapter 5

SCREENING AND SURVEILLANCE: HEPATOCELLULAR CARCINOMA

Russello Maurizio*

Director Division of Hepatology, Centro di Riferimento Regionale per le Malattie del Fegato, ARNAS Garibaldi Hospital, Catania, Italy

ABSTRACT

The HCC has all the requirements to be considered a very affordable program of screening and surveillance. In fact, the incidence and prevalence of HCC is increasing in almost all regions of the world. The results obtained from most studies have confirmed that, in patients undergoing cancer surveillance, vascular invasion is less frequently present and, consequently, patients are more often eligible for curative treatment. As refers to target population, patients with cirrhosis in class A and B of Child-Pugh are the ideal candidates for a screening program, because of the high incidence of HCC and the possibility of treatment that is able to reduce the mortality. Nevertheless, there has been one main randomized clinical trial in literature that has demonstrated the benefit of surveillance (with by performing alphafetoprotein and ultrasound scan twice a year). All strategies are convenient in opposition to non-surveillance: the biannual surveillance with Ultrasound scan + Alphafetoprotein detection resulted as the most effective (irrespective of the etiology), being able to triple the number of the operable HCC diagnosis, and to reduce the tumor-related mortality. The evidence that a more aggressive ecographic surveillance program (3-4 months) allows the diagnosis of small tumors (<2 cm) in a high percentage of cases, was not confirmed subsequently. In literature there is no evidence that screening and surveillance with computerized tomography or magnetic resonance imaging present any cost-effectiveness advantages compared with US, with the exception of the patients in the transplant waiting list, and the cases where the ultrasonographic exploration is limited by physical and anatomic conditions.

* E-mail m.russello@ao-garibaldi.ct.it.

INTRODUCTION

Hepatocellular carcinoma (HCC) is one the highest mortality types of cancer found in humans.

Despite the progress made in the field of treatment in the last decade, the incidence and mortality due to HCC are globally overlapping each other [1]. This daunting result is due to a diagnosis that is still performed today, often too late, during a period when the tumors are not very susceptible to a treatment that would, otherwise, be able to modify their natural history.

In fact, the prognosis of hepatocellular carcinoma is closely related to the stage it is at during diagnosis.

According to the classification of the Barcelona Clinic Liver Cancer (BCLC), which is universally accepted, the diagnosis of HCC performed in stage 0 (Very Early Stage, patient in Child-Pugh class A, with single nodule diameter less than 2 cm) and in stage A (Early Stage, Child-Pugh class AB, single nodule <5 cm or up to 3 nodules, of which the greater ≤ 3 cm), allows treatment, "Healthy," with five-year survival rate of 40-70% (median overall survival >60 months). Patients with more advanced stages of the tumor, such as stage B (multifocal HCC) and stage C (cancer patients with symptomatic portal invasion and/or extrahepatic spread) are eligible for "palliative" treatment, with a very low median survival (20 and 11 months, respectively). Finally, patients in the terminal stage (D) are not amenable to treatment, having a median survival of <3 months [2].

It is evident that only the implementation of screening and surveillance programs in the population at risk may allow early diagnosis. However, even in the most advanced countries, this only occurs in 30-40% of cases.

For screening we mean the application of one or more tests for subjects with an increased risk, in order to diagnose the tumor before the onset of symptoms, while surveillance is defined as the repetition of tests at regular intervals [3].

The World Health Organization (WHO) has indicated that because of the advantages a screening program offers it should also have a certain criteria:

- The tumor must be a public health problem, in terms of mortality and morbidity;
- The target population must be identified;
- There must be an effective treatment that would be able to increase the survival of cases diagnosed;
- Costs must be sustainable;
- Tests must have a high diagnostic accuracy;
- The tests must be accepted by the target population as well as the N.H.S. staff;
- Standardized recall procedures must exist for the repetition of tests.

The HCC has all the requirements to be considered a very affordable program of screening and surveillance. In fact, the incidence and prevalence of HCC is increasing in almost all regions of the world. According to recent data from the International Agency for Research on Cancer, the primary liver cancer in humans is in 5th place for age- standardized incidence (after lung, prostate, colorectal and stomach), and second only to lung cancer for mortality rates; while in women it represents 9th to tumor incidence, and 6th for mortality [4].

The population at risk is easily identifiable: it is known that over 90% of patients with HCC are suffering from cirrhosis of the liver [5]. There are effective treatments that can significantly increase the survival of cases diagnosed at an early stage of the tumor. There are tests such as liver ultrasonography (US) in serum alpha-fetoprotein (AFP) and des-gamma-carboxy prothrombin (DCP), with good sensitivity and specificity, high diagnostic accuracy, non-invasive (and therefore easily acceptable to the target population and physicians), relatively inexpensive. Finally, recall procedures have been defined for cases with hepatic nodules, detected at screening, thus, implementing diagnostic algorithms (CT and MR contrast, biopsy), which have demonstrated high effectiveness and accuracy [6].

The diffusion of guidelines by authoritative scientific societies has led to a large and rapid introduction of surveillance programs in many countries, but without the solid evidence of prolonging survival.

In order to demonstrate the effectiveness of screening and surveillance programs, it is necessary to make an early diagnosis, doing so means a greater possibility of curative treatment and, therefore, a greater survival rate. It would be scientifically more correct to demonstrate the validity of the program by comparing patients who were monitored with those who were not as part of a randomized clinical trial (RCT).

So far, there has been only one RCT in literature that has demonstrated the benefit of surveillance (with a dose of AFP and ultrasound twice a year), the study involved over 18,000 subjects in Shanghai, suffering from HBV-related chronic liver disease. They were compared with patients undergoing surveillance, HCC patients who were diagnosed at the onset of symptoms [7]. Moreover, follow –up also proved to be an advantage in surveillance programs, in terms of:

a) Overall survival of 1,3 and 5 years,
b) HCC- related mortality,
c) Stage of disease at diagnosis,
d) Possibility of curative treatment.

However, the main obstacle to the study was represented by the high percentage of rejections towards the screening (41.8%), but it is conceivable that a greater adherence would increase the overall benefit.

A contrary result emerges from a second RCT [8]. carried out on a sample of 5581 Chinese patients, who were also carriers of HBsAg, being a randomized 6 monthly surveillance, with AFP versus no surveillance at all. The five-year survival and overall mortality between the two groups did not show any statistical difference, although in the monitored group the proportion of patients with early diagnosis was significantly higher (29.6% vs. 6%). Unfortunately, the main problem with this study is represented by the fact that patients with an early diagnosis of HCC were not subjected to curative treatments, thereby negating the advantage of an early diagnosis.

As screening programs have spread rapidly around the world, today it is not ethically feasible to carry out a randomized trial without a control arm, yet adequately informed patients, would never agree to participate in such trials [9]. Therefore, the guideline recommendations are based on the evidence which emerged from several published cohort studies that compared the survival of cirrhotic patients with HCC, who were asked to take part in the surveillance programs, with those patients diagnosed at the onset of symptoms [10-

15]. The results obtained from these studies have confirmed that, in patients undergoing cancer surveillance, vascular invasion is less frequently present and, consequently, patients are more often eligible for curative treatment (transplantation, resection, ablation), with a significant increase in overall survival The major limitation of the non-randomized studies is the so-called lead- time bias, represented by an artificial increase in survival related to time of diagnosis in patients undergoing screening or surveillance [16].

A study has recently been published based on mathematical analysis and probability estimates, evaluating the effect of bias -free surveillance on prognosis and survival of patients with HCC [17]. The data were obtained from a database of 1,380 patients with hepatocellular carcinoma from different Italian centers, with liver cirrhosis of varying etiology, in Child-Pugh class AB, undergoing ultrasound screening and surveillance (with or without dose AFP) every six months (850 cases), annually (234 cases) or no monitoring (296 patients diagnosed with HCC at the onset of symptoms). This study also confirmed that patients undergoing surveillance showed a tumor in the earliest stage which was, more often than not, in class A of CP, and so they could be subjected to curative treatments more frequently and, ultimately, their overall survival rate was significantly higher. Although the best results were obtained with a six-month surveillance, the annual repetition of the tests gave better results than the non- surveillance The most interesting result of this study is the demonstration that the lead-time bias vanishes when the follow-up is longer than the third year after diagnosis, in cases of HCC with rapid growth (tumor doubling time <3 months), and in those with slow growth (doubling time 12 months).

On the basis of these results, the cost-effectiveness of screening and surveillance programs should be evaluated only in the context of studies that provide an observation period of not less than 3 years after the diagnosis of cancer.

Another study recently published meta-analysis [18] analyzed data from 47 cohort studies (European, American and Oriental), mostly retrospective, with a total of more than 15,000 patients with cirrhosis. Ultrasound analysis (with or without dosage AFP) allows more frequent diagnosis of HCC at an early stage (70.9%, compared with 29.9% of the group diagnosed with or incidental to the onset of symptoms, odds ratio 8.2), increases the proportion of patients eligible for treatment (51.6% vs. 23.7%, OR 2.24) and prolongs overall survival rate to three years (50.8% vs. 27.9%, OR 1.90). While considering that only six studies reported a survival rate connected to lead- time bias, and many did not provide a sufficiently long follow-up to evaluate the survival, the results of this meta- analysis demonstrate a clear advantage of the surveillance (regardless of program strategies) compared to the non- surveillance. These data confirm that an early diagnosis in the course of screening increases the chances of treatment and significantly reduces mortality, supporting guideline recommendations.

Target Population

For a program of screening and surveillance to be effective, it is necessary to identify the target population (i.e., individuals at higher risk of cancer, where the cancer has the highest incidence). It has been calculated that in cirrhotic patients a cancer risk of >1.5% per year makes the program beneficial in terms of cost effectiveness (cost per year of life saved), while in patients with chronic liver disease, the incidence of HCC should be >0.2% / year [6, 19, 20].

HCC occurs in 90-95% of cases in patients with liver cirrhosis, and in this phase it is the leading cause of death [5]. The annual incidence of HCC is increased in cirrhosis related to hepatitis B virus (HBV, 3-8%) and C virus (HCV 3-5%), lower in alcohol- related cirrhosis and steatohepatitis non-alcoholic (2-3%). The incidence in the setting of patients with a rarer cirrhosis etiology (hemochromatosis, alpha-1- antitrypsin deficiency, autoimmune) is less known.

Table 1. Categories at risk of HCC in which surveillance is recommended b American Association for the Study of Liver Diseases (AASLD), European Association for the Study of the Liver (EASL) and Japan Society of Hepatology (SH)

AASLD (2010)	EASL (2012)	JSH (2010)
- Asian male HBV carriers over age 40 - Asian female HBV carriers over age 50 - HBV carriers with family history of HCC - African/North American blacks with hepatitis B - Hepatitis B cirrosi - Hepatitis C cirrhosis - Stage 4 primary biliary cirrosi - Other cirrhosis (6)	- Cirrhotic patients, C-P A and B - Cirrhotic patients, C-P- C on LT waiting list - Non-cirrhotic HBV carriers with active hepatitis or family history of HCC - Non-cirrhotic patients with chronic hepatitis C and advanced liver fibrosis F3 (20)	- Cirrhosis of various etiologies - type B chronic liver disease - type C chronic liver disease (21)

However, a monitoring program that would differentiate the target according to the etiology of cirrhosis, would be more expensive and complex. Therefore, all the major scientific hepatological societies recommended screening and monitoring for all patients with cirrhosis, regardless of etiology (Table 1) [6, 20, 21].

One of the essential requirements of a surveillance program is the ability to provide effective care at the time of diagnosis. Therefore, it is considered unnecessary to screen patients with cirrhosis in Child-Pugh class C (CP C), with the exception of candidates for liver transplantation (OLT).

In fact, in the most advanced stages of the hepatic disease, no treatment proved itself superior to the support medical therapy, and death is often related to hepatic insufficiency rather than the tumor.

For the patients in the transplant list, even if in class C of C-P, it is necessary to maintain the surveillance because the eventual appearance of a tumor could: a) raise the priority in the list, b) modify the therapeutic strategy, c) cause an exclusion from the list if the tumor exceeds the transplantability criteria adopted by the centre.

Patients with cirrhosis in class A and B of Child-Pugh are the ideal candidates for a screening program, because of the high incidence of HCC and the possibility of treatment that is able to reduce the mortality.

In non-cirrhotic patients, the yearly risk of cancer onset is considerably lower and different depending on the etiology. The screening program in this category is cost/effective if this risk is not lower than 0.2%. Such a condition applies in chronic HBV carriers with familiarity for HCC, in black Africans/ North Americans, over-40 years old male Asians and females over the age of 50 [6].

Recently the European Association for the Study of the Liver (EASL) included patients with chronic virus C hepatitis with advanced fibrosis ($F \geq 3$) among the categories at risk worthy of screening, on the basis of the results of an important prospective cohort study (HALT-C), involving over 1000 patients: the cumulative risk of HCC onset at 5 years was substantial also in patients with advanced fibrosis, despite being lower than that of cirrhotic patients (4.1% vs. 7%) [22].

Moreover, it was shown how the eradication of HCV infection after an antiviral therapy, when obtained in patients with advanced fibrosis, reduces but does not remove the risk of HCC [23].

It was similarly proved for the suppression of the replication of HBV during the therapy, with nucleosidic analogues [24]. Therefore, both these categories of patients must be admitted into the surveillance programs, even in the absence of viraemia.

Caucasian patients with a chronic HBV infection, without severe fibrosis or cirrhosis, have a very low yearly risk of hepatic tumor (0.1-0.4%) [25]. therefore they do not fall within the target populations, with the exception of people who have familiarity/ a family history of HCC [20].

In the Asiatic countries, where the virus of Hepatitis B has an epidemic diffusion, it is transmitted vertically, and it represents the main cause of hepatocellular carcinomas, there is a risk of HCC even in the absence of cirrhosis, and it is higher in over-40 males and over-50 females [26], it raises in the presence of familiarity [27] and is related to the HBV DNA levels [28].

The genotype influence is less evident, despite some studies related the main oncogene risk to genotype C [29]. In Africa the transmission of virus B happens in the neonatal and perinatal period, causing a reduction of the HCC onset age, thanks to oncogene cofactors, such as B1 aflatoxin. For these reasons, the American Association for the Study of Liver Diseases (AASLD) added Asian, African and African-North American patients to the target populations, even in the absence of cirrhosis [6].

In China, despite the fact that hepatic tumor has a very high incidence and mortality, there are no national surveillance guidelines for the population at risk, hence the diagnosis is almost always late and, consequently, the survival rate is very low [30].

The chronic HBV infection represents the first cause of HCC: it was calculated that over 90 million people in China are virus B bearers, so it is easy to understand how the screening methods that are recommended in countries with a less numerous target population cannot apply to the Chinese reality.

However, even in this country the need to identify some guidelines and start a national screening program in order to make an earlier diagnosis to reduce the mortality is emerging [30].

A recent update of the Japanese guidelines recommends extending the surveillance to all those patients with a chronic hepatitis [31], even though these conclusions seem to have no solid clinical evidence.

Recently, several studies have been carried out in order to stratify the risk of hepatocellular carcinomas in the patients with a chronic HBV infection, thus aiming to reduce the target population and the costs of surveillance.

In a prospective study that was published in 2009, Yuen et al., basing their research on some parameters (age, gender, serum HBV DNA levels, core promoter mutations), were able to identify, in a cohort of cirrhotic patients, the ones at a higher risk of developing HCC, in order to intensify the surveillance strategy on them.

More recently, the results of an analogue research conducted by Lee et al., [32] on a population of chronic HBV carriers, who had taken part to the R.E.V.E.A.L. (Risk Evaluation of Viral Load Elevation and Associated liver disease/cancer in HBV) study, have been published. The 3340 HbsAg-positive patients from Taiwan, of an age between 30 and 65 years, were involved. At the end of the follow-up 164 new HCC cases were diagnosed (with an incidence of 306.3/100,000 people/year). Some predictive factors (age, gender, familiarity with HCC, ALT levels) were then identified, and others related to the virus (HbeAg positivity, HbsAg and DNA levels, genotype C), with which a new model of risk-stratification (high, medium and low) was built, demonstrating an excellent accuracy in comparison with the validation model (AUROC 0.86-0.89 at 5.10 and 15 years).

If these results can be confirmed in Western populations as well, we will be able to locate, thanks to these results, patients with a chronic liver disease at a higher oncological risk, in order to apply the screening and surveillance programs.

Similar attempts have been made on patients with an HCV infection. The R.E.V.E.A.L.-HCV cohort consists of 1095 asymptomatic patients from Taiwan, with positivity towards anti-HCV, HbsAg-negative, between 30 and 65 years, recruited in the years 1991-92. At the end of the observation period (2008) 91 cases of hepatic tumor were notified, with an incidence of 614/100,000/year. Age, presence of cirrhosis, AST levels, AST/ALT ratio, serum RNA concentrations and genotype 1 proved to be factors at risk irrespective of the HCC onset.

The subjects with a more elevated score risk (calculated on the simple sum of the different factors) presented a tumor onset probability at 5,10 and 15 years, considerably higher in comparison with the low score group. These results have been internally validated on a cohort of 572 anti-HCV positive with supposable characteristics [33].

This model, if externally validated, could have an important impact on clinical practice, thanks to its handiness.

Screening and Surveillance Tests

The essential features of a screening-fit test are sensitivity (that is, the ability to diagnose a tumor in those who are actually ill, as early as possible), and specificity (that is, the probability for the test to be negative in those who have no tumor). In clinical practice, a high sensitivity avoids the loss or the delay of the diagnosis on the patients who have the tumor (true positive), whereas a high specificity reduces the costs of further unnecessary research (true negative).

The success of a screening and surveillance program also depends on the choice of tests being sufficiently diffused in the territory and the ease with which these tests can be carried out with accuracy), the evaluation of usefulness and sustainability of a screening program is based not only on the costs and effectiveness of the suggested tests, but also on the diffusion of the tumor in the target population.

Following the Markov models, it was calculated that a program is cost-effective when able to extend the survival of at least 3 months, at the price of 50,000 USD per life-year gained [19].

The AASLD and EASL guidelines exclusively recommend the use of ultrasonography (US) as a test for screening and surveillance on the target population [6, 20].

US is a worldwide image technique, radiation-free, relatively inexpensive, and the patients accept it well. Thanks to these reasons it is the most recommended test of all the screening and surveillance guidelines.

Nevertheless, US has some limits: diagnostic accuracy depends greatly on the quality of the equipment and on the experience of the operator; it is limited by the level of collaboration and the physical characteristics of the patient (obesity, flatulence, ascites). Moreover, a cirrhotic liver often presents an echo coarse pattern that can make it difficult, for an inexpert operator, to distinguish a macroregenerative nodule from an early HCC.

For these reasons the sensitivity of US sensibly varies in the several published studies, in relation with the dimension of the tumor and the experience of the operator.

A recent meta-analysis showed that ultrasonography has a 94% sensitivity for tumors with a >5 cm diameter or multifocal, which reduces to 63% in the early diagnosis, and a specificity that is higher than 90% [34].

For HCC with a ≤2cm diameter the reported sensitivity is 20.5% according to a study made on explanted livers [35], whereas in a similar study of over 1000 Japanese patients, subjected to an ecographic surveillance by expert operators, over 90% of the diagnosed tumors presented an average diameter of less than 2 cm [36].

This heterogeneity of results confirms the importance of an ecographic surveillance on cirrhotic patients that should be carried out in specialized centers with expert operators and technologically advanced equipment [6, 20]. In case that the exam results limited because of patient's specific physical circumstances, it is necessary that US be replaces by other image techniques, such as the computed tomography (CT) or magnetic resonance (MRI), even though the high costs and the limited availability of equipment for MRI, and the exposure to radiations for CT, make these techniques unsuitable for prolonged surveillance [20].

Thanks to its simple execution and very low cost, the most used marker in surveillance is serum alpha-fetoprotein. Nevertheless, when establishing a 20 ng/mL cut off, sensitivity is less than 60%, and specificity is lower than the one of ultrasound [6]. In an observational, multicentric study, carried out in Italy, 57.9% patients, in their HCC diagnosis presented values that were higher than 20 ng/mL, while only 18% of them presented highly concerning values (>400 ng/mL).

Also, cirrhotic patients, especially the ones with high transaminase levels, often present AFP values over 20 ng/mL.

Hence, the use of this low cut off marker significantly increases the surveillance costs for useless diagnostic exams.

But then again, when the cut off is brought to 200 ng/mL, AFP specificity increases, but sensitivity decreases to 22% [6]. Several studies proved the AFP ineffectiveness for an early HCC diagnosis, showing that high values are often related to large tumors and to a more aggressive behavior [37-40].

It was recently suggested to use the AFP variations over time, rather than the simple absolute values, to increase the sensitivity of this marker in the early diagnose [41].

The combined use of US and AFP raises, slightly, the screening sensitivity, as opposed to US alone [34], but, when the number of false-positives increases, the costs do too (2000 to 3000 USD for each diagnosed tumor) [42].

Therefore, in the American and European guidelines, ultrasonography is the only recommended screening and surveillance test [6, 20].

Two other tumor markers were suggested for an early HCC diagnose: Des-gamma-carboxy Prothrombin (DCP, also called protein induced by vitamin k absence or antagonist II, PIVKA-II) [43] and AFP-lectin fraction (AFP-L3) [44]. DCP is an anomalous prothrombin produced by liver neoplastic cells. A survey carried out by Marrero and co. in the USA proved that, at a 125 mAU/mL cut off, DCP has a sensitivity (89%) and specificity (95%) higher than AFP in the early HCC diagnose [45]; Nakamura and co. obtained partly conflicting results, that on a population of over 1000 Japanese patients, found a diagnostic accuracy higher than AFP on tumors bigger than 5 cm, but definitely lower for low-dimension HCC [46].

In a <3 cm diameter HCC, DCP shows a very low sensitivity (27.6% at a 40 mAU/mL cut off, 23.7% at a 100 mAU/mL cut off) [21]. This marker's high values seem to be closely related to the presence of vascular invasion and metastasis [47].

According to these characteristics, DCP does not appear to be a surveillance-fit test. Furthermore, false-positives can be observed on patients with a deficit in synthesizing vitamin K or on those who are taking vitamin k antagonists.

A new immunoassay in chemiluminescence (NX-DCP) was recently suggested, and it only seems higher in patients with deficits or in a therapy involving vitamin k antagonists, in the absence of HCC. The serum DCP/NX-DCP ratio would allow to significantly raise the test specificity compared with the conventional DCP calculation [48].

AFP-L3 is a fraction of alpha-fetoprotein with affinity for lens-culinaris agglutinin. It is able to increase the AFP specificity (beyond 95%), but not the sensitivity, especially in early HCC [49]. The combined calculation of DCP and AFP-L3 increases sensitivity relatively to the individual tests, decreasing its specificity.

Japan Society of Hepatology (JSH) in its guidelines recommends the use of ultrasonography combined with two serum markers (AFP and DCP); for patients with AFP >20 ng/mL the calculation of AFP-L3 fraction is suggested as well [21].

Anyway, this screening and surveillance program cost/effectiveness needs further validation.

SURVEILLANCE INTERVAL

The regular repetition of the test has a key role for the effectiveness of the screening program, because it increases the probability of diagnosing a single, small (<3 cm), easily treatable tumor.

The subject of the ideal surveillance interval has been discussed for years.

The most important variable to take into consideration is the doubling time (DT) of the tumor. Although the fact that the HCC growth speed is heterogeneous (the DT can change from less than 3 months to more than 12 months) is common knowledge, and also that it can change through time, several studies agree to establish an average DT of 6 months [50, 51].

The biannual ecographic surveillance proved to be more effective than the annual one, in a prospective study carried out in Italy on 649 patients with cirrhosis (in most cases related to virus C), in C-P class A or B, with an average follow-up of about ten years [52]. Ten patients received the HCC diagnosis after a biannual surveillance, 139 after an interval of one year. The first ones had a five times higher probability to have a ≤2cm diameter tumor than the second ones (24.1% vs 5.1%); also, the average diameter of the tumor was significantly lower (2.5 vs. 3.3 cm), a higher percentage of patients could be subjected to effective treatments, and the average survival rate, following the time bias, was longer (45 vs. 30 months, $p = 0.001$).

Only half of the observed patients showed AFP values that could not be considered standard, which confirms the low sensitivity of this marker. The majority of the patients studied were put through an ultrasonographic surveillance in peripheral centers; this explains the low number of very early HCC diagnosis, but it allows us to evaluate the potentiality of a surveillance program in the "real world."

The results of this study confirm the first observations published in favor of the biannual surveillance [34, 53].

The evidence that a more aggressive ecographic surveillance program (3-4 months) allows the diagnosis of small tumors (<2 cm) in a high percentage of cases [54], was not confirmed in patients with a three-month surveillance, as opposed to a group undergoing a biannual US [55].

This is why the western guidelines recommend the biannual ultrasonographic surveillance [6, 20, 56].

Contrary to this position, JSH suggests a surveillance algorithm based on the risk of HCC, patients with a very high risk (HBV and HCV cirrhosis related) are suggested a 3-4 months surveillance interval (with ultrasonography and serum markers), while all the other categories are recommended to have a 6 months interval [21].

This lack of agreement could be justified by the different biology of the tumor in the eastern population.

A cost/efficacy analysis was recently carried out in the United Kingdom, which compared the non-surveillance, the biannual and annual surveillance (through US or without AFP), in groups of cirrhotic patients with different etiology (virus and alcohol related) [57].

All strategies are convenient in opposition to non-surveillance: the biannual surveillance with US + AFP resulted as the most effective (irrespective of the etiology), being able to triple the number of the operable HCC diagnosis, and to reduce the tumor-related mortality. In the cost/efficacy analysis this strategy, despite being the most expensive one (34,200 £ against the non-surveillance 26,900 £), proved to be more advantageous (especially in patients with HBV-related cirrhosis), with an increased cost-effectiveness ratio (ICER) of 26,800 £ per QUALY gained.

In literature there is no evidence that screening and surveillance with CT or MRI present any cost-effectiveness advantages compared with US, with the exception of the patients in the transplant waiting list, and the cases where the ultrasonographic exploration is limited by physical and anatomic characteristics [20].

Despite the fact that the efficacy of screening and surveillance programs has been generously demonstrated, their effectiveness (the benefit of its appliance in the field of clinical practice) is not well known.

The aspects limiting the screening and surveillance effectiveness for HCC are the following:

1. Chronic liver disease is often completely asymptomatic, even in the case of full-blown cirrhosis, so the patients do not know that they belong to a category at risk. In clinical practice, an accidental HCC diagnosis in patients who did not know they had it is not rare. This case particularly recurs in diabetic and obese patients with non-alcoholic liver cirrhosis, a condition that is becoming one of the most frequent causes of hepatocellular tumor in the western world [58, 59]. In this group of patients the ecographic exam is often limited by physical conditions, and even non-invasive fibrosis evaluation methods, such as transient elastography (Fibroscan), can be influenced by the presence of moderate to severe steatosis [60]. Hence, it is often difficult to distinguish the cirrhotic patients (who must be subjected to a screening according to the guidelines), from the ones with a non-advanced stage of fibrosis.

The surveillance of patients with NAFLD is even more complex because HCC is not rare even in the absence of cirrhosis [61, 62]. It was demonstrated that patients with HCC with a metabolic aetiology are diagnosed in a more advanced stage in comparison with HCC on HCV-related cirrhosis, they are less frequently prone to the treatment and have a lower average survival rate [63], since they elude surveillance.

2. The acceptance and application of the screening and surveillance program by the medical personnel is insufficient, especially by the primary care physicians. According to a recently published American study, the patients who are followed by hepatologists or gastroenterologists in reference centers in urban areas, had much more chances to be correctly put into surveillance programs as opposed to patients who are followed in peripheral geographic areas by non-specialist doctors [64].

A retrospective study carried out in the USA by the National Veterans Administration on a large cohort of patients with an HCV infection, proved that 42% of patients at risk underwent at least one surveillance test (US or AFP) in the year following the cirrhosis diagnosis; anyway, from the second year on, this percentage decreased progressively, and only 12% of the patients underwent a regular surveillance [65].

A similar result emerged from a study which evaluated the respect of the guidelines by AASLD in 30 non-reference Italian centers: only 54% of the 536 recruited patients underwent a regular surveillance [66].

In conclusion, a recent meta-analysis of 9 published studies on the use of surveillance in American cirrhotic confirmed that only 18.4% of the total number of studied patients goes to regular clinic exams as recommended by the guidelines, with a remarkable discrepancy between the patients followed in a specific field and the ones followed by primary care (51.7% vs. 16.9%) [67].

3. The patients' subscription to the screening and surveillance program is suboptimal for several reasons. The patient does not always understand, for cultural reasons or because of a communication deficit, the importance of the execution of tests that, as simple as they are, require time and eventually the loss of some working days. Furthermore, not every health program can provide free and fast services for the required exams. For instance, in Italy the ecographic surveillance for cirrhotic patients is completely offered by the National Health Service, but each Region has its own rules on the possibility to obtain this service at the time

intended by the surveillance program. The realization of the program in specialized reference centers, with a trained staff and with technologically advanced equipment, would permit to overcome all the above-mentioned limits, allowing a higher efficacy and effectiveness of the surveillance. Channeling some economic resources to this area of interest would give a general advantage to the whole system, both in terms of economy and health.

RECALL POLICY

A surveillance program lacking an adequate recall policy is useless.

Acknowledging an anomalous test imperatively starts the diagnostic algorithm needed to provide in a short time a reliable diagnosis followed by the customized therapy based on each patient's personal needs.

According to the AASLD [6] and EASL [20] guidelines, the ecographic evidence of a <10 mm diameter nodule just requires the repetition of the test every 3-4 months, and, if it does not grow bigger after one year, the patient can return to a biannual surveillance. In fact, focal lesions of this dimension are rarely malignant and they rarely have vascular characteristics to such an extent that allows diagnosis, not even with sophisticated imaging technologies. Echo-guided biopsy is not indicated because of a high possibility of false-negatives.

Nodules bigger than 10 mm must be examined with CT or MRI, and if they present the typical HCC contrastographic pattern, there is no need for further investigation.

In the event of nodules with an anomalous vascular behaviour, the use of an echo-guided biopsy is suggested. The AISF [56] and JSH [21] guidelines have put the contrast-enhanced ultrasonography among the image techniques that can be used for the diagnosis of tumors with a diameter bigger than 1-2 cm.

It stands to reason how the recall strategies require the use of expert radiologists and pathologists, hence they must be practiced in reference centers.

FUTURE PERSPECTIVES

The current screening and surveillance programs allowed an increasing of the early diagnosed tumors, with a higher probability of effective treatments, with a general increasing of the survival rate.

Nevertheless, in the following years an effort must be made in order to overtake the current limits, synthetically presented in the following list:

- The current target population is extremely numerous and heterogeneous. Several risk-stratification modalities have been suggested, but they still need a validation. The highest expectations are on the identification of molecular biomarkers able to detect the patients at a higher oncological risk who need an intensified surveillance program, in order to reduce the general cost and increasing its effectiveness. By means of some genome wide association (GWAS) studies, several single nucleotide polimorphisms (SNPs) were identified, associated to a higher risk of HCC;

incorporated on specific panels, they will allow the evaluation of the individual risk on selected patients. In the HALT-C cohort, a close association with an epidermal growth factor gene polimorphism was documented [68].

- The possibility to apply on a large scale these results, which were often obtained in single centers and on not very large groups of patients, will have to be demonstrated.
- It is necessary to find serum screening and surveillance tests with a higher sensitivity and specificity than the current ones. New biomarkers have been proposed, such as Glypican-3 [69], HSP70 [70], Osteopontin [71], circulating microRNAs [72] and several others. Their use, combined with the historic markers, could probably increase their diagnostic accuracy [73].
- Ultrasonography still is the ideal surveillance image technique; nevertheless, sensitivity and specificity can be enhanced with a specific training for the operators and the technological update of the equipment. The best results will be ideally obtained with surveillance programs that are conducted in hepatologic/ gastroenterologic reference centers, where the patients at risk are guaranteed an easy access to the tests.
- Recall policy requires a careful application of the diagnostic and therapeutic algorithms. The surveillance strategy fails when diagnostic and therapeutic competences are missing, and this is a strong topic in support of the treatment of patients in centers where a multidisciplinary approach to the hepatocellular tumor is possible [6, 20, 56].

Conclusion

The cost of the screening and surveillance programs is well and truly justified by the results they give. They often allow to diagnose the hepatic tumor at an early stage and to perform the necessary therapies thus ultimately increasing the general survival rate.

Screening tests with a good sensitivity and specificity are already available, but in the future it will be possible to improve the results and optimize the program cost/efficacy.

Despite the progress made, today the programs are still not sufficiently used, even in the most advanced countries.

In the following years, increasing the surveillance rates will have to be one of our main objectives, thanks to medical training and patient educational programs, in order to demolish the current geographic, social and economic disparities.

References

[1] Bosch FX, Ribes J, Cleries R, Diaz M. Epidemiology of hepatocellular carcinoma. *Clin Liver Dis* 2005;9:191-211.

[2] Llovet JM, Bru C, Bruix J. Prognosis of hepatocellular carcinoma: the BCLC staging classification. *Sem Liver Dis* 1999;19:329-38.

[3] http://www.who.int/cancer/detection/en/.

[4] International Agency for Research on Cancer. GLOBOCAN 2012: http://globocan.iarc.fr/Pages/fact_sheets_population.aspx.

[5] El Serag HB. Hepatocellular carcinoma. *N Engl J Med* 2011;365:1118-27.

[6] Bruix J, Sherman M. Management of hepatocellular carcinoma: an update. *Hepatology* 2011;53:1020-2.

[7] Zhang BH, Yang BH, Tang Zy. Randomized controlled trial of screening for hepatocellular carcinoma. *J Cancer Res Clin Oncol* 2004;130:417-22.

[8] Chen JG, Parkin DM, Chen QG, et al. Screening for liver cancer: results of a randomized controlled trial in Qidong, China. *J Med Screen* 2003;10(4):204-9.

[9] Poutschi H, Farrell GC, Strasser SI, et al. Feasibility of conducting a randomized controlled trial for liver cancer screening: is a randomized controlled trial for liver cancer screening feasible or still needed? *Hepatology* 2011;54:1998-2004.

[10] Oka H, Kurioka N, Kim K, et al. Prospective study of early detection of hepatocellular carcinoma in patients with cirrhosis. *Hepatology* 1990;12:680-7.

[11] Wong LL, Limm WM, Severino R, et al. Improved survival with screening for hepatocellular carcinoma. Liver Transpl 2000;6:320-5.

[12] Bolondi L, Sofia S, Siringo S, et al. Surveillance programme of cirrhotic patients for early diagnosis and treatment of hepatocellular carcinoma: a cost effectiveness analysis. *Gut* 2001;48:251-9.

[13] Trevisani F, De Notariis S, Rapaccini G, et al. Semiannual and annual surveillance of cirrhotic patients for hepatocellular carcinoma: effects on cancer stage and patient survival (Italian experience). *Am J Gastroenterol* 2002;97:734-44.

[14] Stravitz RT, Heuman DM, Chand N, et al. Surveillnace for hepatocellular carcinoma in patients with cirrhosis improves outcome. *Am J Med* 2008;121:119-26.

[15] Kuo YH, Lu SN, Chen CL, et al. Hepatocellular carcinoma surveillance and appropriate treatment options improve survival for patients with liver cirrhosis. *Eur J Cancer* 2010;46:744-51.

[16] Walter SD, Stitt LW. Evaluating the survival of cancer cases detected by screening. *Stat Med* 1987;6:885-900.

[17] Cucchetti A, Trevisani F, Pecorelli A, et al. Estimation of lead-time bias and its impact on the outcome of surveillance for the early diagnosis of hepatocellular carcinoma. *J Hepatol* 2014;61:333-41.

[18] Singal AG, Pillai A, Tiro J. Early detection, curative treatment, and survival rates for hepatocellular carcinoma surveillance in patients with cirrhosis; a meta-analysis. *PLOS Med* 2014;11(4):e1001624.

[19] Laupacis A, Feeny D, Detsky AS, et al. How attractive does a new technology have to be to warrant adoption and utilization? Tentative guidelines for using clinical and economic evaluations. *CMAJ* 1992;146:473-81.

[20] European Association for the Study of the Liver; European Organisation for Research and Treatment of Cancer. EASL-EORTC clinical practice guidelines: management of hepatocellular carcinoma. *J Hepatol* 2012;56:908-43.

[21] Makuuchi M, Kokudo N, Arii S, et al. Clinical Practice Guidelines for Hepatocellular Carcinoma 2009. *Hepatol Res* 2010;40(Suppl.1):2-144.

[22] Lok AS, Seeff LB, Morgan TR, et al. Incidence of hepatocellular carcinoma and associated risk factors in hepatitis C-related advanced liver disease. *Gastroenterology* 2009;136:138-43.

[23] Bruno S, Stroffolini T, Colombo M, et al. Sustained virological response to interferon-alpha is associated with improved outcome in HCV-related cirrhosis: a retrospective study. *Hepatology* 2007;45:579-87.

[24] Lampertico P, Viganò M, Manenti E, et al. Low resistance to adefovir combined with lamivudine: a 3-year study of 145 lamivudine-resistant hepatitis B patients. *Gastroenterology* 2007;133:1445–51.

[25] Fattovich G, Bortolotti F, Donato F. Natural history of chronic hepatitis B: special emphasis on disease progression and prognostic factor. *J Hepatol* 2008;48:335-52.

[26] Beasley R. Hepatitis B virus as the etiologic agent in hepatocellular carcinoma. *Hepatology* 1982;2:21S-26S.

[27] Yu MW, Chang HC, Liaw YF, et al. Familial risk of hepatocellular carcinoma among chronic hepatitis B carriers and their relatives. *J Natl Cancer Inst* 2000;92:1159-64.

[28] Loeje UH, Yang HI, Su J, et al. Predicting cirrhosis risk based on the level of circulating hepatitis B viral load. *Gastroenterology* 2006,130(3):678-86.

[29] Chan HLY, Hui AY, Wong ML, et al. Genotype C hepatitis B virus infection is associated with an increased risk of hepatocellular carcinoma. *Gut* 2004;53:1494-8.

[30] Song P, Feng X, Zhang K, et al. Screening for and surveillance of high-risk patients with HBV-related chronic liver disease: Promoting the early detection of hepatocellular carcinoma in China. *Bioscience Trends* 2013;7(1):1-6.

[31] Yuen MF, Tanaka Y, Fong DY, et al. Independent risk factors and predictive score for the development of hepatocellular carcinoma in chronic hepatitis B. *J Hepatol* 2009;50:80-8.

[32] Lee M-H, Yang H-I, Liu J, el al. Prediction models of long-term cirrhosis and hepatocellular carcinoma risk in chronic hepatitis B patients: risk scores integrating host and virus profiles. *Hepatology* 2013;58:546-54.

[33] Lee M-H, Lu S-N, Yuan Y, et al. *PLoS ONE* 2014;9(5):e94760.

[34] Singal A, Volk ML, Waljee A, el al. Meta-analysis: surveillance with ultrasound for early-stage hepatocellular carcinoma in patients with cirrhosis. *Aliment Pharmacol Ther* 2009;30:37-47.

[35] Bennett GL, Krinsky GA, Abitbol RJ, et al. Sonographic detection of hepatocellular carcinoma and dysplastic nodules in cirrhosis: correlation of pretransplantation sonography and liver explant pathology in 200 patients. *Am J Roentgenol* 2002;179:75-80.

[36] Sato T, Tateishi R, Yoshida H, et al. Ultrasound surveillance for early detection of hepatocellular carcinoma among patients with chronic hepatitis C. *Hepatol Int* 2009;3:544-50.

[37] Stroffolini T, Andreone P, Andriulli A, et al. Characteristic of hepatocellular carcinoma in italy. *J Hepatol* 1998;29(6):944-52.

[38] Giannini EG, Marenco S, Borgonovo G, et al. Alpha-fetoprotein has no prognostic role in small hepatocellular carcinoma identified during surveillance in compensated cirrhosis. *Hepatology* 2012;56:1371-9.

[39] Farinati F, Marino D, De Giorgio M, et al. Diagnostic and prognostic role of alpha-fetoprotein in hepatocellular carcinoma: both or neither? *Am J Gastroenterol* 2006;101:524-32.

[40] Lok AS, Sterling RK, Everhart JE, et al. Des-gamma-carboxy Prothrombin and alpha-fetoprotein as biomarkers for the early detection of hepatocellular carcinoma. *Gastroenterolgy* 2010;138;493-502.
[41] Lee E, Edward S, Singal AG, et al. Improving screening for hepatocellular carcinoma by incorporating data on levels of alpha-fetoprotein, over time. *Clin Gastroenterol Hepatol* 2013;11:437-40.
[42] Zhang B, Yang B. Combined alpha-fetoprotein testing and ultrasonography as a screening test for primary liver cancer. *J Med Screen* 1999;6:108–10 .
[43] Suheiro T, Sugimachi K, Matsumata T, et al. Protein induced by vitamin K absence or antagonist II as a prognostic marker in hepatocellular carcinoma. Comparison with alpha-fetoprotein. *Cancer* 1994;73:2464-71.
[44] Sato Y, Nakata K, Kato Y, et al. Early recognition of hepatocellular carcinoma based on altered profiles of alpha-fetoprotein. *N Engl J Med* 1993;328:1802-6.
[45] Marrero JA, Su GL, Wei W, et al. Des-gamma carboxy prothrombin can differentiate hepatocellular carcinoma from nonmalignant chronic liver disease in American patients. *Hepatology* 2003;37:1114-21.
[46] Nakamura S, Nouso K, Sakaguchi K, et al. Sensitivity and specificity of de-gamma-carboxy prothrombin for diagnosis of patients with hepatocellular carcinomas varies according to tumor size. *Am J Gastroenterol* 2006;101:2038-43.
[47] Koike Y, Shiratori Y, Sato S, et al. Des-gamma-carboxy prothrombin as a useful predisposing factor for the development of portal venous invasion in patients with hepatocellular carcinoma: a prospective analysis of 277 patients. *Cancer* 2001;91: 561-9.
[48] Tanaka T, Taniguchi T, Sannomiya K, et al. Novel des-γ-carboxy prothrombin in serum for the diagnosis of hepatocellular carcinoma. *J Gastroenterol Hepatol* 2013;28:1348-55.
[49] Oka H, Saito A, Ito K, et al. Multicenter prospective analysis of newly diagnosed hepatocellular carcinoma with respect to the percentage of Lens culinaris agglutinin-reactive alpha-fetoprotein. *J Gastroenterol Hepatol* 2001;16:1378-83.
[50] Barbara L, Benzi G, Gaiani S, et al. Natural history of small untreated hepatocellular carcinoma in cirrhosis: a multivariate analysis of prognostic factors of tumor growth rate and patient survival. *Hepatology* 1992;16:132-7.
[51] Sheu JC, Sung JL, Chen DS, et al. Growth rate of asymptomatic hepatocellular carcinoma and its clinical implications. *Gastroenterology* 1985;89:259-66.
[52] Santi V, Trevisani F, Gramenzi A, et al. Semiannual surveillance is superior to annual surveillance for the detection of early hepatocellular carcinoma and patient survival. *J Hepatol* 2010;53:291-7.
[53] Santagostino E, Colombo M, Rivi M, et al. A 6-month versus a 12-month surveillance for hepatocellular carcinoma in 559 haemophiliacs infected with the hepatitis C virus. *Blood* 2003;102:78-82.
[54] Oka H, Kurioka N, Kim K, et al. Prospective study of early detection of hepatocellular carcinoma in patients with cirrhosis. *Hepatology* 1990;12:680-7.
[55] Trinchet JC, Chaffaut C, Bourcier V, et al. Ultrasonographic surveillance of hepatocellular carcinoma in cirrhosis: a randomized trial comparing 3-and 6-mo periodicities. *Hepatology* 2011;54:1987-97.

[56] Italian Association for the Study of the Liver (AISF). Position Paper of the Italian Association for the Study of the Liver (AISF): the multidisciplinary clinical approach to hepatocellular carcinoma. *Dig Liver Dis* 2013;45:712-23.
[57] Coon JT, Rogers G, Hewson P, et al. Surveillance of cirrhosis for hepatocellular carcinoma: a cost-utiliy analysis. *Br J Cancer* 2008;98:1166-75.
[58] Marrero JA, Fontana Rj, Su GL, et al. NAFLD may be a common underlying liver disease in patients hepatocellular carcinoma in the United States. *Hepatology* 2002;36:1349-54.
[59] Santi V, Buccione D, Di Micoli A, et al. The changing scenario of hepatocellular carcinoma over the last two decades in Italy. *J Hepatol* 2012;56:397-405.
[60] Macaluso FS, Maida M, Cammà C, et al. Steatosis affect the performance of liver stiffness measurement for fibrosis assessment in patients with genotype 1 chronic hepatitis C. *J Hepatol* 2014;61:523-9.
[61] Hashimoto E, Yatsuji S. Tobari M, et al. Hepatocellular carcinoma in patients with nonalcoholic steatohepatitis. *J Gastroenterol* 2009;44:89-95.
[62] Takuma Y, Nouso K. Nonalcoholic steatohepatitis-associated hepatocellular carcinoma: our case series and literature review. *World J Gatroenterol* 2010;16: 1436-41.
[63] Giannini EG, Marabotto E, Savarino V, et al. Hepatocellular carcinoma in patients with cryptogenic cirrhosis. *Clin Gastroenterol Hepatol* 2009;7:580-5.
[64] Davila JA, Morgan RO, Richardson PA, et al. Use of surveillance for hepatocellular carcinoma among patients with cirrhosis in the United States. *Hepatology* 2010;52:132-41.
[65] Davila JA, Henderson L, Kramer JR, et al. Utilization of surveillance for hepatocellular carcinoma among hepatitis C virus-infected veterans in the United States. *Ann Intern Med* 2011;154:85-93.
[66] Borzio M, Fornari F, De Sio I, et al. Adherence to American Association for the Study of Liver Diseases guidelines for the management of hepatocellular carcinoma: results of an Italian field practice multicenter study. *Future Oncol.* 2013;9:283-94.
[67] Singal AG, Yopp A, Skinner CS, et al. Utilization of hepatocellular carcinoma surveillance among american patients: a sistematic review. *J Gen Intern Med* 2012,27:861-7.
[68] Abu Dayyeh BK, Yang M, Fuchs BC, et al. A functional polymorphism in the epidermal growth factor gene is associated with risk for hepatocellular carcinoma. *Gastroenterology* 2011;141:141-9.
[69] Capurro M, Wanless IR, Sherman M, et al. Glypican-3: a novel serum and hisochemical marker for hepatocellular carcinoma. *Gastroenterology* 2003;125:89-97.
[70] Di Tommaso L, Destro A, Seok JY, et al. The application of markers (HSP70 GPC3 and GS) in liver biopsies is useful for detection of hepatocellular carcinoma. *J Hepatol* 2009;50:746-54.
[71] Shang S, Plymoth A, Ge S, et al. Identification of osteopontin as a novel marker for early hepatocellular carcinoma. *Hepatology* 2012;55:483-90.
[72] Qu KZ, Zhang K, Li H, et al. Circulating microRNAs as biomarkers for hepatocellular carcinoma. *J Clin Gastroenterol* 2011;45:355-60.

[73] Xu C, Yan Z, Zhou L, et al. A comparison of glypican-3 with alpha-fetoprotein as a serum marker for hepatocellular carcinoma: a meta-analysis. *J Cancer Res Clin Oncol* 2013;139:1417-24.

In: Hepatocellular Carcinoma in the 3rd Millennium
Editors: M. Berretta and B. Cacopardo
ISBN: 978-1-63484-025-5

Chapter 6

PRIMARY PREVENTION OF HEPATOCELLULAR CARCINOMA

Rossella Fontana Del Vecchio and Bruno Cacopardo*
Department of Clinical and Experimental Medicine,
University of Catania, Italy

ABSTRACT

Primary prevention of cancer consists in all the interventions that keep a cancerogenic agent from initiating the carcinogenic process. This is achieved by eliminating, avoiding, or neutralizing the carcinogen, or by stopping the *in vivo* conversion of a pre-carcinogen into a carcinogen. Prevention is the only realistic approach for reducing mortality rates associated with hepatocellular carcinoma (HCC) worldwide. Primary prevention of HCC is made through the prevention of its major risk factors, i.e., hepatitis B (HBV) and hepatitis C (HCV) infection. Vaccination against HBV and screening of blood donations are well-known and effective measures of primary prevention.

Primary prevention also includes antiviral treatments, which may slow or definitively stop the progression of liver disease towards cirrhosis. Primary prevention seems to work successfully against HBV and its complications. In those areas where a nationwide HBV universal vaccination program was implemented, the incidence of HCC declined significantly. Also, in HBV-infected subjects, long-term suppression of HBV with antiviral therapies can slow the progression of liver disease or even reverse liver damage, therefore, preventing HCC formation. In HCV-infected subjects, a yet controversial strategy to reduce HCC incidence, is based on viral eradication by Interferon (IFN)-based or IFN-free treatments. In the latter case, the cost of new antiviral drugs for primary prevention of HCC remains a remarkable obstacle to such a strategy.

* Corresponding author: Bruno Cacopardo, cacopardobruno@inwind.it

INTRODUCTION

Hepatocarcinogenesis is a multistep process mainly associated with persistent infection with hepatitis B virus (HBV) and/or hepatitis C virus (HCV) [1, 2]. This is the reason why hepatocellular carcinoma (HCC) is highly prevalent in regions endemic for chronic HBV and HCV infection, especially in Africa and East Asia (China), where more than 80% of cases are recorded [1].

On the other hand, HCC rising incidence in Western countries is mostly related to the "cohort effect" of HCV epidemic and the increase in prevalence of non-alcoholic fatty liver disease (NAFLD) [3]. HCC usually affects people in their fifties, although it has an earlier onset in Africa where the mean age of the affected population ranges between 25 and 40 years. The youngest age of affected population is likely due to longer exposure to HBV and HCV. Men have been reported to have a three- to eight-fold greater risk of developing HCC compared to women.

Primary prevention of cancer consists in all the interventions that keep a cancerogenic agent from initiating the carcinogenic process. This is achieved by eliminating, avoiding, or neutralizing the carcinogen, or by stopping the *in vivo* conversion of a pre-carcinogen into a carcinogen. Prevention is the only realistic approach for reducing mortality rates associated with HCC. Primary prevention of HCC is made through the prevention of its major risk factors, i.e., by reducing the incidence of HBV and HCV [2]. Vaccination against HBV and screening of blood donations are well-known and effective measures of primary prevention. Screening of blood donations has led to a substantial reduction in viral hepatitis transmission among the general population; moreover, in Taiwan vaccination against HBV caused a significant reduction in HCC incidence among infants [2]. Primary prevention also includes antiviral treatments, which may slow or definitively stop the progression of liver disease towards cirrhosis [2].

PREVENTION OF HBV-RELATED HCC

The main known risk factors for HBV-related HCC can be distinguished into host- and virus-related [3]. Host factors include: male gender, Asian race, age older than 40 years, habitual smoking or alcohol consumption and a family history of HCC [4-6]. Virus-related factors include coinfections with HCV or Hepatitis Delta Virus (HDV), pre-core (Pre-C) or basal core promoter mutations, HBV genotype C[5] and high HBV DNA serum levels [3]. In particular, elevated HBV DNA serum level (≥2000 IU/mL) is a strong predictive factor for HCC development, independent of serum alanine aminotransferase (ALT) levels and presence of liver cirrhosis [7].

Hepatocarcinogenesis sustained by HBV infection is still not completely known, although it is a multistep process involving direct and indirect components, some of which may act synergistically [3]. HBx protein has an important role in activating HBV transcription and replication, and consequently stimulating the expression of genes implicated in cell cycle control, oncogenesis, proliferation, inflammation and apoptosis [3]. A key mechanism for hepatocarcinogenesis is also represented by the integration of HBV DNA into the host genome, forming a covalently closed circular DNA (cccDNA), responsible for the persistence of viral replication [3].

Primary prevention seems to work successfully against HBV and its complications. HBV vaccine has been incorporated into the Expanded Program of Immunization in 181 countries, including most countries in Eastern and South-eastern Asia [8]. Nevertheless, because of the long interval between HBV infection and HCC development, it will take several decades to appreciate a consistent decrease in incidence of HBV-related HCC in these countries. A relevant experience comes from the nationwide HBV universal vaccination program for infants in Taiwan, which started in 1984. From 1981 to 1994, the incidence of HCC in 6- to 9-year old children declined significantly [8].

In HBV-infected subjects, long-term suppression of HBV might improve or even reverse fibrosis or cirrhosis [3]. Actually, there is abundant evidence that antiviral therapies can slow progression or even reverse liver damage, therefore, preventing HCC formation. The retrospective evaluation of studies designed to assess the antiviral activity of Interferon and Nucleoside analogues suggested a reduced incidence of HCC in responders [9]. Nevertheless, most of these studies are subject to criticisms because of a number of biases, such as heterogeneity of patient referral, adoption of surrogate end points and lack of control arms [9]. A systematic review and meta-analysis on the role of antiviral therapy for prevention of HCC showed that in cohort studies antiviral therapy increased the risk of HCC, whereas case-control studies found a decreased risk of HCC in the intervention group, with a clear-cut difference between the results of randomized trials and observational studies [10].

A Chinese study demonstrated that IFN (interferon)-α was not effective in preventing HCC and other cirrhosis-related complications [2]. Also, the clinical benefit of first generation nucleoside analogues used in HBV therapy, such as lamivudine, was also limited because of the potential development of resistance and virological relapse after treatment cessation [3]. The main drugs currently used to prevent HCC in HBV-infected people are currently two second generation nucleos(t)ide analogue reverse transcriptase inhibitors, which hold potent activity against HBV and high genetic barrier to resistance: entecavir and tenofovir dipivoxil [3, 11].

With regard to entecavir, some studies demonstrated that it significantly reduces the 5-year risk of HCC in treatment-naïve patients [5]. However, in a multicenter Italian study, cirrhotic patients were still at risk of development HCC over time, despite profound and durable viral suppression obtained with entecavir, which was administered for up to 66 months [12]. Clinical decompensation did not occur during follow up among the 164 cirrhotic patients, showing that entecavir is effective in preventing the progression of cirrhosis.

But these patients had still a 14% risk of HCC at the fifth year, indicating that some premalignant cellular clones had probably developed before starting therapy [12]. The long-term effect tenofovir on HCC incidence was recently evaluated using a predictive model know as REACH-B: the results indicated that the incidence of HCC in patients on tenofovir was lower than predicted by the REACH-B model both in non-cirrhotic and in cirrhotic patients [13]. In non-cirrhotic patients, the effect of tenofovir became significant after 6 years of therapy, whereas the impact of tenofovir was less pronounced in cirrhotic patients [13].

Two main targets need to be achieved when administering potent antiviral drugs with elevated genetic barrier (such as entecavir and tenofovir) for HCC prevention: histological amelioration and cccDNA elimination. Since cirrhosis is an important risk factor itself for HCC, the improvement in histology achieved with entecavir and tenofovir may partly explain a reduction in HCC development in high-risk patients [3, 11]. Moreover, long-term therapy is necessary to eliminate intrahepatic cccDNA: a 48-week treatment with entecavir monotherapy has recently shown to significantly reduce hepatic HBV cccDNA levels in comparison with lamivudine [3].

PREVENTION OF HCV-RELATED HCC

In HCV-infected subjects, a yet controversial strategy to reduce HCC incidence is based on viral eradication by IFN-based or IFN-free treatments. Combination of pegylated (PEG)-IFN and ribavirin is an IFN-based therapy recommended worldwide as effective in reducing HCV-related HCC incidence rate, especially in cirrhotic patients[2]. Several observational studies and randomized controlled trials have shown that clearance of viremia with achievement of Sustained Virologic Response (SVR) using IFN-based treatments is associated with a remarkable decline in the risk of developing HCC [14]. Zhang et al. [15] in a meta-analytic study on 9 randomized clinical trials in 1614 patients with HCV infection, observed that patients treated with IFN had a lower risk of HCC, compared with untreated patients: nevertheless, the decline was remarkable only in those cases who achieved SVR. In the HALT-C trial [16], the adjusted cumulative incidence of HCC eight years after enrolment was 1.1% in the SVR group, whereas it was higher (5.5% and 8.8%, respectively) in relapsers and nonresponders. In a pooled analysis of 30 observational studies, Morgan et al. [17] observed that the rate of HCC was 1.6% among those patients who reached SVR by IFN-based therapy and 6.1% among patients who failed or missed therapy. The risk reduction was similar for all stages of HCV disease. New oral agents increase the endpoint of SVR (up to 90%) and reduce the duration of treatment to 12-24 weeks. Their safety profile is better than the IFN-based therapy one, but their use is limited by their cost. IFN-free treatments might result in a greater rate of HCV-infected patients being treated successfully [14]. On this basis, a relevant decline of HCC rates due to HCV infection is expected over time. However, the costs of these new drugs for primary prevention of HCC remain a remarkable obstacle to this strategy.

Other Strategies of Prevention

Contamination of staple foodstuffs by aflatoxin B1 might represent a relevant cause of HCC in countries with limited resources. This is due to contamination by Aspergillus flavus or A. parasiticus during growth of the crops or improper storage. Methods of primary prevention include sun drying of the crops before storage or drying on cloth rather than directly on earth, rainproof storage facilities, storage in jute, removal of moldly plants, use of insecticides and fungicides [18]. Also, a number of substances and drugs are under investigation for their capacity of inhibiting HCC development. Aspirin has been associated with a 41% lower risk of HCC in a large population-based study in the NIH-AARP Diet and Health Study cohort. Aspirin probably inhibits or delays immune-mediated hepatocarcinogenesis, suggesting that platelets may have a central role in the pathogenesis of HCC, especially HBV-related [19]. Likewise, statins may decrease HCC risk in HBV-infected patients in a dose-dependent manner, maybe by reducing fat accumulation in the liver [2]. Some natural polyphenols, such as resveratrol, seem to be effective in preventing HCC, by downregulating lipogenesis, promoting transient liver regeneration, and stimulating antioxidant activity [2]. Propranolol has antioxidant, anti-inflammatory, anti-angiogenic and anti-tumoral properties; therefore, it can be potentially active in the prevention of HCC [2]. One of the major risk factor for HCC, especially in decompensated cirrhotic patients, is metabolic syndrome, which is closely related to obesity, insulin resistance and diabetes mellitus. Some studies conducted on animal models such as mice have shown that dietary intake of branched-chain amino acids, may significantly reduce the risk of hepatocarcinogenesis [20]. Therefore, all the benefits of a healthy lifestyle, including decreased body weight and adipose mass as well as improved glucose homeostasis and dyslipidemia, are important not only for reducing cardiovascular risk, but also to decrease the risk of liver cancer. In this regard, metformin has been demonstrated to be effective in primary prevention of HCC risk [21]. Several observational studies have reported an association between metformin and decreased risk of HCC in patients with diabetes. This effect of metformin was dose-dependent: in fact, every additional year of metformin use was associated with a 7% decrease in HCC risk. More recent data have shown that certain dietary factors, such as coffee, green tea, unsaturated fatty acids and fish can be considered protective against HCC [2, 20].

REFERENCES

[1] Brian I. Carr, *Tumori del fegato e delle vie biliari*, Harrison principi di medicina interna, Fauci et al., 17th edition, vol. I, 573 – 578.

[2] Tao Lu, Wai-Kay Seto, Ran-Xu Zhu, Ching-Lung Lai, Man-Fung Yuen. Prevention of hepatocellular carcinoma in chronic viral hepatitis B and C infection. *World J Gastroenterol* 2013 December 21; 19(47): 8887-8894.

[3] Conrado M Fernàndez – Rodrìguez, Marìa Luisa Gutiérrez – Garcìa. Prevention of hepatocellular carcinoma in patients with chronic hepatitis B. *World J Gastrointest Pharmacol Ther* 2014 August 6; 5 (3): 175-182.

[4] Gao Y, Jiang Q, Zhou X, Ding B, Wang R, Zhao G, Chen Y. *HBV* infection and familial aggregation of liver cancer: an analysis of case-control family study. *Cancer Causes Control* 2004; 15: 845-850.

[5] Park CH, Jeong SH, Yim HW, Kim JD, Bae SH, Choi JY, Yoon SK. Family history influences the early onset of hepatocellular carcinoma. *World J Gastroenterol* 2012; 18: 2661-2667.

[6] Yu MW, Chang HC, Liaw YF, Lin SM, Lee SD, Liu CJ, Chen PJ, Hsiao TJ, Lee PH, Chen CJ. Familial risk of hepatocellular carcinoma among chronic hepatitis B carriers and their relatives. *J Natl Cancer Inst* 2000; 92: 1159-1164.

[7] Chen CJ, Yang HI, Su J, Jen CL, You SL, Lu SN, Huang GT, Iloeje UH. Risk of hepatocellular carcinoma across a biologi cal gradient of serum hepatitis B virus DNA level. *JAMA* 2006; 295: 65-73.

[8] Ni YH, Chen DS. Hepatitis B vaccination in children:the Taiwan experience. *Pathol Biol* (Paris) 2010 Aug;58(4):296-300.

[9] Colombo M. Does chemotherapy prevent HBV related hepatocellular carcinoma? Cons. Dig Liver Dis 2010Jul;42 Suppl3:S298-301.

[10] Thiele M., Gluud LL, Dahl EK, Kraq A. Antiviral therapy for prevention of hepatocellular carcinoma and mortality in chronic hepatitis B: systematic review and meta-analysis *BMJ Open* 2013;Aug 14;pii:e003265.

[11] Liaw YF Does chemotherapy prevent HBV related hepatocellular carcinoma? *Pros. Dig Liver Dis* 2010 Jul;42 Suppl3:S293-7.

[12] Lampertico P, Soffredini R, Vigano M, Minola E, Cologni G, Rizzi M, Zaltron S, Vavassori A, Carosi G, Angeli E. Entecavir treatment for NUC naïve, field practice patients with chronic hepatitis B: excellent viral suppression and safety profile over 5 years of treatment. 63rd *Annual Meeting of the American Association for the Study of Liver Diseases (AASLD)* 2012; 2012 November 9-13, 2012; Boston, MA, USA: Wiley-Blackwell 111 *River St, Hoboken* 07030-5774, NJ USA: 370A-371A .

[13] Kim W, Berg T, Loomba R, Schall RA, Dinh P, Yee L, Mar- tins E, Flaherty J, Gurel S, Buti M. Long term tenofovir diso- proxil fumarate (TDF) therapy and the risk of hepatocellular carcinoma [Abstract]. 48th *Annual Meeting of the European Association for the Study of the Liver (EASL 2013);* 2013 April 24-28; Amsterdam, The Netherlands: S19.

[14] Kohli A, Shaffer A, Sherman A, Kottilil S. Treatment of hepatitis C: a systematic review. *JAMA*. 2014;312:631-40.

[15] Zhang CH, Xu GL, Jia WD, Li JS, Ma JL, Ge YS. Effects of interferon treatment on development and progression of hepatocellular carcinoma in patients with chronic virus infection: a meta-analysis of randomized controlled trials *Int J Cancer*. 2011 Sep 1;129(5):1254-64.

[16] Singal AG, Nehra M, Adams-Huet B, Yopp AC, Tiro JA, Marrero JA, Lok AS, Lee WM Detection of hepatocellular carcinoma at advanced stages among patients in the HALT-C trial: where did surveillance fail? *Am J Gastroenterol* 2013 Mar; 108(3):425-32.

[17] Morgan TR. Chemoprevention of hepatocellular carcinoma in chronic hepatitis *C Recent Results Cancer Res.* 2011;188:85-99.

[18] Kew MC Hepatocellular carcinoma in developing countries: prevention, diagnosis and treatment. *World J Hepatol*. 2012 Mar 27;4(3):99-104.

[19] Sahasrabuddhe VV, Gunja MZ, Graubard BI, Trabert B, Schwartz LM, Park Y, Hollenbeck AR, Freedman ND, McGlynn KA. Nonsteroidal anti-inflammatory drug use, chronic liver disease, and hepatocellular carcinoma *J Natl Cancer Inst.* 2012 Dec 5;104(23):1808-14.

[20] M. Shimizu, Y. Shirakami, H. Sakai, M. Kubota, T. Kochi, T. Ideta, T. Miyazaki, H. Moriwaki. Chemopreventive Potential of Green Tea Catechins in Hepatocellular Carcinoma. *Int. J. Mol. Sci*. 2015, 16, 6124-6139.

[21] J. Kasznicki, A. Sliwinska, J. Drzewoski. Metformin in cancer prevention and therapy. *Ann Transl Med* 2014, 2 (6): 57.

In: Hepatocellular Carcinoma in the 3rd Millennium
Editors: M. Berretta and B. Cacopardo ISBN: 978-1-63484-025-5

Chapter 7

NATURAL HISTORY OF HEPATOCELLULAR CARCINOMA

***Alessandra Mataloni Paggi*[1], *Anna Marigliano*[1] and *Marcello Tavio*[1,*]**
[1]Division of Infectious Disease "Ospedali Riuniti delle Marche," Pescara, Italy

ABSTRACT

The natural history of Hepatocellular Carcinoma (HCC) is complex and severe because of the coexistence of liver inflammatory disease, often cirrhosis, which worsens the clinical progress causing the patient death and generally limiting the therapy choices. HCC natural history has been divided in 4 evolutionary stages, following Barcelona Clinic Liver Cancer classification, based on volume and number of tumor nodules, relationship of the tumour with portal vascular system, level of liver failure and presence/absence of general symptoms of neoplasm. Cirrhosis is the most important single risk factor for HCC. The risk for HCC differs depending on numerous factors such as sex, patients age, etiology and cirrhosis clinical stage, level of hepatocellular proliferation and presence/absence of hepatocellular dysplasia.

The understanding of HCC natural history has been possible because of perspective studies of patients at risk, in particular of patients with cirrhosis and chronic HBV infection. In most cases, HCC is unicentric, allowing clinically early diagnosis, with positive repercussion on treatment outcome. Since HCC is essentially a tumor that growths just inside the liver for years, it is successfully treatable with surgery resection or local ablation.

Dividing patients in different clinical stages with different prognosis levels, allowed different treatments and proven efficacy also for patients with intermediate and advanced tumour. Depending on geographic differences of HCC epidemiology and natural history, it is not clear if it would be necessary following a unique HCC staging system. Nevertheless, staging systems as BCLC, used by the most important international scientific society, allowed multicentric studies finalized to validating new therapeutic options.

[*] E-mail: m.tavio@ospedaliriuniti.marche.it.

INTRODUCTION

The natural history of Hepatocellular Carcinoma (HCC) is complex and severe, as shown by the overlapping high incidence and mortality rate [1]. This overlapping rate reflects the prevalence of HCC cases with late diagnosis, especially frequent in the geographical areas with high incidence of tumour, where there is a constant lack of screening program for HCC early diagnosis. In the countries adopting screening programs, 30-50% of the patients with HCC diagnosis has an early-diagnosed HCC, it means potentially treatable [2]. The patients precluded from early diagnosis are the patients from geographical areas without screening programs and surveillance, and rare patients (5%) with HCC in a healthy liver, when lack of risk factor hinders surveillance [3].

The natural history of HCC is complex and severe because of the coexistence of liver inflammatory disease, often cirrhosis, which worsens the clinical progress; in several cases, it is the cause of patient death and generally limits the therapy possibilities.

The prospective study of the cirrhotic patients with early-diagnosed tumor, under surveillance with abdominal echography, explained the natural history of HCC. Recently, the tumor natural history was divided in 4 evolutionary stages, following Barcelona Clinic Liver Cancer classification, based on volume and number of tumor nodules, relationship of the tumor with portal vascular system, level of liver failure and presence/absence of general symptoms of neoplasm [4].

THE TUMOR ASSOCIATED TO CHRONIC HEPATIC DISEASE

Cirrhosis is the most important single risk factor for HCC; it develops in annual rate between 3% and 8% [5]. The risk for HCC differs depending on numerous factors, as sex, patient age, etiology and cirrhosis clinical stage, level of hepatocellular proliferation and presence/absence of hepatocellular dysplasia [6-9]. Even if the etiology prognostic meaning is controversial, in 30% of cases related to hepatitis B, the tumor anticipates cirrhosis. It is possible that this rate is going to increase in patients with chronic therapy with drugs for hepatitis B, which can stop the progression of the chronic infection to cirrhosis. On the other hand, HCV related HCC is usually associated to cirrhosis and differs from HBV-related tumor, because it develops 10 years earlier, as a consequence of different ways of transmission. The HBV is often sexually transmitted or early familiar transmitted, while the HCV related hepatitis is late transmitted, iatrogenic or drug user related.

In addition, alcohol associated HCC is usually related to cirrhosis and is often the first cause of clinical liver failure, worsening the prognosis and the possibility of radical treatment. In most cases, cirrhosis related HCC is a single nodular lesion, developing from regenerating parenchymal foci rich of dysplastic hepatocytes [10].

EARLY TUMOR

There is not a precise definition of early HCC. In the seventies, early diagnosis was considered a nodule equal or inferior to 5 cm of diameter, diagnosed in a compensated cirrhotic patient, since these patients showed satisfactory survival rates after surgical resection compared to patents with wider nodules or decompensate cirrhosis. In 1996, early diagnosis was extended to patients with 3 nodules equal or inferior to 3 cm of diameter, after the demonstration of satisfactory survival rate after 5 years after liver transplantation [11]. After the BCLC classification [4], adopted by EASL and AASLD, early diagnosis is considered 3 nodules equal or inferior to 3 cm or a single nodule inferior to 5 cm, in patients with no portal invasion or neoplastic symptoms (performance status = 0) and with satisfactory liver function (Child-Pugh A or B).

Even if the small neoplasm is considered early neoplasm, just a minimal number of tumors with volume between 1,0 and 1,5 cm are biologically and clinically low aggressive. Just 20% of all tumors with this volume range, identified by ultrasound surveillance, have a nodular shape, reflecting a tissue organization close to the one typical of the cirrhotic liver [12]. These tumors are nowadays defined "very early," to be differentiated from the "early" tumors of the same size. The "early" tumors have by ultrasound a better-defined nodular shape with peritumoral capsule, and produce micro-metastasis in the cirrhotic liver and in the tumor vases. The contrastographic imaging techniques, unable to identify the very early tumor, because poor of arteriole, are on the other hand able to identify the early tumor of nodular aspect, rich of arteriole compared to portal venule. In a perspective study, it was seen that of 60 tumoral nodules not identified with contrastographic techniques, 2/3rd after 3 years were visible, getting the aspect of classical early tumor [14]. In general, the diagnostic contrastographic sensibility depends on the volume of the nodular tumor, since the number of supernumerary arteriole compared to portal venule increases together with the tumor volume [10]. The difference between very early HCC and early HCC is clinically very important, since the survival rate after 5 years after surgical resection in patients with the first type of tumor is 90% compared to 50% in patients with the second type [13]. For this reason, surgical resection is the elective treatment for very early tumor.

The natural history of the early HCC, following the BCLC classification, varies depending on the possibility of applying a radical treatment.

The survival rate after 5 years of selected patients can reach 75% after resection, transplantation and thermal ablation; while in patients treated with the same cures, with negative predictor response, the survival rate can be around 50%. The survival rate in the various categories of patients in stage A (BCLC) depends on the volume and number of tumors and the level of portal hypertension and bilirubin values.

The survival rate after surgical resection in a patient with early HCC measuring 5 cm is better than the one of a patient in the same stage with 3 nodules, each equal or inferior to 3 cm. The same happens in the patients with a single nodule and low portal hypertension (HVPG < 10 mmHg) compared to the ones with HVPG >10 mmHg [15]. The survival rate of patients with a single nodule depends on the HCC recurrence risk that relates to macroscopic vascular invasion prevalence: 5% in the nodules inferior to 2 cm and rises to 22% for the ones of 5 cm [15] (Table 1).

The vascular metastasis is a histological marker with negative predictor value also in patients inserted in transplantation waiting list. The HCC growth speed varies from nodules to nodules and in this way, it's an important variable in the tumor natural history and makes difficult defining patient prognosis.

Several perspective studies in cirrhosis patients with periodic ultrasound exams demonstrated important differences in the doubling time of HCC nodule volume.

Table 1. Pathological classification of hepatocellular carcinoma early diagnosed

Characteristics	Very early	Early	p
Number of tumors	15	52	-
Diameter of tumor, mm	14 ± 3	17 ± 4	=0.02
Portal spaces	15(100%)	3(6%)	<0.001
Edmonson, grade 1	15(100%)	0	<0.001
Capsular formation	0	36 (69%)	<0.001
Locoregional spread	1 (7%)	22 (42%)	-
Vascular invasion	1 (7%)	15 (29%)	-
Intrahepatic metastasis	0	11 (21%)	<0.01

Takayama et al., modified.

The doubling time of HCC volume varies from 1 to 20 months, with a median of 6 months. This frequency is used in the Western countries for ecographic surveillance of cirrhotic patients risking HCC [16]. The ecographic surveillance of patients at risk for HCC is clinically very important, since it betters the patient survival due to early diagnosis. A randomized controlled study in Shanghai [17], demonstrated a significant reduction of liver-specific mortality in chronic viral hepatitis patients that were screened with abdominal ultrasound every 6 months, compared to control subjects not performing the screening (83 vs. 131 x 100.000 inhabitants, rate = 0.63). On the other hand, the liver-specific mortality of the patients with HCC early diagnosis depends on the therapeutic progress of these last years. As a matter of fact, it was demonstrated by an Italian study in patients with early HCC, whose survival rate was higher in the last 5 years of the study compared to the previous 5 years (90% vs 55%, $p = 0.0009$) [8]. The higher survival rate was connected to significant mortality reduction in treated patients (from 34% to 5%, $p = 0.003$), due to more effective cures and a better patient selection undergoing surgery, while untreated patient mortality was substantially the same (69% vs 92%, ns). In a small percentage (<20%) of early-diagnosed patients, HCC has a multinodular presentation. The natural history of these patients is controversial. Old studies in surgery resection selected patients, and more recent studies dealing with global expression of HCC genes, confirmed the existence of two types of multiple nodules, with a different prognosis. Actually, there are nodules caused by intrahepatic early metastatic dissemination and at the same time multicentric nodules, which means nodules genetically different one from the other, caused by different foci of cirrhotic tissue [18, 19] (Figure 1). There are different evidences that HCC with early local metastatization, causing also early recurrence after surgical resection, has often the phenotype of progenitor stem cells [20]. Due to this chemo-resistance, these cells explain also the unsuccessful tertiary prophylaxis of HCC with classic antitumoral chemotherapy.

INTERMEDIATE TUMOR

Since a few years ago, the HCC patients were classified in 3 evolutive stages: a) early tumor b) terminal tumor and in between c) unresectable tumor.

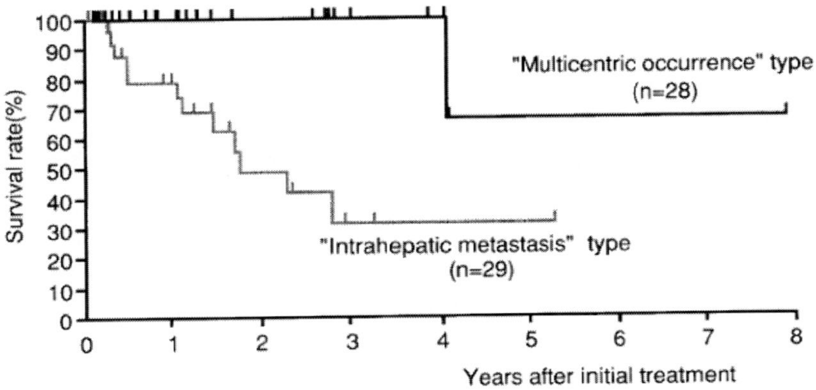

From Kumada et al., modified.

Figure 1. Type of recurrences of hepatocellular carcinoma after surgery.

A group of researchers in Barcelona studied in a retrospective analysis, the natural history of this heterogeneous group of patients with not resectable, not alcohol- percutaneous-treatable HCC, distinguishing the patients with intermediate HCC from advanced HCC, equally distributed in the group. The patients with intermediate tumor are peculiar for the presence of a tumor that exceeds Milano criteria for liver transplantation, with no portal/extra hepatic invasion, or neoplastic disease symptoms, with a good compensation and good general performance (PS=0). The spontaneous survival rate of these patients is 50% after 3 years, correspondent to a median of 16 months.

Since the limited number of patients included in the original study, it is not clear if these patients natural history could be stratified in relationship to liver failure level, it means between Child-Pugh A and Child-Pugh B cirrhosis patients. The spontaneous survival rate of intermediate HCC patients was confirmed by an international, controlled, multicentric study, enrolling 747 non-resectable tumor patients [21].

Advanced Tumor

These patients have tumors of various dimensions, which invade the portal system and/or diffuse in lymph nodes or in other organs. Even if in a condition of good compensation of cirrhotic liver (Child-Pugh A and B), these patients have a significant deterioration of the general performance status (PS=1 or 2) or the neoplastic disease symptoms. The spontaneous survival rate after 3 years is just of 8%, corresponding to a median of 6 months. The spontaneous survival rate of these patients was also confirmed in this controlled multicentric international study [21].

Terminal Tumor

The terminal study is characterized by the presence of an advanced tumor but also by the severe clinical decompensation (Child-Pugh C) and the general performance impairment (PS = 3 or 4).

The life expectancy is around 3 months, and could be shorter in patients with portal hypertension complications like digestive hemorrhage and spontaneous bacterial peritonitis.

The Causes of Death

In a perspective study of early-diagnosed tumor, the principal cause of death was intrahepatic progression of tumor (67% of cases), followed by hepatic failure (9%), digestive hemorrhage (8%) and other than hepatic death factors (9%) [8]. (Table 2). The extra hepatic localization of tumor, frequent in the HCC advanced and terminal phases, in most cases has not an important role in the patient death.

The Predictive Factors of Death

The HCC patient prognosis depends strictly on the possibility of receiving curative treatments and is in this way, bounded to the HCC staging. For this reason, the multidimensional staging systems, which combine more parameters, like volume, tumor aggressivity and liver impairment, are more accurate and clinically more useful than uni dimensional parameters like bilirubin, creatinine, and coagulation tests in evaluating the HCC patient prognosis. These last parameters, considered in combination, have a high predictive value in the short term in the cirrhotic patients, regardless the HCC presence/absence, as in the case of MELD score (Model for End-Stage Liver Disease) to list the patients for liver transplantation. Recently, several studies on the HCC global expression genes, identified groups of patients sharing a gene expression pattern, typical of fetal human and murine hepatocytes, characterized by a reduced survival rate and higher rate of tumor recurrence after surgical resection [21]. The same studies demonstrated that the patients with reduced survival rate, presented gene markers of high cellular proliferation and apoptosis. While in the group of hepatitis B- associated HCC, a particular molecular sequence composed by 153 genes help identifying a small number of patients with reduced survival rate [22].

Table 2. Causes of death in 76 patients with compensated cirrhosis that developed a hepatocellular carcinoma under surveillance. Cohort prospective study of 447 patients began in 1986 in Milan

Cause of death	N° of patients
Tumor progression	51 (67%)
Hepatic failure	7 (9%)
Gastrointestinal hemorrhage	6 (8%)
Other conditions not liver-related	7 (9%)
Unknown causes	5 (7%)
Total	76 (100%)

From Sangiovanni et al., modified.

Due to these studies, a new approach to HCC prognosis was possible by using molecular techniques. As a matter of fact, nowadays, they seem to be of limited utility, since these studies were performed on tumoral tissue obtained with surgical resection and not by perioperative needle-biopsy, representing a small and favorably selected minority of HCC patients.

Tumor on Healthy Liver

The natural history of this tumor is severe, since the patients are late identified, when they present symptoms like hepatomegaly, fever, fatigue or weight loss, typical of advanced tumor.

A consistent quote of patients presents portal invasion and/or neoplastic thrombosis of portal main vases, which hinders from applying successful treatments. In a cohort of 330 HCC patients, treated with liver resection at Hopital Beaujon of Clichy (France), 52 (16%) presented minimal fibrosis in the not neoplastic liver, while 28 (8%) presented a perfectly healthy liver [3]. Since the patients with liver resection represented a selected group of HCC patients, it is possible that the percentage of cases with HCC healthy-liver-associated is actually inferior to the one presented in Hospital Beaujon study. 75% of patients with healthy liver do not present any known risk factor for HCC, this is the reason why these patients are not screened in any surveillance program and can rarely undergo an early diagnosis.

Fibrolammellar Carcinoma

The patients with fibrolamellar carcinoma are different from the HCC patients, because of young age (median age 23 years), same sex distribution, absence of underlying liver disease and known risk factors for HCC. In most cases (90%), the tumor presents as a single mass, well defined, lobulated, non-encapsulated, with slow progression [23].

The most frequent clinical presentation is abdominal pain associated to hepatomegaly and to the presence of palpable abdominal mass, with normal values of Alfa-fetoprotein. The absence of underlying liver disease makes easier the tumor surgical resection, even if it is often complicated by recurrence, due to advanced stage of tumor in the symptomatic identified patients. The survival rate of the patients after 5 years is 70% [23] and in half cases, the tumor responds to systemic and intra/artherious chemotherapy.

Conclusion

Understanding the HCC natural history was possible because of perspective studies of patients at risk, in particular of patients with cirrhosis and chronic HBV infection. In most cases, the HCC is unicentric, allowing clinically early diagnosis, with positive repercussion on treatment outcome. Since the HCC is essentially a tumour that growths just inside the liver for years, it is successfully treatable with surgery resection or local ablation. By dividing patients in different clinical stages, with different prognosis levels, it was possible to diversify treatments with proven efficacy also for patients with intermediate and advanced tumour.

Depending on the geographic differences of the HCC epidemiology and natural history, it is not clear if it would be necessary following a unique HCC staging system. Nevertheless, staging systems as BCLC, used by the most important international scientific society, allowed muticentric studies finalized to validating new therapeutic options.

REFERENCES

[1] Bosch F. X., Ribes J., Cléries R., Díaz M. Epidemiology of hepatocellular carcinoma. *Clin. Liver Dis.,* 2005 May; 9(2):191-211.

[2] Toyoda H., Kumada T., Kiriyama S., Sone Y., Tanikawa M., Hisanaga Y., Yamaguchi A., Isogai M., Kaneoka Y., Washizu J. Impact of surveillance on survival of patients with initial hepatocellular carcinoma: a study from Japan. *Clin. Gastroenterol. Hepatol.*, 2006 Sep.; 4(9):1170-6.

[3] Bralet M. P., Régimbeau J. M., Pineau P., Dubois S., Loas G., Degos F., Valla D., Belghiti J., Degott C., Terris B. Hepatocellular carcinoma occurring in nonfibrotic liver: epidemiologic and histopathologic analysis of 80 French cases. *Hepatology*, 2000 Aug.; 32(2):200-4.

[4] Llovet J. M., Brú C., Bruix J. Prognosis of hepatocellular carcinoma: the BCLC staging classification. *Semin. Liver Dis.*, 1999; 19(3):329-38.

[5] Fattovich G., Stroffolini T., Zagni I., Donato F. Hepatocellular carcinoma in cirrhosis: incidence and risk factors. *Gastroenterology,* 2004 Nov.; 127(5 Suppl. 1):S35-50.

[6] Colombo M. Treatment of hepatocellular carcinoma. *Antiviral Res.,* 2001 Nov.; 52(2):209-15.

[7] Donato M. F., Arosio E., Del Ninno E., Ronchi G., Lampertico P., Morabito A., Balestrieri M. R., Colombo M. High rates of hepatocellular carcinoma in cirrhotic patients with high liver cell proliferative activity. *Hepatology*, 2001 Sep.; 34(3):523-8.

[8] Sangiovanni A., Del Ninno E., Fasani P., De Fazio C., Ronchi G., Romeo R., Morabito A., De Franchis R., Colombo M. Increased survival of cirrhotic patients with a hepatocellular carcinoma detected during surveillance. *Gastroenterology,* 2004 Apr.; 126(4):1005-14.

[9] Degos F. 1., Christidis C., Ganne-Carrie N., Farmachidi J. P., Degott C., Guettier C., Trinchet J. C., Beaugrand M., Chevret S. Hepatitis C virus related cirrhosis: time to occurrence of hepatocellular carcinoma and death. *Gut,* 2000 Jul.; 47(1):131-6.

[10] Kojiro M. Pathological evolution of early hepatocellular carcinoma. *Oncology*, 2002; 62 Suppl. 1:43-7.

[11] Mazzaferro V., Regalia E., Doci R., Andreola S., Pulvirenti A., Bozzetti F., Montalto F., Ammatuna M., Morabito A., Gennari L. Liver transplantation for the treatment of small hepatocellular carcinomas in patients with cirrhosis. *N Engl. J. Med.,* 1996 Mar. 14; 334(11):693-9.

[12] Kojiro M., Roskams T. Early hepatocellular carcinoma and dysplastic nodules. *Semin. Liver Dis.*, 2005; 25(2):133-42.

[13] Takayama T., Makuuchi M., Hirohashi S., Sakamoto M., Yamamoto J., Shimada K., Kosuge T., Okada S., Takayasu K., Yamasaki S. Early hepatocellular carcinoma as an entity with a high rate of surgical cure. *Hepatology,* 1998 Nov.; 28(5):1241-6.

[14] Takayasu K., Muramatsu Y., Mizuguchi Y., Okusaka T., Shimada K., Takayama T., Sakamoto M. CT Evaluation of the progression of hypoattenuating nodular lesions in virus-related chronic liver disease. *AJR Am. J. Roentgenol.*, 2006 Aug.; 187(2):454-63.

[15] Llovet J. M., Schwartz M., Mazzaferro V. Resection and liver transplantation for hepatocellular carcinoma. *Semin. Liver Dis.*, 2005; 25 (2):181-200.

[16] Bruix J., Sherman M. Management of hepatocellular carcinoma. *Hepatology,* 2005 Nov.; 42(5):1208-36.

[17] Zhang B. H., Yang B. H., Tang Z. Y. Randomized controlled trial of screening for hepatocellular carcinoma. *J. Cancer Res. Clin. Oncol.*, 2004 Jul.; 130(7):417-22.

[18] Kumada T., Nakano S., Takeda I., Sugiyama K., Osada T., Kiriyama S., Sone Y., Toyoda H., Shimada S., Takahashi M., Sassa T. Patterns of recurrence after initial treatment in patients with small hepatocellular carcinoma. *Hepatology,* 1997 Jan.; 25(1):87-92.

[19] Llovet J. M., Chen Y., Wurmbach E., Roayaie S., Fiel M. I., Schwartz M., Thung S. N., Khitrov G., Zhang W., Villanueva A., Battiston C., Mazzaferro V., Bruix J., Waxman S., Friedman S. L. A molecular signature to discriminate dysplastic nodules from early hepatocellular carcinoma in HCV cirrhosis. *Gastroenterology,* 2006 Dec.; 131(6):1758-67. Epub 2006 Sep. 19.

[20] Lee J. S., Heo J., Libbrecht L., Chu I. S., Kaposi-Novak P., Calvisi D. F., Mikaelyan A., Roberts L. R., Demetris A. J., Sun Z., Nevens F., Roskams T., Thorgeirsson S. S. A novel prognostic subtype of human hepatocellular carcinoma derived from hepatic progenitor cells. *Nat. Med.*, 2006 Apr.; 12(4):410-6.

[21] Beaugrand M., Sala M., Degos F., et al. Treatment of advanced hepatocellular carcinoma (HCC) by seocalcitol (a vit D analogue): An International randomized double-blind placebo-controlled study in 747 patients. *J. Hepatol.*, 2005; 42 (Suppl. 2):17.

[22] Ye Q. H. 1., Qin L. X., Forgues M., He P., Kim J. W., Peng A. C., Simon R., Li Y., Robles A. I., Chen Y., Ma Z. C., Wu Z. Q., Ye S. L., Liu Y. K., Tang Z. Y., Wang X. W. Predicting hepatitis B virus-positive metastatic hepatocellular carcinomas using gene expression profiling and supervised machine learning. *Nat. Med.*, 2003 Apr.; 9(4):416-23. Epub 2003 Mar. 17.

[23] Stevens W. R. 1., Johnson C. D., Stephens D. H., Nagorney D. M. Fibrolamellar hepatocellular carcinoma: stage at presentation and results of aggressive surgical management. *AJR Am. J. Roentgenol.*, 1995 May; 164(5):1153-8.

In: Hepatocellular Carcinoma in the 3rd Millennium
Editors: M. Berretta and B. Cacopardo

ISBN: 978-1-63484-025-5

Chapter 8

CLINICO-PATHOLOGICAL AND MOLECULAR FINDINGS IN HEPATOCELLULAR CARCINOMA

***Vincenzo Canzonieri*[1]*, Lara Alessandrini*[1]*, Laura Caggiari*[2]*, Tiziana Perin*[1]*, Massimiliano Berretta*[3]*, Renato Cannizzaro*[4] *and Valli De Re*[2]**

[1]Pathology Unit, Centro di Riferimento Oncologico (CRO), Aviano National Cancer Institute, IRCCS, Aviano (PN) Italy
[2] Facility of Bio-Proteomics, Centro di Riferimento Oncologico (CRO), Aviano National Cancer Institute, IRCCS, Aviano (PN) Italy
[3]Medical Oncology A Unit, CRO Centro di Riferimento Oncologico (CRO), Aviano National Cancer Institute, IRCCS, Aviano (PN) Italy
[4]Gastroenterology Unit , CRO Centro di Riferimento Oncologico (CRO), Aviano National Cancer Institute, IRCCS, Aviano (PN) Italy

ABSTRACT

Hepatocellular carcinoma (HCC) is a major health problem with a high incidence and mortality all over the world. The current ability to increase the survival of patients with HCC relies upon clinical surveillance, which allows HCC precursors and malignant tumors to be recognized at an earlier stage, making cure possible. In this report we describe the main histopathological criteria to discriminate between HCC precursors and well differentiated HCC, with attention to the role of immunohistochemical markers.

Over time, many staging and scoring systems have been proposed for the classification and prognosis of patients with HCC. A complete system for HCC classification nowadays should include multifunctional and phenotypic characteristics of the tumor, the general health of the patient and the potential therapeutic approaches available. The second part of the paper is devoted to an overview of the current staging systems for HCC.

Genetic studies of tumor samples and the use of newer molecular approaches such as non-coding RNA and genome-wide association studies, according to immunohistochemistry, proteomics and clinical criteria are highlighting the variability that exists among diverse HCC. Identification of new target pathways for the treatment of

HCC by more personalized and targeted regimens are the main goals of the current translational medical research.

Introduction

The criteria for the diagnosis of Hepatocellular carcinoma (HCC) have been defined at the Barcelona-2000 EASL (European Association for the Study of the Liver) conference [1]. Not so defined were the staging criteria, a useful tool to the physician to choose the most appropriate form of care. Since the choice for treatment is influenced by the tumor stage, it is obvious that a good classification is able also to predict the prognosis of the patient with HCC. Unlike most other cancers, for which the staging systems are well codified and universally accepted, the HCC staging systems proposed are not by all shared. One of the reasons that make the staging of HCC difficult is that in almost all cases the HCC occurs in patients suffering from liver cirrhosis.

Therefore, the staging of the tumor does not take into account the severity of the underlying liver disease that most often is the factor conditioning the prognosis of HCC. In other words, a complete system for HCC classification nowadays should include multifunctional and phenotypic characteristics of the tumor, the general health of the patient and the potential therapeutic approaches available.

Pathology

Surveillance and Clinical Aspects for Early Detection of HCC

The population groups at risk for HCC have traditionally included those with chronic hepatitis and cirrhosis. Recently, also non-alcoholic fatty liver disease (NAFLD), when progressed to cirrhosis, has been indicated as a risk factor for HCC. Less certain is whether diabetes and/or the metabolic syndrome causes HCC in the absence of NAFLD or cirrhosis. Surveillance should be undertaken if the risk of HCC is high enough, if an appropriate treatment is available and if surveillance is cost-effective. The latter parameter seems to be strongly influenced by the incidence of HCC. The American Association for the Study of Liver Disease (AASLD) identified different groups for whom surveillance is recommended, according to specific threshold incidence per year (0.2% for hepatitis B and 1.5-2% for cirrhosis from other causes, for instance) [2].

The occurrence of hepatocellular nodules (hyperplastic, benign, dysplastic and malignant) is substantially different according to the liver background. In the hepatitic liver HCC and nodular precursors such as regenerative /dysplastic nodules related to hepatocarcinogenesis, far outnumber all the other lesions. Conversely in non-hepatitic liver, metastases are more common than primary benign and malignant neoplasms. The prevalence of malignancy among hepatocellular nodules in the hepatitic/cirrhotic liver under surveillance for early HCC detection is largely dependent on the size of the lesion: most of <1 cm lesions are non-malignant whereas the large majority of lesions exceeding 2 cm are HCC. (Figure 1) Only a minority of regenerative/dysplastic nodules convert to malignancy (mostly in the group high-grade dysplasia), doing so in a relatively short interval, while 40–60% stabilize and a few definitely disappear during follow-up [3, 4].

HCC is fed by a neoarterial supply which is of major importance for its imaging detection. Because of HCC specific radiologic features, biopsy is only required when the radiologic appearance is not typical. Indeed, current international guidelines indicate that nodules greater than 2 cm arising in cirrhotic patients, with typical features for HCC at one dynamic technique, do not require biopsy confirmation. On the contrary, if lesions reveal atypical features, which occurs in 10–15% of the cases [5], biopsy is required. For nodules between 1 and 2 cm, two concordant radiological tests are needed for a non-invasive diagnosis of HCC, otherwise biopsy is recommended and this occurs in about 60–70% of the cases. Thus, most of small incident nodules in cirrhosis, suspicious but not conclusive for HCC, are currently biopsied.

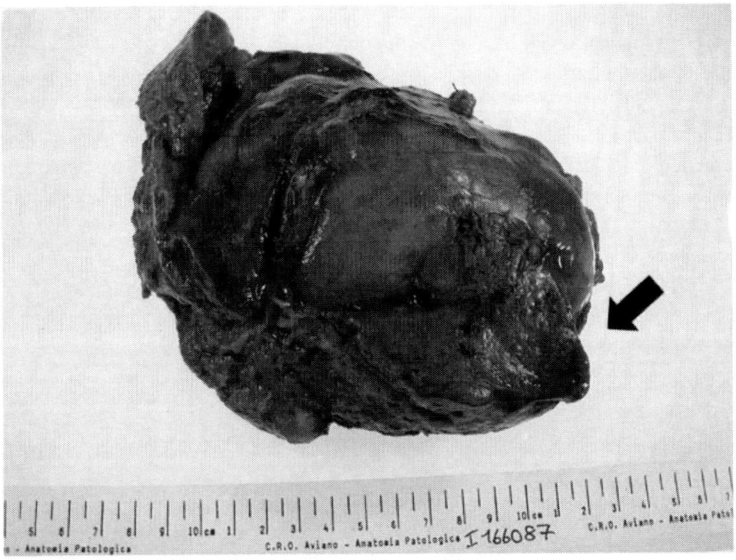

Figure 1. Surgical specimen from a partial hepatectomy. A multinodular, dark brown area, measuring 7 cm in maximum diameter in evident on the right. Central cystic colliquation (arrow), due to necrosis, in frequently detected in larger HCCs.

Nomenclature of Small Hepatocellular Nodules

An International Consensus has recently been obtained on the classification of small (≤2 cm) hepatocellular nodules [6]. Nodular lesions found in chronic liver disease are classified into large regenerative nodule (LRN), low-grade dysplastic nodule (LGDN), high-grade dysplastic nodule (HGDN), and HCC. In addition, the concept of dysplastic focus (a cluster of hepatocytes with features of early neoplasia - in particular small cell change or iron-free foci in a siderotic background- measuring less than 0.1 cm) was introduced, and small HCC was defined as a tumor measuring less than 2 cm. More recent studies support the division of small HCC into two clinico-pathological groups that have been termed early HCC and progressed HCC. Early HCC has a vaguely nodular appearance and is well differentiated.

Progressed HCC has a distinctly nodular pattern and is mostly moderately differentiated, often with evidence of microvascular invasion (see Table 1 for details).

Table 1. Nomenclature of small hepatocellular nodules/lesions

Displastic foci A cluster of hepatocytes with features of early neoplasia (small- and large-cell change or iron-free foci in a siderotic background) measuring less than 0.1 cm
Displastic nodule Gross features: these nodules have different color, size, texture and bulging from the adiacent liver paranchyma and have distinct margins Histologic features: a. *low-grade (LGDN)*: mild increase in cell density with a monotonous pattern, no cytologic atypia, detectable portal tracts inside the nodule, large cell change/dysplasia may be present; b. *high-grade (HGDN)*: increased cell density, architectural and cytologic atypia, but insufficient for a diagnosis of HCC, unpaired arteries in most lesions, detectable portal tracts inside the nodule, large cell change/dysplasia and small cell change/dysplasia (most frequent) may be present
Small HCC (≤ 2 cm) a. *early HCC*: a vaguely nodular lesion with indistinct margins, incomplete/absent capsule, increased cell density (>2x the surrounding non tumoral liver), well differentiated (G1), mild cellular/architectural atypia, scattered intratumoral portal tracts, variable number of unpaired arteries, fatty change, absence of microvascular invasion; b. *Progressed HCC*: distinctly nodular lesion rimmed by condensed fibrosis/pseudocapsule, well to moderately differentiated (G1/G2), portal tracts are no longer identified, rare steatosis for more complete neoarterialization (unpaired arteries), microvascular invasion is seen in 25% of cases.

Small and Early HCC

This lesion, also termed *HCC of vaguely nodular type or HCC with indistinct margins*, is characterized by the small size, the pushing margins and expansile growth pattern, the incomplete or absent perilesional fibrous capsule, mild cellular and structural atypia, the presence of some acinar/pseudoglandular structures (i.e., a very well differentiated histology), the presence of scattered intratumoral portal tracts, the variable number of unpaired arteries, the absence of microvascular invasion and the frequent (40%) steatosis. The most difficult differential diagnosis is with HGDN. Morphology alone is often not sufficient and requires additional techniques.

Extensive neovascularization process could be detected by immunohistochemical staining with endothelial marker CD34 and the Actin Smooth Muscle antigen (SMA) for muscolarized unpaired arteries. Stromal invasion of well differentiated hepatocytes into portal tracts or fibrous septa could be a useful diagnostic clue for malignancy: this histological aspect can be highlighted by immunostaining for cytokeratins CK7/19 depicting the ductular reaction which takes place around non-malignant nodules but is absent around HCC. In malignant lesions, reticulin framework, depicted by appropriate istochemical techniques, may be lost or overtly reduced as compared to surrounding tissue; however, this characteristic is not always present in the earliest phases of malignant transformation.

Finally, the overexpression of three specific immunomarkers (Glypican 3- GPC3; Heat Shock protein 70- HSP70; Glutamine synthetase – GS) in the neoplastic cell population, has been recognized as able to selectively label small and early HCC as compared to non-malignant counterparts. GPC3, a cell surface heparin sulphate proteoglycan, is an HCC serum and tissue marker with a sensitivity of 77% and specificity of 96%. GPC3 staining must be interpreted in the clinical context because it may also be seen in regenerating hepatocytes in a chronic hepatitis setting [6]. HSP70 is a stress protein implicated in cell-cycle progression, apoptosis and tumorigenesis. It was reported as the most abundantly upregulated gene in early HCC where it can be detected in up to 78% of the cases with 95% specificity [6]. GS catalyzes the synthesis of glutamine from glutamate and ammonia and it is the main source of energy for hepatocytes located in pericentral areas. However, it is also a target gene of ß-catenin, a major driver of human HCC, where GS overexpression is able to mirror ß-catenin mutation. In malignant hepatocytes GS immunostaining should be diffuse and strong, a pattern that can be seen in 50% of HCC [6]. In the appropriate clinico-pathological context, the finding of 2 unequivocal positive immunomarker (out of 3 among GPC3, HSP70, and GS) can detect early HCC with a sensitivity of 72% and a specificity of 100% [7].

Small and Progressed HCC

Also known as *HCC of distinctly nodular type or HCC with distinct margins,* progressed HCC may develop from a pre-existing dysplastic focus or nodule or from an early HCC. In the latter two cases, it can take the gross and radiological appearance of the so-called "nodule in nodule" (Figure 2) which is highly suspicious for malignancy, especially in a cirrhotic setting.

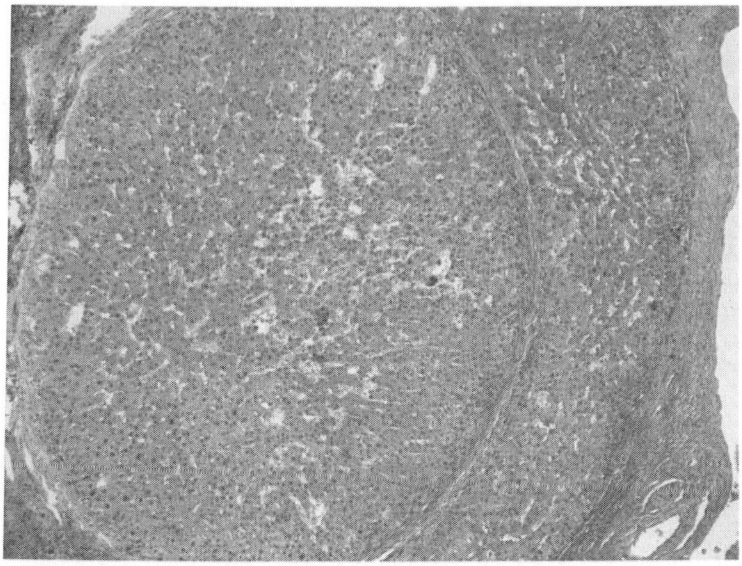

Figure 2. "Nodule in nodule" appearance of nodules highly suspicious for malignancy. This morphology is particularly evident in a cirrhotic setting. In these cases the parent outer nodule may be dysplastic or well differentiated HCC while the smaller, inner subnodule is invariably malignant and less differentiated (hematoxylin& eosin – original magnification 10x).

In these cases the parent outer nodule may be dysplastic or well differentiated HCC while the smaller, inner subnodule is invariably malignant and less differentiated. Similar to early HCC, progressed HCC can be small, less than 2 cm. At variance with the latter, however, progressed HCC is morphologically characterized by a destructive and expansile growth pattern with complete neoarterialization and frequent vascular invasion. Portal tracts are no longer detected, and the expansile round border of the tumour is generally rimmed by a condensed fibrosis showing up as a tumour capsule. Histologically small but progressed HCC is usually moderately differentiated (G2), rarely steatotic for more complete and advanced neoarterialization, but it can be poorly differentiated (G3) with size enlargement.

Role of Biopsy Sampling in HCC Diagnosis

As an increasing number of HCCs are diagnosed without pathologic examination (see paragraph "Surveillance and clinical aspects for early detection of HCC"), pathologists examine fewer cases of HCCs with the typical cytoarchitectural features: most cases are small well-differentiated hepatocellular nodules for which the differential diagnosis between early HCC and precursor lesions should be considered. The first step to characterize hepatocellular nodules in biopsy specimens is to evaluate the adequacy of the specimen itself. The ideal liver biopsy should contain sufficient tissue from both the tumour and the adjacent non-neoplastic liver. If there is no histological evidence of the target lesion, serial or deeper sections should be performed prior to recommending a repeat biopsy or follow up. If there is a suspected target on the biopsy but the lesion is too small for morphological evaluation or accompanied by a marked crushing artifact, an immunohistochemical stain could be performed with the 3-HCC marker panel (GPC3/HSP70/GS), as already stated [6]. The morphological features are recommended to be interpreted in context with the clinico-radiological findings, especially as the gross features of the nodule cannot be evaluated on biopsy specimens.

The replacement of biopsy evaluation as the gold standard for the diagnosis of HCC >2 cm does not imply that all atypical cases in a cirrhotic liver represent HCC or its precursors: other lesions, such as large regenerative nodules (> 2cm), may be detected in a cirrhotic liver (e.g., in autoimmune epatitis cirrhosis).

In the setting of non-cirrhotic livers, the possibility of hepatocellular adenoma (HCA) or focal nodular hyperplasia (FNH) should be considered in the differential diagnosis of hepatocellular nodules. HCA is characterized by proliferation of bland-looking hepatocytes. The trabeculae are irregularly and mildly thickened, numerous thin-walled arteries are present without accompanying bile ducts, and pseudoglandular structures can occasionally be seen, especially in□□-catenin-activated HCAs. Therefore, the differential diagnosis between HCA and well-differentiated HCC may be challenging on a liver biopsy. It is even more problematic when there is evidence of focal cytologic or architectural atypia and in clinical settings unusual for HCA (atypical age/sex/ morphology): terms such as 'atypical HCA-like neoplasms' and 'well-differentiated hepatocellular neoplasm of uncertain malignant potential (HUMP)' have been proposed for similar tumors, which have shown aggressive behavior. GPC3 and HSP70 immunostains may be helpful in distinguishing between HCAs and HCC; whereas GS, also part of the 3-marker HCC panel, is not always helpful in the differential diagnosis between HCC and HCA, as it is diffusely expressed in b-catenin-activated HCAs.

In all of these patterns, cytologic features of HCC tend to resemble those of normal hepatocytes, with variable degree of nuclear atypia. Neoplastic cells often maintain their polygonal shape, with a slightly basophilic cytoplasm, and have round vesicular nuclei and prominent nucleoli (Figure 3A). Poorly differentiated tumors, however, have also pleomorphic/bizarre mono-multinucleated giant cells. Intranuclear vacuoles and glycogenation of nuclei, both features seen in normal liver, are fairly common in HCCs. Cytoplasmic inclusions, such as Mallory bodies, or globular acidophilic bodies, composed of proteins (including albumin, fibrinogen, alpha $_1$-antitrypsin or ferritin) may be present, as well. Also fat and glycogen may be prominent in HCCs, providing tumor with a clear cell appearance. Other, less frequent, cytoplasmic changes include: pale bodies (round to oval, lightly eosinophilic or clear cytoplasmic structures, characteristically seen in fibrolamellar variant of HCC), ground-glass cells containing hepatitis B surface antigen (HBsAg), and dark brown to black pigment. In rare cases, HCC displays a spindle-cell component.

Special Types of HCC

Fibrolamellar carcinoma: overall, fibrolamellar carcinoma accounts for 0.5-9% of all primary liver cancers, with a peak incidence around 25 years. It typically arises in non-cirrhotic liver and, in two-third of the cases, it occurs in the left lobe. Gross appearance is yellow to pale tan with a firm texture and a central scar. Histologically, fibrolamellar carcinoma has pushing margins and is made up of large polygonal cells, with abundant eosinophilic cytoplasm, large nuclei and nucleoli.

The latter, along with lamellar fibrosis, are its distinctive features. Pale and hyaline bodies may be seen. Prognosis is more favourable than HCC arising in cirrhosis, but similar to HCC in non-cirrhotic liver.

Scirrhous HCC: about 5% of HCCs showed marked fibrosis along sinusoid-like spaces associated with varying degree of atrophy of neoplastic trabeculae. They typically arise below liver capsule. Similar changes occur after chemotherapy, radiation and transarterial chemoembolization. Due to its morphology and less frequent Hep Par-1 staining (see below) scirrhous HCC must be distinguished from fibrolamellar HCC, cholangiocarcinoma and metastatic adenocarcinoma. Glypican 3 and arginase have yielded a 100% sensitivity to identify scirrhous HCC variant in this context [11].

Undifferentiated carcinoma: it is a rare primary liver tumor that can be diagnosed as carcinoma on the basis of immunohistochemical findings alone, but cannot be further classified. It shares similar clinical manifestations and imaging data with classic HCC, but prognosis is supposed to be worse.

Lymphoepihelioma-like carcinoma: It is a very rare tumor featuring pleomorphic tumor cells, occasionally organized in a syncytial growth, intermixed with numerous lymphocytes. In some cases, neoplastic cells are positive for Epstein-Barr virus (EBV).

Sarcomatoid HCC: HCC could be partially or fully composed of malignant spindle cells. When such sarcomatoid transformation is prominent, the tumor is defined sarcomatoid HCC. Areas of more typical morphology usually emerge after adequate sampling. Sarcomatoid change is more frequent after chemotherapy and transarterial chemoembolization.

Recently Discovered Subtypes

HCC with stem/progenitor cell immunophenotype: there is a recently proposed subtype of progressed HCC (mostly G2/G3), not otherwise recognizable by hematoxylin and eosin stain, in which a fraction of tumour cells (>5%) expresses stem/progenitor cell markers such as CK19 (cytokeratin 19), epithelial cell adhesion molecule (EpCAM), CD133, etc. It has been suggested to be a peculiar HCC linked to a stem/progenitor cell phenotype, and this subtype has also been suggested to be a biliary phenotype, as CK19 is expressed in biliary epithelium as well as in stem/progenitor cell. It is still unaddressed whether this phenotype reflects an origin from a stem/progenitor cells or dedifferentiation from mature hepatocytes [12, 13].These tumours have been reported to be more aggressive as compared to usual HCC without stem/progenitor markers, with increased likelihood of recurrence following resection, resistance to chemotherapy, and radiotherapy, and increased likelihood of metastasis [12, 13]. It has, therefore, been suggested that the application of these specific immunomarkers on the biopsied or resected HCC tissue may be helpful to select patients with more aggressive HCC, in order to provide useful information for optimal management and treatment of patients.

Mixed hepatobiliary carcinoma, classical type: mixed hepatobiliary carcinoma, classical type, accounts for about 2.5% of primary liver cancers. The most typical form is combined hepatocellular and cholangiocarcinoma, which has areas of typical HCC and areas of typical cholangiocarcinoma. This definition has not to be applied to collision tumours in which HCC and cholangiocarcinoma arise separately. These tumours can be defined morphologically. Confirmation of hepatocellular differentiation can be supported by immunostaining for hepatocyte specific antigen (Hep Par1), polyclonal anti-carcinoembryonic antigen (pCEA), and CD10. Cholangiocarcinoma components are usually positive for CK7 and CK19. Small areas of intermediate morphology at the interface between HCC and cholangiocarcinoma areas can be detected at careful examination. They are composed of small cells with a high nuclear cytoplasmic ratio and hyperchromatic nuclei, and the expression of CK7 and CK19, nuclear cell adhesion molecule (NCAM, CD56), c-kit, or EpCAM. Therefore, these small tumour cells at the interface suggest a recapitulation of stem/progenitor cells [14]. The prognosis of this subtype has been reported to be poorer as compared to the usual progressed HCC. Mixed hepatobiliary carcinoma, with stem/progenitor cell phenotype and immunophenotype: recently a rare subtype has been reported, in which the majority of tumour cells show stem/progenitor like cells or intermediate features between hepatocyte and cholangiocyte. The prognosis of this subtype is uncertain given the absence of large cohorts of patients. The large sized "cholangiolocellular carcinomas" (>4.0 cm) had higher recurrence rates following treatment [15], and the overall survival of intermediate carcinoma was intermediate between those of typical HCCs and typical cholangiocarcinoma, whereas small sized mixed hepatobiliary carcinomas with stem/progenitor cell phenotype and immunophenotype in explanted livers showed no recurrence [16].

Grading

Grading of HCC has relied for many years on Edmondson and Steiner system, which divided HCC into four grades from I to IV on the basis of histological differentiation [17].

Grade I is the best differentiated consisting of small tumor cells, with regular nuclei, arranged in thin trabeculae. Cells in grade II are larger with abnormal nuclei, some hyperchromatism, nucleoli, >N/C ratio and glandular structures may be present. In grade III nuclei are larger and more hyperchromatic than grade II cells and cytoplasm is granular and acidophilic, but less than grade II. In grade IV, tumor cells are much less differentiated with hyperchromatic nuclei and loss of trabecular pattern. Marked anaplasia with giant and pleomorphic cells are evident.

HCC versus Metastatic Neoplasms

Metastases are by far the most common malignant neoplasms in non-hepatitic/cirrhotic liver. Without antecedent liver disease, HCC seems to account for about 2% of malignant neoplasms in the liver.

Because of the wide spectrum of histologic appearance of HCC, the differential diagnosis between HCC and other tumors involving the liver can be challenging. Lung, colon, pancreas and breast are the most common primary sites of hepatic metastases, but malignant tumors from almost any site can metastasize to the liver. Some tumors such as melanoma, neuroendocrine carcinoma, neuroblastoma and adenocarcinoma of gastrointestinal tract, pancreas and biliary tract, breast and lung often metastasize to the liver, other tumors as squamous cell carcinoma of head and neck, prostate adenocarcinoma and most sarcomas seldom do. Secondary carcinomas may be difficult to assign to their origin but immunohistochemistry may be very helpful to distinguish between primary and metastatic tumors and, among metastases, to identify their primaries [18].

Immunoistochemistry

Hepatocyte paraffin 1 (Hep Par 1): is a monoclonal antibody against an urea cycle enzyme located in mitochondria. It has emerged as the most sensitive (around 80% to 100%) and specific immunohistochemical marker for HCC and reflects hepatocyte differentiation in hepatic as well as extra-hepatic tumors. Hep Par 1 yields a diffuse cytoplasmic granular staining pattern in normal and neoplastic hepatocytes, sparing bile duct epithelium and inflammatory cells (Figure 3B). Variation in staining may occur, particularly when there is fatty, clear cell or oncocytic change. Staining is also probably inversely related to the differentiation grade of the hepatocellular tumor.

Polyclonal carcinoembryonic antigen (pCEA): is a glycoprotein present in the glycocalix of fetal epithelial cells and in small amounts in normal adults cells. This antibody stains a cross-reactive substance called biliary glycoprotein present in bile canaliculi and ductal epithelium but not in hepatocytes. Diffuse cytoplasmic expression is observed in most adenocarcinomas (>90%). In HCC, pCEA staining reveals a characteristic and specific "chicken-wire fence" canalicular pattern (Figure 3C), not observed in adenocarcinomas. As already noted for Hep Par 1, the sensitivity of this marker given by the canalicular staining, decreases with increasing anaplasia. Monoclonal CEA is not reactive in HCC.

Alpha-fetoprotein (AFP): is an oncofetal protein expressed mainly in fetal gut, liver and yolk sac. Its expression in a tumor is specific for hepatocellular differentiation if germ cell tumors can be excluded. Normal livers do not express AFP. Staining tends to be focal and sensitivity is about 30%.

Common Acute Lymphoblastic Leukemia Antigen (CD10): is a zinc-dependent 90 to 110 kDa cell membrane metallopeptidase normally expressed in several normal tissues, including kidney, liver, small intestine, placenta, gonads, adrenal gland and brain. CD10 in HCC typically shows a canalicular pattern similar to that of pCEA, not seen in adenocarcinoma, but displaying a lower sensitivity (50%) compared to pCEA.

MOC-31: is a monoclonal antibodieses that reacts with membrane glycoproteins expressed in benign and malignant glandular epithelia of multiple sites, but not in lymphomas, melanomas and HCC. 50% to 98% of cases of adenocarcinoma stain with a cytoplasmic pattern.

Cytokeratins: normal and neoplastic hepatocytes express cytokeratins CK 8 and 18 and about 70% of HCC are negative for CK7, CK19, and CK20. Therefore, CK7 and CK20 are more helpful in determining the primary site once the diagnosis of adenocarcinoma has been established.

The role of immunohistochemistry in the differential diagnosis of HCC versus metastases is highlighted in Table 2.

Table 2. Immunoistochemistry of primary HCC and metastastic carcinoma

Differential diagnosis between HCC and...	Most useful Panel of antibodies	Profile and comments
metastatic adenocarcinoma (MA); cholangiocarcinoma (CC)	HepPar1, pCEA,MOC-31	HCC: HepPar 1+ pCEA +, MOC-31- MA and C: HepPar 1- pCEA -, MOC-31+ Additional HCC markers: GPC3, CD10 Additional MA and CC markers: CK7/CK20, TTF-1 (lung, thyroid), CDX2 (colon, small intestina, ampulla Vater), PSA (prostate), ER, PgR (breast, endometrium) Not useful markers: CK19, AE1/AE3, CAM5.2
Renal cell carcinoma (RCC)	HepPar1, pCEA, RCC Ag, PAX-2	HCC: HepPar 1+, PAX-2 -, RCC Ag- RCC: HepPar 1-, PAX-2 +, RCC Ag+ Additional RCC marker: vimentin Additional HCC markers: GPC3, pCEA Not useful marker: CD10
Neuroendocrine carcinoma (NE)	HepPar1, pCEA,MOC-31, Synaptophysin (Syn), Chromogranin (CG)	HCC: HepPar1+, pCEA+, Syn-, CG-,MOC-31- NE: HepPar1-, pCEA-, Syn+, CG+,MOC-31+ CDX2 and TTF-1 can be useful to identify primary site of NE
Adrenocortical carcinoma (ACC)	HepPar1, pCEA, Inhibin, Melan-A	HCC: HepPar1+, pCEA+,Inhibin-, Melan-A- ACC: HepPar1-, pCEA-,Inhibin+, Melan-A+
Melanoma	HepPar1, pCEA, HMB-45, Melan-A, S100	HCC: HepPar1+, pCEA+, Melan-A-, HMB-45-, S100- Melanoma: HepPar1-, pCEA-, Melan-A+, HMB-45+, S100+ Not useful marker: GPC3

Overview of Current HCC Staging Systems

The goal of a tumor staging system is to estimate a patient's prognosis, which allows for appropriate therapy to be selected. In HCC the importance to measure the contribution of both the cancer and the impaired liver function – due to metabolic and/or viral conditions at the roots of cancer itself- was early recognized. To be effective and widely used, a staging system has to be reliable, reproducible and simple, using data elements that can be obtained as part of standard clinical practice across a wide range of treatment sites. Most HCC staging systems have identified prognostic factors through multivariate analyses of large cohorts of patients to weight the different variables according to prognostic impact. Once proposed, a classification system must be validated across the spectrum of HCC cohorts.

TNM

The TNM system assesses primary tumor features (T), the presence or absence of nodal involvement (N) and distant metastasis (M). The criteria are developed jointly by the American Joint Committee on Cancer (AJCC) and the International Union for Cancer Control (UICC) and have been lastly updated in 2010, when the Seventh Edition took effect [19]. Recent versions of the TNM staging have been influenced largely by data from patients who underwent curative resections.

Different authors proposed that the T-component focused on vascular invasion, tumor number/s and tumor size [20] and found that the key prognostic factors for 5-year survival were major vascular invasion, microvascular invasion and involvement of surrounding tissues [21]. The TNM system is based on histopathology and is applicable in prognosticating survival for the distinct minority of patients who have undergone curative surgery. By itself, the TNM T-stage does not offer guidance on resectability and therefore adds very little discriminatory value to patients' assessment. It has little relevance to patients presenting with advanced disease because of the model's inability to reflect the prognosis of underlying liver disease.

Okuda Score

The Okuda system is a prognostic score introduced in 1985 [22] and incorporates both tumor features as well as the degree of underlying cirrhosis. Okuda and colleagues devised a staging system based on four factors representing advanced disease: tumor occupying greater or less than 50% of the liver, the presence or absence of ascites, and serum albumin and bilirubin levels. Despite the absence of a prospective validation and its crude classification of early stage patients, the Okuda system is still in use. The evolution of imaging and surveillance make it extraordinary nowadays to discover a tumor when it occupies more than half the liver.

BCLC Staging Classification

Derived from a single institution experience, the BCLC classification was first published in 1999 [23] and is considered the standard HCC system by the American Association of for the Study of Liver Disease (AASLD) and European Association for the Study of the Liver. BCLC considered parameters are: size and extent of the primary tumor, liver function and physiological factors and incorporates the Okuda stage and Child-Pugh score. Each stage has a corresponding treatment schedule, ranging from curative therapies such as resection or transplant for early stage patients to best supportive care for end-stage patients.

CLIP Score

Cancer of the Liver Italian Program (CLIP) is a simple scoring system designed by an Italian group with the aim of overcoming the main limitations of the TNM and Okuda. It has been derived from a retrospective cohort study of 435 patients [24] and then externally validated by a randomized trial that prospectively enrolled patients with cirrhosis and HCC. The CLIP includes the liver function according to Child-Pugh score, the morphology of the tumor (uninodular, multinodular, massive), its extension in the liver, the levels of Alpha-fetoprotein and the eventual presence of PVT. This score presents some limits, including the absence of general well-being assessment of the patient, and the inability to identify the early stages, which may benefit from percutaneous or surgical therapies.

Japan Integrated Staging (JIS)

In 2003, the Liver Cancer Study Group of Japan (LCSGJ) proposed the JIS score, which incorporates the LCSGJ's modification of the TNM system and the Child-Pugh score [25]. Arguing that the CLIP score did not provide sufficiently accurate prognostication for the early stage patients commonly diagnosed in Japanese centers due to screening programs and increased awareness of HCC, these investigators emphasized this very favorable group from other early-stage patients. Patients with a JIS score of 0 had a 10-year survival rate of 65% while patients with a CLIP score of 0 had 10-year survival rates of only 23%. It is widely used in Japan but it lacks external validation in Western countries.

Chinese University Prognostic Index (CUPI)

The CUPI [26] was designed in 2002 by the analysis of a cohort of 926 Chinese patients with HCC, adding five prognostic factors (total bilirubin, presence of ascites, alkaline phosphatase, alpha fetoprotein, and asymptomatic disease on presentation) to the TNM, in order to set up 3 classes of risk with highly significant differences in survival. This score was obtained from a monocentric and mono-ethnic cohort of patients, it was not validated in studies involving Western populations and most of the patients had a liver disease secondary to HBV infection. Therefore, the transportability of data of this score could be limited to this specific subset of patients.

Groupe d'Etude et de Traitement du Carcinome Hépatocellulaire (GRETCH)

The French scoring system, proposed by GRETCH in 1999 [27], uses objective measures and an estimate of performance status to predict survival. A cohort of 761consecutive patients across 24 institutions in Europe and Canada were randomly assigned to a training or a validation sample. Five predictors able to affect 1-year survival were identified using univariate analysis with Kaplan-Meier estimates and then included in a Cox proportional hazards model: performance status by Karnofsky score, serum bilirubin, serum alkaline phosphatase, AFP, and presence or absence of portal obstruction by ultrasonography. An advantage of the French classification is that its variables are generally available at the time of initial diagnosis and do not require invasive procedures or sophisticated imaging. The increasing use of cross-sectional imaging as a diagnostic modality could impact the prognostic value of this scoring system by modifying the sensitivity for diagnosis of portal obstruction.

Clinical Staging Comments

Several studies comparing the predictive power of different models have shown conflicting results, both in the general population and in specific subsets of patients receiving different class of treatments [28]. Currently, there is not an ideal staging and prognostic system for HCC. The BCLC seems to be the most comprehensive, since it integrates information about tumor extension, liver function and the presence of constitutional symptoms. It also provides prognostic information and guidance to the therapeutic choices, and it has been endorsed by EASL and AASLD as standard for patients with HCC. Anyway, it does not represent a perfect model and still it has several unmet points. First, unlike CLIP, GRETCH and CUPI, the BCLC was not derived from a cohort of HCC patients by a multivariate analysis, and therefore it is not a prognostic model able to predict the mortality of HCC patients, being internally and externally validated just as a staging system. Second, as a classification model, it presents itself some inherent drawbacks. BCLC stage B encompasses a great variety of clinical situations, from four small tumors to near complete replacement of the liver by tumor, provided liver function is preserved and there is no vascular invasion, extrahepatic spread, or compromised performance status, which would upstage to BCLC stage C or D. Consequently, some BCLB-B patients may no longer be eligible for liver directed therapies, and are in practice treated following BCLC-C algorithms. The different conditions included in the BCLC-B stage also introduce the potential for prognostic heterogeneity within clinical research protocols employing BCLC stage for eligibility or stratification.

Third, as a treatment algorithm, the main limitations of the BCLC is represented by its rigidity: some prognostic factors are outlined as contraindications that preclude a therapy, whereas evidence suggests the contrary. Moreover, BCLC algorithm does not provide indications concerning second-line therapies, retreatment choices or combined treatments.

THERAPEUTIC MARKERS FOR HCC

AKT and Wnt/Β-Catenin Pathways

HCC develops in a liver suffering from a chronic disease with addition of multifactorial processes characterized by the accumulation of genetic alterations and progressive chromosomal instability, caused at least in part from chronic inflammatory processes associated to pre-neoplastic stages of the disease. To date, it is not yet possible to identify a unique panel of molecular markers to detect in a uniform and satisfactory way the HCC disease. By analyzing the multitude of genetic profiles originating from HCC of different etiology reported in the literature in the last years, the most important emerging element is the common over-expression and/or genetic alteration of genes involved in cell proliferation and in mitosis. The HCC identified with such "highly proliferative" profiles are characterized by a poorer prognosis with a decreased patient survival and regardless of cancer etiology.

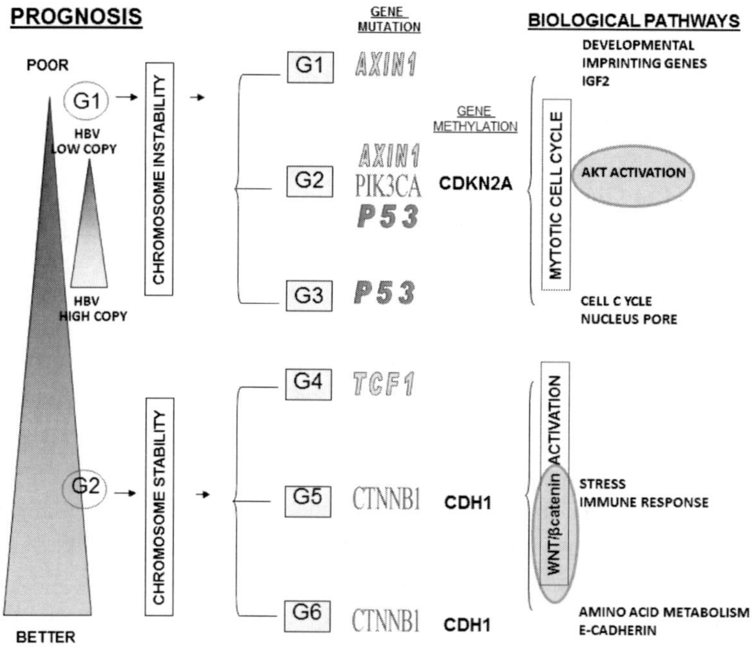

Figure 4. Principal genetic and transcriptomic characteristics of the different G1 to G6 HCC subgroups taken from published data [31]. G1 tumors were associated with low copy number of HBV and overexpression of genes expressed in fetal liver and controlled by parental imprinting. G2 included HCCs infected with a high copy number of HBV and mutations in PIK3CA and TP53. Both G1 and G2 correlated with an activation of the AKT pathway. G3 showed mutation of TP53 and overexpression of genes controlling the cell cycle. G4 showed TCF1-mutated HCC. G5 and G6 were strongly related to β-catenin mutations that lead to Wnt pathway activation; and in particular associated in G6 to E-cadherin expression.

The more indicative genetic alterations include mutation acquisition or chromosome loss (LOH) leading to an inactivation of p53 and activation of the Wnt / β-catenin pathways mainly through Axin1 or CTNNB1gene alterations, activation of RB1, p16 or IGF2 genes or inactivation of IGFR2 receptor by mutation and methylation of the promoter region of the CDKN2A gene.

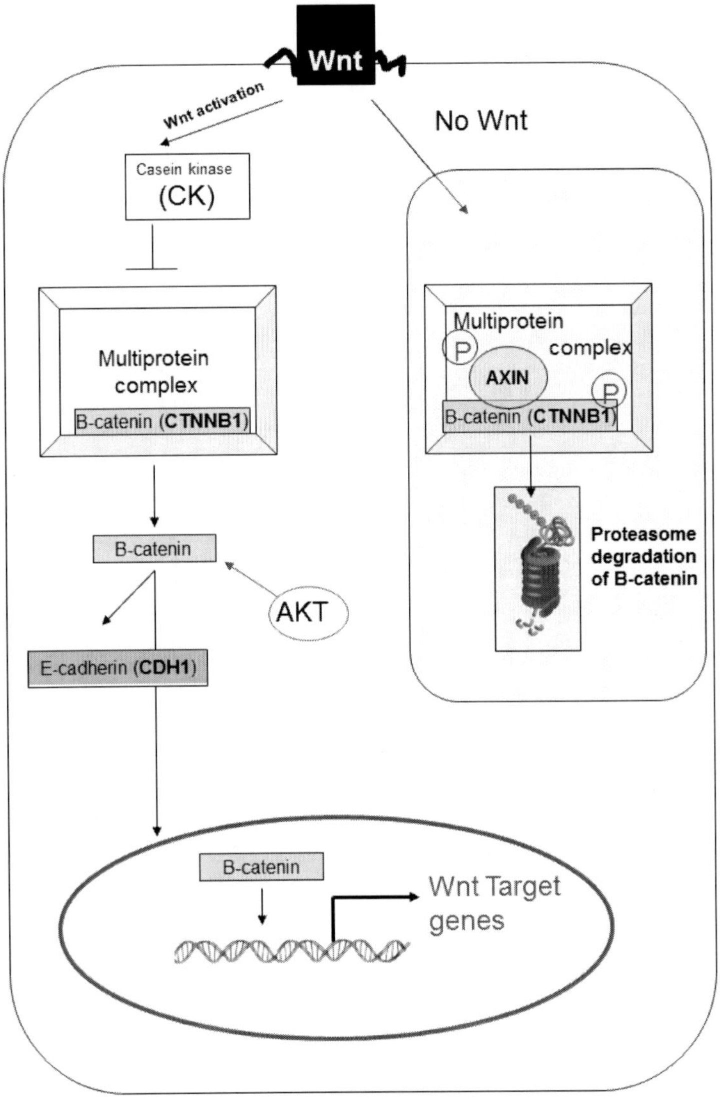

Figure 5. Wnt/β-catenin pathway. A) In the presence of a Wnt ligand, Wnt through casein kinase (CK) activity, inhibits the activity of the multiprotein complex (β-catenin-Axin-adenomatous polyposis coli (APC)-glycogen synthase kinase (GSK)-3b), which targets β-catenin by phosphorilation, and thereby indirectly inhibit β-catenin phosphorilation. The overall results culminate an accumulation of β-catenin that in part links to the E-cadherin and in part translocates into the nucleus where it leads to transcription of Wnt target genes. B) Without activation of Wnt the multiprotein complex phosphorilates β-catenin, and this can be now degradated by the proteasome complex.

Based on the chromosome instability Laurent-Puig and Zucman-Rossi indicated 2 different HCC classes occurring from a different pathogenetic way [29, 30]: a pathogenetic way that lead to poorly differentiated and HBV positive tumors with a high chromosomal instability, mutations of p53 and Axin1 genes; and a second way that leads to well-differentiated tumors, negative for HBV infection and chromosomal instability and with an altered activation of the WNT/β-catenin pathway through CTNNB1 gene alteration (Figure 4). A subsequent study [31] not only confirmed this distinction but further subdivided these 2 groups into 6 groups basing on their transcriptomic profile. Groups 1-3 and groups 4-6, for chromosomal instability and stability, respectively (Figure 4).

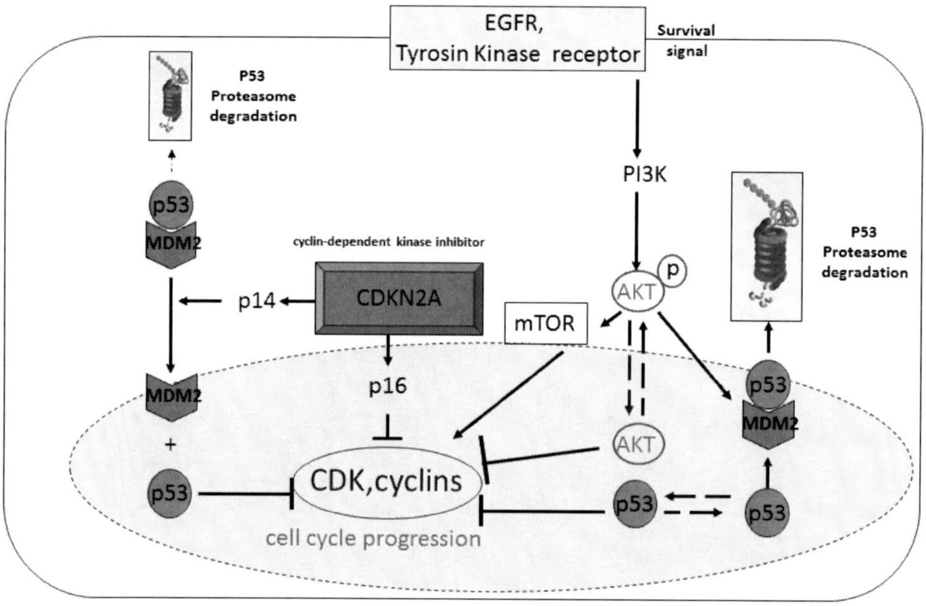

Figure 6. AKT pathway regulates cell cycle proliferation. Binding to tyrosin kinase receptor activates PI3K and then Akt. Activated Akt translocates to the nucleus and shuttles back to the cytoplasm. The transient nuclear Akt phosphorylates cyclin-dependent kinase (CDK) in the nucleus and leads to the temporary CDK relocation to the cytoplasm. When Akt is shuttled back to the cytoplasm, CDK rapidly translocates to the nucleus and helps in the cell cycle progression. AKT phosphorilates MDM2, this results in MDM2 translocation into the nucleus where it binds to P53, and targets it for degradation by the proteasome. Cyclin-dependent kinase inhibitor (CDKN2A) had a role in the cell cycle regulation directly by the tradition of p16 that inhibits cyclin-dependent kinase, and indirectly by producing p16 protein that blocks MDM2 and the consequent degradation of p53.

A summary of the main pathways, AKT and Wnt/B catenin, involved in HCC are reported in Figure 5 and Figure 6. According with this model it appeared that the “high proliferation index” showed in HCC with a worse prognosis was associated with an increased activity of genes involved in the AKT pathway and suggested that the activation of molecules with tyrosine kinase activity could be a trigger to counteract the high proliferation of tumor cells observed in HCC. Nowadays for advanced-stage HCC the only systemic treatment available is based on the inhibition of multichinase inhibitors, the sorafenib. The prolongation in survival of patients have encouraged to persist the studies in this direction with the development of other drugs targeted to protein kinases and confirmed the predictive value of the molecular signals identified.

p-RPS6 Protein and mTOR Pathway

However, sorafenib treatment had demonstrated limited benefit and moreover not all patients are responsive.

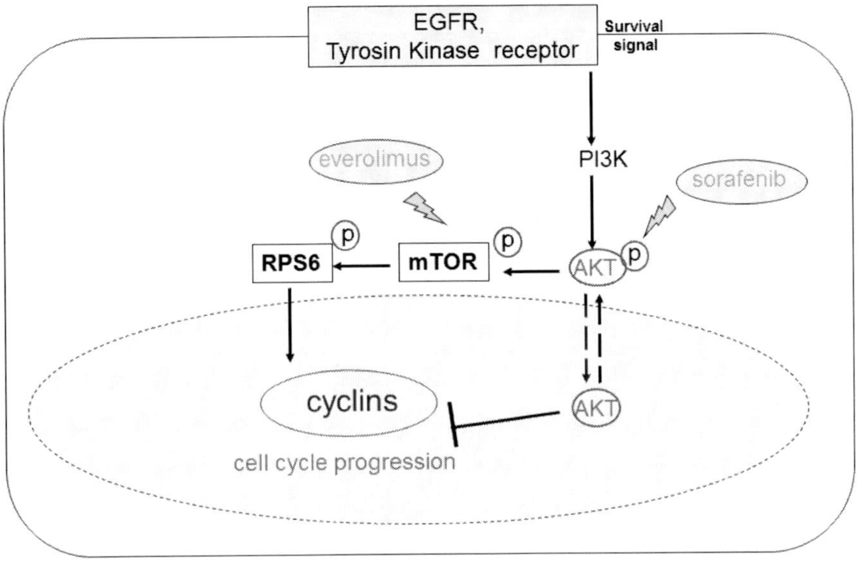

Figure 7. RPS6 is considered a molecular marker for the activation of mTOR signaling pathway and a marker for everolimus treatment. HCC who did not respond to sorafenib showed a significant correlation between the phosphorilated form of the RPS6 protein, a component of the 40S ribosomal subunit regulating the protein synthesis, and the resistance to treatment. AKT and mTOR pathways were both involved on cell cycle progression deregulated in HCC, thus sorafenib and everolimus have being proposed in advanced HCC treatment.

Subsequent studies by using array-based pathway profiling has identified a significant correlation between the phosphorilated form of the RPS6 (p-RPS6) protein, a component of the 40S ribosomal subunit regulating the protein synthesis, and the resistance to sorafenib treatment [32]. Since, p-RPS6 is considered a molecular marker for the activation of mTOR signaling pathway (Figure 7) [33]. These experimental data have led to the use of mTOR inhibitors, such as everolimus, in patients with HCC resistant or not responsive to sorafenib. Partial success of sorafenib and everolimus in clinical phase I and II supports the pivotal role of mTOR signaling in HCC and highlights the importance of reliable biomarkers discovery to set best therapeutic options [34]. Identification of p-RSP6 like a predictive marker for response to sorafenib treatment is particularly important since at today several prognostic markers, like Ang2, VEGF, HGF, and IGF-2, were proved unable to predict a response to sorafenib [35].

Expression Profiling

Molecular expression profiling has also demonstrated a utility for prognostication of patients with HCC. To this an HCC five-gene score (HN1, RAN, RAMP3, KRT19 and

TAF9) rigorously validated has been strongly proposed as prognostic markers for survival of patients after liver resection [36]. These genes are not functionally related, but for the first time, they represent a useful tool to stratify patients for various therapeutic decisions. In particular HCC with KRT19 expression could be used to identify a subtype of HCC originated from a common progenitor between hepatocytes and cholangiocytes and thus perhaps to be managed differently [13].

Epigenetics

With the advent of new techniques like the genome-sequencing, epigenetics and proteomics analyses, new perspectives regarding prognostic markers are now appearing. Genome-sequencing had highlighted that about 5% of all HCC had not mutation in any protein kinase genes, thus suggesting that any kinase inhibitors, as sorafenib, would be effective in these cases. In the remaining 95% of cases mutations of CTNNB1 (11–32%) and AXIN1 (15%), and alteration of genes involved in cell cycle regulation such as p53 (18-35%) and CDKN2A (7-10%) were confirmed as previously found [37-40]. In addition, by studying noncoding RNA, new insights in HCC tumorigenesis has been found. According to their size, non coding RNAs are divided into two groups: small (<200 nucleotides, miRNA) and long (>200 nucleotides, LncRNA). On the basis of overall miRNA profiles and integrating them with gene expression analysis and assessment of cellular pathway activation previously reported, a classification of HCC based on miRNA profiles has been proposed [36]. Moreover, it was found that lncRNA-UFC1 by interacting with b-catenin promotes the tumor progression when overexpressed [41]. Thus, lncRNA-UFC1 has been identified as both a prognostic marker and a potential new therapeutic target associated with the WNT/β-catenin pathway in HCC.

Epigenetic studies in HCC emphaticizes an important role of chromatin remodelling proteins in hepatocarcinogenesis. These studies are interesting because they shifted HCC therapeutic targets from coding tumor sequences of AKT and WNT/β-catenin pathways towards the area of chromatin-regulatory enzymes [42-49]. Telomerase (TERT) is a RNA polymerase that added telomere repeat sequences at the end of chromosomes and it is normally repressed in postnatal somatic cells. Telomeres shorten progressively with each round of cell division up to the death of the cell. A worst prognostic factor and aggressive behavior of HCC had been associated with long telomeres and increased telomerase activity [42]. Moreover, HBV genome integration was recurrently found into the promoter region of the TERT gene, and this correlated with the increased TERT activity [43]. Genes involved in chromatin remodeling are the histone methyltransferase (MLL), human AT-rich interaction domain (ARID) family of genes, SWI/SNF complex [39, 40, 48, 49]. Key proteins that mediate epigenetic signalling through the acetylation and methylation of histones and through chromatin remodelling represent a new frontier for the development of future therapeutics [46, 47]. The clinical characteristics of tumors harboring these types of gene mutation suggest that their inactivation may be associated with an aggressive tumor phenotype and reinforce the link between cancer genome defects and epigenetic alterations in liver tumorigenesis.

Metabolomics

HCC metabolite profiling (metabolomics), the global view of aminoacids end products of cellular processes, is another promising new approach to underlying patients classification by using a rapid sensitive measure of cellular phenotype. Integration of both proteomics and genomics data will lead to a more accurate and precise known of cellular processes, which will move to the identification of key biomarkers for a personalized prognostic classification of HCC. A preliminary study of Budhu and col. by using a complex integrated metabolic and transcriptome analyses highlighted metabolites coding some enzymes that catalyzed the biosynthesis of monounsaturated fatty acid with the HCC proliferation [50]. They hypothesed that a reduction in lipid bioavailibility, which affect the liver microenvironment may promote the HCC aggressiveness, since expression of these metabolites were significantly and independently associated with survival times and HCC recurrence. This study is interesting because it shifts the focus from tumor cells to the microenvironment. Accordantly, an analog study by combining HCC pathway classification with metabolomic results showed that HCC tumor with a good prognosis harbored a diminished concentration of certain statured lipids, consistent with an up-regulation of lipid catabolism in HCC [51].

Table 3. Contribution to the definition of some among the key markers for HCC

Type of analysis	Main Results	Comments
Genomics studies	AKT and Wnt/B-catenin pathways	The main pathways involved in HCC
Molecular expression profiling	five- gene score	Expression of unrelated genes associated with the prognosis
Epigenetics studies	TERT and chromatin remodeling	A new therapeutic target based on epigenetic factors
	lncRNA-UFC1 related to Wnt/B-catenin pathways	An epigenetic factor associated to the Wnt/B-catenin pathway
	miRNA for HCC classification	A classification of HCC based on miRNA
Proteomics studies	up-regulation of lipid catabolism	Markers associated with the tumor microenvironment

Altogether, these data (Table 3) appear to be promising, but it must be remembered that genome-sequencing and genomic expression require further investigation to establish the real clinical utility of these assays. Moreover, further studies are needed to elaborate how disrupted histone and chromatin regulators cooperate with alterations in known signaling pathways, such as AKT, Wnt/b-catenin, and gene expression alteration in HCC progression.

CONCLUSION

There is increasing need for reliable pathological classifications of HCC based on morphological and immunophenotypic grounds. New pathological entities are constantly recognized and defined by using multiparametric characterization. Data generated by massive genome sequencing offers new possibilities for better taxonomy and advanced therapeutic approaches. Results could be integrated with transcriptomic, methylome analysis, proteomic, and metabolomic in order to capture the full complexity of liver cancer and heterogeneous patient's response. Over the past years, several therapeutic trials of newer tirosin kinase targeting pathways have been developed, but, in this category of systemic drug, sorafenib remains the only drug currently approved to treat advanced HCC. Genetic studies of tumor samples and the use of newer molecular approaches such as non coding RNA and genome-wide association studies, according to immunohistochemistry, proteomics and clinical criteria are highlighting the variability that exists among diverse HCC. Identification of new target pathways for the treatment of HCC by more personalized and targeted regimens are the main goals of the current translational medical research.

REFERENCES

[1] Bruix J, Sherman M, Llovet JM, Beaugrand M, Lencioni R, Burroughs AK, Christensen E, Pagliaro L, Colombo M, Rodés J; EASL Panel of Experts on HCC. Clinical management of hepatocellular carcinoma. Conclusions of the Barcelona-2000 EASL conference. European Association for the Study of the Liver. *J. Hepatol.* 2001; 35: 421-430.

[2] Sherman M. Modern approach to hepatocellular carcinoma. *Curr. Gastroenterol. Rep.* 2011; 13: 49-55.

[3] Borzio M, Fargion S, Borzio F, Fracanzani AL, Croce AM, Stroffolini T, Oldani S, Cotichini R, Roncalli M. Impact of large regenerative, low grade and high grade dysplastic nodules in hepatocellular carcinoma development. *J. Hepatol.* 2003; 39: 208–214.

[4] Kobayashi M, Ikeda K, Hosaka T, Sezaki H, Someya T, Akuta N, Suzuki F, Suzuki Y, Saitoh S, Arase Y, Kumada H. Dysplastic nodules frequently develop into hepatocellular carcinoma in patients with chronic viral hepatitis and cirrhosis. *Cancer* 2006; 106: 636–647.

[5] Forner A, Vilana R, Ayuso C, Bianchi L, Solé M, Ayuso JR, Boix L, Sala M, Varela M, Llovet JM, Brú C, Bruix J. Diagnosis of hepatic nodules 20 mm or smaller in cirrhosis: prospective validation of the noninvasive diagnostic criteria for hepatocellular carcinoma. *Hepatology* 2008; 47: 97–104.

[6] International Consensus Group for Hepatocellular Neoplasia. Pathologic diagnosis of early hepatocellular carcinoma: A Report of the International Consensus Group for Hepatocellular Neoplasia. *Hepatology* 2009; 49: 658–664.

[7] Di Tommaso L, Franchi G, Park YN, Fiamengo B, Destro A, Morenghi E, Montorsi M, Torzilli G, Tommasini M, Terracciano L, Tornillo L, Vecchione R, Roncalli M. Diagnostic value of HSP70, glypican 3 and glutamine synthetase in hepatocellular nodules in cirrhosis. *Hepatology* 2007; 45: 725-734.

[8] Eggel H. Ueber das primare Carcinom der Leber (in German). *Beitz Pathol. Anat.* 1901; 30: 506-604.

[9] Hui AM, Takayama T, Sano K, Kubota K, Akahane M, Ohtomo K, Makuuchi M. Predictive value of gross classification of hepatocellular carcinoma on recurrence and survival after hepatectomy. *J. Hepatol.* 2000; 33: 975-979.

[10] Roayaie S, Blume IN, Thung SN, Guido M, Fiel MI, Hiotis S, Labow DM, Llovet JM, Schwartz ME. A system of classifying microvascular invasion to predict outcome after resection in patients with hepatocellular carcinoma. *Gastroenterology* 2009; 137: 850–855.

[11] Krings G, Ramachandran R, Jain D, Wu TT, Yeh MM, Torbenson M, Kakar S. Immunohistochemical pitfalls and the importance of glypican 3 and arginase inthe diagnosis of scirrhous hepatocellular carcinoma. *Modern Pathology* 2013; 26: 782–791.

[12] Durnez A, Verslype C, Nevens F, Fevery J, Aerts R, Pirenne J, Lesaffre E, Libbrecht L, Desmet V, Roskams T. The clinicopathological and prognostic relevance of cytokeratin 7 and 19 expression in hepatocellular carcinoma. A possible progenitor cell origin. *Histopathology* 2006; 49: 138–151.

[13] Lee JS, Heo J, Libbrecht L, Chu IS, Kaposi-Novak P, Calvisi DF, Mikaelyan A, Roberts LR, Demetris AJ, Sun Z, Nevens F, Roskams T, Thorgeirsson SS. A novel prognostic subtype of human hepatocellular carcinoma derived from hepatic progenitor cells. *Nat. Med.* 2006; 12: 410–416.

[14] Roncalli M, Park YN, Di Tommaso. Histopathological classification of hepatocellular carcinoma. *Dig & Liver Disease* 2010; 42S: S228-S234.

[15] Komuta M, Spee B, Vander Borght S, De Vos R, Verslype C, Aerts R, Yano H, Suzuki T, Matsuda M, Fujii H, Desmet VJ, Kojiro M, Roskams T. Clinicopathological study on cholangiolocellular carcinoma suggesting hepatic progenitor cell origin. *Hepatology* 2008;47: 1544–1556.

[16] Fujii T, Zen Y, Harada K, Niwa H, Masuda S, Kaizaki Y, Watanabe K, Kawashima A, Nakanuma Y. Participation of liver cancer stem/progenitor cells in tumorigenesis of scirrhous hepatocellular carcinoma-human and cell culture study. *Hum. Pathol.* 2008; 39: 1185–1196.

[17] Edmondson HA, Steiner PE. Primary carcinoma of the liver: a study of 100 cases among 48,900 necropsies. *Cancer* 1954; 7: 462–503.

[18] Kakar S, Gown AM, Goodman ZD, Ferrell LD. Best practices in diagnostic immunohistochemistry: hepatocellular carcinoma versus metastatic neoplasms. *Arch. Pathol. Lab. Med.* 2007; 131: 1648–1654.

[19] Sobin LH, Gospodariwicz M, Wittekind C, eds. TNM classification of malignant tumors. ed.7th. Hoboken, NJ: Wiley-Blackwell, 2009.

[20] Vauthey JN, Lauwers GY, Esnaola NF, Do KA, Belghiti J, Mirza N, Curley SA, Ellis LM, Regimbeau JM, Rashid A, Cleary KR, Nagorney DM. Simplified staging for hepatocellular carcinoma. *J. Clin. Oncol.* 2002; 20: 1527-1536.

[21] Poon RT, Fan ST. Evaluation of the new AJCC/UICC staging system for hepatocellular carcinoma after hepatic resection in Chinese patients. *Surg. Oncol. Clin. N. Am.* 2003; 12: 35-50.

[22] Okuda K, Ohtsuki T, Obata H, Tomimatsu M, Okazaki N, Hasegawa H, Nakajima Y, Ohnishi K. Natural history of hepatocellular carcinoma and prognosis in relation to treatment. Study of 850 patients. *Cancer* 1985; 56: 918-928.

[23] Llovet JM, Brú C, Bruix J. Prognosis of hepatocellular carcinoma:the BCLC staging classification. *Semin Liver Dis.* 1999; 19: 329-338.

[24] The Cancer of the Liver Italian Program (CLIP) investigators. A new prognostic system for hepatocellular carcinoma: a retrospective study of 435 patients. *Hepatology* 1998; 28: 751-755.

[25] Kudo M, Chung H, Osaki Y. Prognostic staging system for hepatocellular carcinoma (CLIP score): its value and limitations, and a proposal for a new staging system, the Japan Integrated Staging Score (JIS score). *J. Gastroenterol.* 2003; 38: 207-215.

[26] Leung TW, Tang AM, Zee B, Lau WY, Lai PB, Leung KL, Lau JT, Yu SC, Johnson PJ. Construction of the Chinese University Prognostic Index for hepatocellular carcinoma and comparison with the TNM staging system, the Okuda staging system, and the Cancer of the Liver Italian Program staging system: a study based on 926 patients. *Cancer* 2002; 94: 1760-1769.

[27] Chevret S, Trinchet JC, Mathieu D, Rached AA, Beaugrand M, Chastang C. A new prognostic classification for predicting survival in patients with hepatocellular carcinoma. Groupe d'Etude et de Traitement du Carcinome Hépatocellulaire. *J. Hepatol.* 1999; 31: 133-141.

[28] Maida M, Orlando E, Cammà C, Cabibbo G. Staging systems of hepatocellular carcinoma: A review of literature. *World J. Gastroenterol.* 2014; 20: 4141-4150.

[29] Zucman-Rossi J, Jeannot E, Nhieu JT, Scoazec JY, Guettier C, Rebouissou S, Bacq Y, Leteurtre E, Paradis V, Michalak S, Wendum D, Chiche L, Fabre M, Mellottee L, Laurent C, Partensky C, Castaing D, Zafrani ES, Laurent-Puig P, Balabaud C, Bioulac-Sage P. Genotype-phenotype correlation in hepatocellular adenoma: new classification and relationship with HCC. *Hepatology* 2006; 43: 515-524.

[30] Laurent-Puig P, Legoix P, Bluteau O, Belghiti J, Franco D, Binot F, Monges G, Thomas G, Bioulac-Sage P, Zucman-Rossi J. Genetic alterations associated with hepatocellular carcinomas define distinct pathways of hepatocarcinogenesis. *Gastroenterology* 2001; 120: 1763-1773.

[31] Boyault S, Rickman DS, de Reyniès A, Balabaud C, Rebouissou S, Jeannot E, Hérault A, Saric J, Belghiti J, Franco D, Bioulac-Sage P, Laurent-Puig P, Zucman-Rossi J. Transcriptome classification of HCC is related to gene alterations and to new therapeutic targets. *Hepatology* 2007; 45: 42-52.

[32] Masuda M, Chen WY, Miyanaga A, Nakamura Y, Kawasaki K, Sakuma T, Ono M, Chen CL, Honda K, Yamada T. Alternative mTOR signal activation in sorafenib-resistant hepatocellular carcinoma cells revealed by array-based pathway profiling. *Mol. Cell Proteomics*. 2014; 13: 1429-1438.

[33] Steelman LS, Chappell WH, Abrams SL, Kempf RC, Long J, Laidler P, Mijatovic S, Maksimovic-Ivanic D, Stivala F, Mazzarino MC, Donia M, Fagone P, Malaponte G, Nicoletti F, Libra M, Milella M, Tafuri A, Bonati A, Bäsecke J, Cocco L, Evangelisti C, Martelli AM, Montalto G, Cervello M, McCubrey JA. Roles of the Raf/MEK/ERK and PI3K/PTEN/Akt/mTOR pathways in controlling growth and sensitivity to therapy-implications for cancer and aging. *Aging* (Albany NY) 2011; 3: 192-222.

[34] Bhoori S, Toffanin S, Sposito C, Germini A, Pellegrinelli A, Lampis A, Mazzaferro V. Personalized molecular targeted therapy in advanced, recurrent hepatocellular carcinoma after liver transplantation: a proof of principle. *J. Hepatol.* 2010; 52: 771-775.

[35] Llovet JM, Peña CE, Lathia CD, Shan M, Meinhardt G, Bruix J; SHARP Investigators Study Group. Plasma biomarkers as predictors of outcome in patients with advanced hepatocellular carcinoma. *Clin. Cancer Res.* 2012; 18: 2290-2300.

[36] Nault JC, De Reyniès A, Villanueva A, Calderaro J, Rebouissou S, Couchy G, Decaens T, Franco D, Imbeaud S, Rousseau F, Azoulay D, Saric J, Blanc JF, Balabaud C,

Bioulac-Sage P, Laurent A, Laurent-Puig P, Llovet JM, Zucman-Rossi J. A hepatocellular carcinoma 5-gene score associated with survival of patients after liver resection. *Gastroenterology* 2013; Jul; 145: 176-187.

[37] Guichard C, Amaddeo G, Imbeaud S, Ladeiro Y, Pelletier L, Maad IB, Calderaro J, Bioulac-Sage P, Letexier M, Degos F, Clément B, Balabaud C, Chevet E, Laurent A, Couchy G, Letouzé E, Calvo F, Zucman-Rossi J.Integrated analysis of somatic mutations and focal copy-number changes identifies key genes and pathways in hepatocellular carcinoma. *Nat. Genet.* 2012; 44: 694-698.

[38] Fujimoto A, Totoki Y, Abe T, Boroevich KA, Hosoda F, Nguyen HH, Aoki M, Hosono N, Kubo M, Miya F, Arai Y, Takahashi H, Shirakihara T, Nagasaki M, Shibuya T, Nakano K, Watanabe-Makino K, Tanaka H, Nakamura H, Kusuda J, Ojima H, Shimada K, Okusaka T, Ueno M, Shigekawa Y, Kawakami Y, Arihiro K, Ohdan H, Gotoh K, Ishikawa O, Ariizumi S, Yamamoto M, Yamada T, Chayama K, Kosuge T, Yamaue H, Kamatani N, Miyano S, Nakagama H, Nakamura Y, Tsunoda T, Shibata T, Nakagawa H. Whole-genome sequencing of liver cancers identifies etiological influences on mutation patterns and recurrent mutations in chromatin regulators. *Nat. Genet.* 2012; 44: 760-764.

[39] Huang J, Deng Q, Wang Q, Li KY, Dai JH, Li N, Zhu ZD, Zhou B, Liu XY, Liu RF, Fei QL, Chen H, Cai B, Zhou B, Xiao HS, Qin LX, Han ZG. Exome sequencing of hepatitis B virus-associated hepatocellular carcinoma. *Nat. Genet.* 2012; 44: 1117-1121.

[40] Nault JC, Zucman-Rossi J.Genetics of hepatocellular carcinoma: the next generation. *J. Hepatol.* 2014; 60: 224-226.

[41] Collins JF.Long noncoding RNAs and hepatocellular carcinoma. *Gastroenterology* 2015; 148: 291-294.

[42] Nault JC, Mallet M, Pilati C, Calderaro J, Bioulac-Sage P, Laurent C, Laurent A, Cherqui D, Balabaud C, Zucman-Rossi J. High frequency of telomerase reverse-transcriptase promoter somatic mutations in hepatocellular carcinoma and preneoplastic lesions. *Nat. Commun.* 2013; 4: 2218.

[43] Cleary SP, Jeck WR, Zhao X, Chen K, Selitsky SR, Savich GL, Tan TX, Wu MC, Getz G, Lawrence MS, Parker JS, Li J, Powers S, Kim H, Fischer S, Guindi M, Ghanekar A, Chiang DY. Identification of driver genes in hepatocellular carcinoma by exome sequencing. *Hepatology* 2013; 58: 1693-1702.

[44] Oh BK, Kim H, Park YN, Yoo JE, Choi J, Kim KS, Lee JJ, Park C. High telomerase activity and long telomeres in advanced hepatocellular carcinomas with poor prognosis. *Lab. Invest.* 2008; 88: 144-152.

[45] Kim H, Yoo JE, Cho JY, Oh BK, Yoon YS, Han HS, Lee HS, Jang JJ, Jeong SH, Kim JW, Park YN. Telomere length, TERT and shelterin complex proteins in hepatocellular carcinomas expressing "stemness"-related markers. *J. Hepatol.* 2013; 59: 746-752.

[46] Toh ST, Jin Y, Liu L, Wang J, Babrzadeh F, Gharizadeh B, Ronaghi M, Toh HC, Chow PK, Chung AY, Ooi LL, Lee CG. Deep sequencing of the hepatitis B virus in hepatocellular carcinoma patients reveals enriched integration events, structural alterations and sequence variations. *Carcinogenesis* 2013; 34: 787-798.

[47] Sung WK, Zheng H, Li S, Chen R, Liu X, Li Y, Lee NP, Lee WH, Ariyaratne PN, Tennakoon C, Mulawadi FH, Wong KF, Liu AM, Poon RT, Fan ST, Chan KL, Gong Z, Hu Y, Lin Z, Wang G, Zhang Q, Barber TD, Chou WC, Aggarwal A, Hao K, Zhou W, Zhang C, Hardwick J, Buser C, Xu J, Kan Z, Dai H, Mao M, Reinhard C, Wang J, Luk

JM. Genome-wide survey of recurrent HBV integration in hepatocellular carcinoma. *Nat. Genet.* 2012; 44: 765-769.

[48] Arrowsmith CH, Bountra C, Fish PV, Lee K, Schapira M. Epigenetic protein families: a new frontier for drug discovery. *Nat. Rev. Drug Discov.* 2012; 11: 384-400.

[49] Lin C, Song W, Bi X, Zhao J, Huang Z, Li Z, Zhou J, Cai J, Zhao H. Recent advances in the ARID family: focusing on roles in human cancer. *Onco. Targets Ther.* 2014; 7: 315-324.

[50] Budhu A, Roessler S, Zhao X, Yu Z, Forgues M, Ji J, Karoly E, Qin LX, Ye QH, Jia HL, Fan J, Sun HC, Tang ZY, Wang XW. Integrated metabolite and gene expression profiles identify lipid biomarkers associated with progression of hepatocellular carcinoma and patient outcomes. *Gastroenterology* 2013; 144: 1066-1075.

[51] Beyoglu D, Imbeaud S, Maurhofer O, Bioulac-Sage P, Zucman-Rossi J, Dufour JF, Idle JR. Tissue metabolomics of hepatocellular carcinoma: tumor energy metabolism and the role of transcriptomic classification. *Hepatology* 2013; 58: 229-238.

In: Hepatocellular Carcinoma in the 3rd Millennium
Editors: M. Berretta and B. Cacopardo

ISBN: 978-1-63484-025-5

Chapter 9

TREATMENT APPROACH OF HCC

Andrea Ruzzenente, Alessandro Valdegamberi, Simone Conci and Alfredo Guglielmi*

Department of Surgery,
Division of General and Hepatobiliary Surgery,
Unit of Hepato-Pancreatico-Biliary surgery,
University of Verona Medical School,
Verona, Italy

ABSTRACT

Many options are available for the treatment of hepatocellular carcinoma (HCC). The selection among different treatment options varies in relation to the tumor stage and the degree of hepatic dysfunction. Treatments can be divided into curative treatments (liver transplantation, liver resection, local ablation) and palliative treatments (trans-arterial therapies and systemic chemotherapy). The best results have been reported after surgical resection in patients with single tumors and good liver function (no portal hypertension, normal bilirubin), after liver transplantation in single tumors ≤5 cm or three nodules ≤3 cm, and after ablative treatments for single tumors ≤3 cm in Child-Pugh A patients[1]. In these patients a 5-years survival of 50–70% can be achieved [1].

Among the different treatments allocation algorithms described in literature, the Barcelona Cancer Liver Center (BCLC) is the most widely utilized in the Western Countries. Although this allocation system is criticized for the excessive decisional rigidity it is useful to give a guideline among the different treatments. This system divides HCCs in four different stages: very early stage; early stage, intermediate stage, advance stage and end stage (Figure 1).

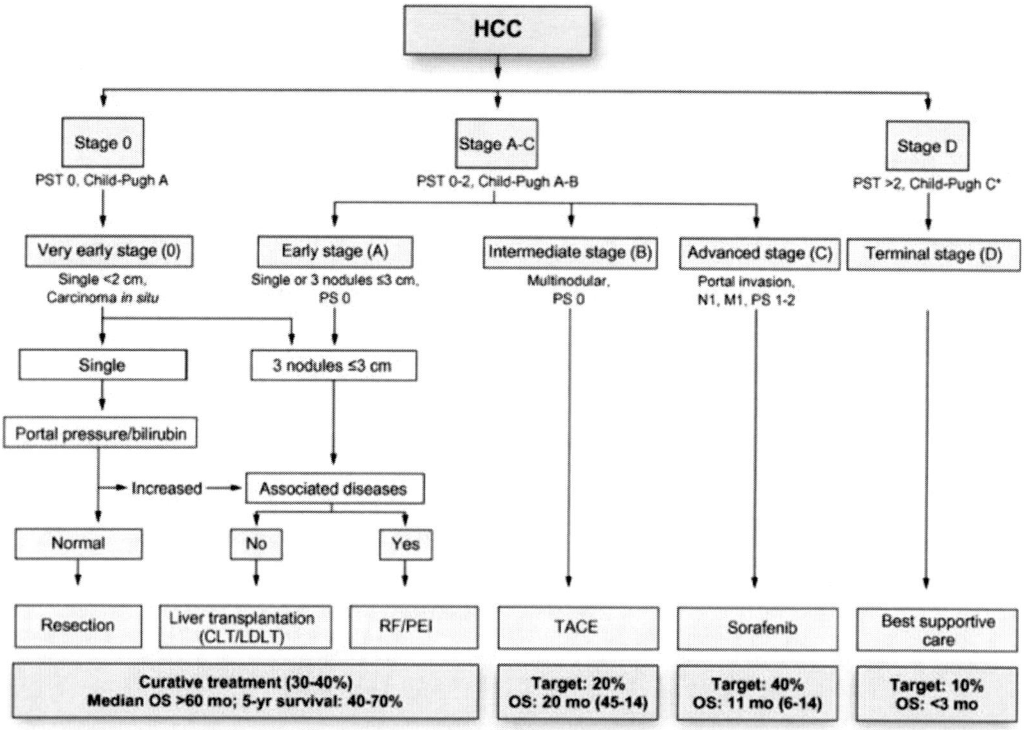

Figure 1. BCLC algorithm for treatment allocation for patients with HCC[2].

Very Early Stage

In the latest revised version of the BCLC system [2], a further classification of early stage HCC was introduced; it is defined "very early" HCC when a Child-Pugh A class patient present a single node HCC, smaller than 2 cm. On the contrary the term "early stage" HCC is referred to a single node of HCC, smaller than 5 cm, or up to 3 nodes <3 cm each, in Child-Pugh A-B class.

In the AASLD guidelines, patients with "very early" HCC are candidates for resection, unless they have portal hypertension and/or increased bilirubin levels, in these cases either liver transplantation or locoregional percutaneous treatments are recommended, depending on associated diseases.

Whether resection or ablation is considered as the first line treatment has been addressed in two randomized studies. In the first study, 140 patients with HCC <3 cm, with Child–Pugh stages A and B were randomized to resection (n = 70) or ablation (n = 70). There was no survival difference with 50–55% survival with both modalities [3]. Another study randomized 160 HCC patients to resection or ablation (n = 80 in each arm) and found similar 3-year survival of 70–80% [4]. In a meta-analysis of fifteen studies, including the abovementioned two randomized studies, comparing resection (n = 1,233) and ablation (n = 1,302), the survival was higher among resected patients. However, the complication rate was about six-fold higher with resection compared to ablation [5]. Similar data were reported in a national survey on more than 54,000 patients with HCC treated in Japan [6]. Based on these data, ablation may be considered as the first-line option for very early HCC with favorable location and adequate distance from major vessels [7, 8].

Early HCC

In the Early stage HCC (single nodule smaller than 5 cm or up to 3 nodules smaller than 3 cm) the three recommended treatment options are: liver transplantation, liver resection and local ablation. When applied in early stages HCC, liver transplantation (LT) allows excellent 5-year survival (70-75%) and is associated with low rates of recurrence (10-15%) [9]. Unfortunately, due to shortage of organs and the strict selection criteria, this resource is limited to a small number of patients. Moreover about 30% of patients with HCC are dropped out during the waiting list period due to tumor progression [10, 11]. A higher probability of dropout from the waiting list is directly related to the number of tumors, alpha-fetoprotein levels, tumor biology and biological or calculated MELDD score, moreover these factors are related to a higher risk of recurrence of HCC after LT [12]. Hence, a balanced approach is needed to optimize the use of livers for transplanting HCC patients aiming at maintaining post-transplant survival as well as optimizing the chance of receiving a transplant. In this regard, the concept of dropout equivalent MELD (deMELD) points has been introduced taking into consideration the risk of dropout from the waiting list based on MELD score and other HCC characteristics. For example, two patients with similar MELD scores may be given different exception points based on their dropout risk from the waiting list after considering factors such as the number of tumors, maximum tumor size, age of the patient, etiology of the liver disease and aFP levels. To avoid the delisting from the transplant list, it is recommended that patients with HCC should be transplanted within 6 months of listing [8].

The excellent results yielded by the adoption of Milan Criteria led many Transplant Centers to suggest new strategies to expand the criteria to allow more patients to receive LT. In 2001, a research group from the University of California San Francisco reported a 5-year survival of over 70% by expanding the tumor criteria (1 lesion <6.5 cm or up to 3 lesions <4.5 cm) [13]. This good outcome was confirmed in a more recent comparative series [14] and led to new studies exploring the opportunity of down staging the tumor to bring it back within Milan or UCSF criteria. The down staging treatments, resection and loco regional therapies, have the advantages of expansion of the potential number of candidates for transplantation and the reduction of dropout risk in the waiting list. Among the various retrospective data, only two prospective studies reported comparable survival after LT in patients initially out of Milan criteria compared with patients meeting the Milan criteria at diagnosis [15, 16]. The down staging procedures in these studies included trans-arterial chemo-embolization (TACE) or radiofrequency ablation (RFA) and, to proceed to LT, a total necrosis of the treated lesions had to be diagnosed at the pre-LT imaging. After an imaging evaluation of an effective down staging, a 3-months period before placing the patient in the waiting list was scheduled to exclude the more aggressive tumors with higher risk of recurrence after LT.

The good results of down staging led to a recent consensus conference about LT for HCC to recommend this procedure before LT, although more prospective studies are needed to strengthen these evidences [17]. Similarly, the bridging procedures have been recommended for patients with tumors >2 cm who are likely to wait more than 6 months for transplantation [17]. There are still no recommendations about the preferred bridging treatment [18], although a combination of the different loco regional therapies seems to reduce the progression rate of the tumor and increase the overall survival [19].

Recently, a retrospective multicenter study was performed to evaluate the survival after LT for HCC beyond the Milan criteria; if the rule of "up to seven" was fulfilled (the score was calculated as the sum of the size of the largest tumor and the number of tumors), the 5-year survival could reach 70%. The Metro ticket calculator was then created as a statistical tool that could predict the 5-year survival of any given patient on the basis of morphological and pathologic characteristics: total size of the nodules, size of the largest nodule and presence or absence of vascular invasion (if available) [20]. Although the prediction of survival has recently become more accurate and precise, an agreement among centers has not yet been reached as to which survival rate is considered acceptable in balancing the highest chances of cure with actual organ availability [21].

The other curative treatment option for early HCC is surgical resection that is applicable to approximately 20-30% of patients. Surgical resection is safe and is associated with low rates of mortality (0-3%) and morbidity (25-30%). (Figure 2) In patients with moderate liver impairment, resection requires a careful preoperative assessment of liver function along with tests of biochemical and dynamic parameters, such as the indocyanine green retention test [22]. Surgical resection with radical intent enables good long-term survival: 40-50% at 5 years [23]. In HCCs smaller than 3 cm, the 5-year survival exceeds 60%, with a 10-year survival of 20% [24]. Until few years ago, the presence of portal hypertension was considered an absolute contraindication to surgical resection. However, recent data show that in patients with moderate portal hypertension who were classified as Child-Pugh class A, a limited (up to two segments) liver resection can be performed with results that are comparable to those of patients without portal hypertension [23]. Also the major vascular invasion is an important prognostic factor after resection. Indeed, it is reported that the presence of portal vein tumor thrombus in a patient with hepatocellular carcinoma is one of the most significant factors for a poor prognosis. In patients with portal vein tumor thrombus (PVTT), the median survival was reported to be 2.7 months, whereas survival in those without PVTT was 24.4 months [25]. Other important prognostic factors are the liver function, the pTNM stage, the tumor size, the number of tumor, the degree of cirrhosis and the pathological features of tumor [26-28].

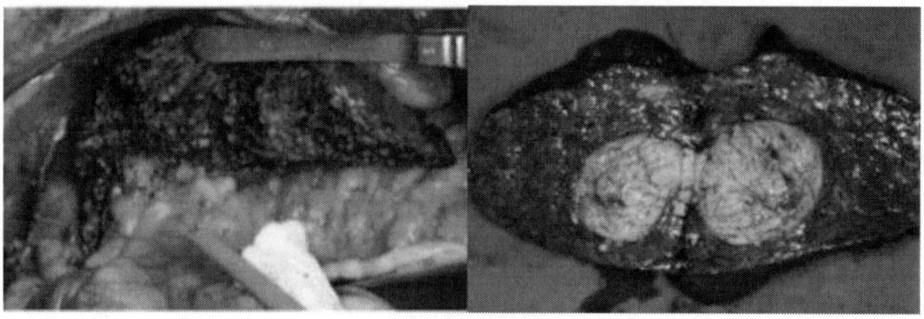

Figure 2. Intraoperative image and surgical specimen of right hepatectomy for 5 cm HCC in a patient with HBV related cirrhosis.

Recurrence of HCC is the major drawback of potentially curative treatments. Even after curative resection, recurrence is very frequent and occurs in approximately 70-100% of cases within 5 years of treatment [29]. Recurrence can be due to the presence of intrahepatic metastases or to neocarcinogenesis in the remnant liver. In the literature, many prognostic factors related to recurrence have been identified, and among these, the most important are the size, the absence of a pseudo capsule, the presence of satellite nodules, vascular invasion, tumor grading and the serum levels of alpha-fetoprotein [30]. The activity of the underlying liver disease, the type of viral infection and the degree of fibrosis are related to the development of recurrence secondary to neocarcinogenesis [31]. New molecular markers that are related to early recurrence have recently been proposed, which may help with the understanding of the biological subclasses and the optimization of benefits from molecular therapies. Actually, no molecular classification has demonstrated its ability to precisely predict survival and recurrence of HCC in a clinical setting. A recent study seemed to prove that *C-MYC* status is an important prognostic factor: the amplified *C-MYC* status was associated with a risk of recurrence that is significantly higher compared to disomic and polysomic status. Additionally, for OS, amplified *C-MYC* status was the strongest prognostic factor in both univariate and multivariate analyses [32].

The third curative treatment options for early HCC are the local ablative treatments. The most widely used is radiofrequency ablation (RFA). According to the data of the literature, RFA offers good long-term results that are comparable to the results after surgery in patients with small HCCs [33]. These data were confirmed by a recent review of the literature in which the authors concluded that it is reasonable to offer radiofrequency ablation to patients with HCCs less than 2 cm. On the contrary, for larger nodules or in tumor locations in which ablation is not expected to be effective or safe, surgical removal is preferred [34]. RFA allows complete response in about 80% of tumors smaller than 3 cm and about 50% for lesions of 3–5 cm in size, with 40–70% survival at 5 years [35]. RFA is associated with about 6% incidence of major complications such as pain, liver abscess, pleural effusion, bowel perforation and hemo-peritoneum [36]. There is no defined follow-up interval; however, it is suggested that dynamic imaging should be done every 3–4 months for the first 2 years. The interval can be increased if there is no evidence of recurrence [21].

Four randomized controlled studies involving 652 patients compared RFA to PEI. The results showed a better 3-year survival with the RFA compared with the PEI (63–81 vs. 48–67%). The benefit of RFA may be substantial in tumors larger than 2 cm [37]. Complete response rates were similar (90–96% with RFA and 80–88% with PEI), but with a fewer number of sessions with RFA as compared to PEI (1.1–2.1 vs. 4.8–6.4) [37]. Based on these data, RFA is considered the ablative modality of choice over PEI [7, 21, 37].

Microwave ablation (MWA) is a relatively new type of ablative approach for the treatment of liver cancer. From a technical point of view the MWA induces higher temperature and should have less heath sink effect compared to RFA. MWA can efficiently induce coagulative necrosis in tumor tissues, and tumors with unfavorable location or those larger than 3 cm reducing the risk of local tumor recurrence [38, 39]. In a recent study, MWA was used to treat 47 patients with 80 tumor nodules (average tumor size 2.6 ± 0.9 cm) in 51 treatment sessions [39]. The treatment was delivered laparoscopically in 20 cases and percutaneously in 31 cases. High-risk conditions (defined as unfavorable tumor location such as those invisible by native trans-abdominal ultrasound, superficial tumors, or risk of heat sink phenomena) were found in 28 cases (53%). Local recurrence rate occurred in 17% of patient and 12% of tumors. One patient died of uncontrollable upper gastrointestinal bleeding during the postoperative hospital stay. No MWA-associated complications occurred. Median follow-up period was 20 mo. By univariate logistic Cox regression, it was revealed that tumor size, procedure access, and high-risk location were significant prognostic factors for local tumor recurrence. The commonly encountered complications of MWA include skin burns, liver capsule bleeding, and severe pain [39].

Intermediate HCC

Approximately 20% of patients with HCC are classified as intermediate-stage HCC (large and/or multi nodular HCC in asymptomatic patients without a neoplastic vascular invasion). The expected 2-year survival rate is 50% [2]. Intermediate-stage HCC includes a heterogeneous population of patients with different tumor burden, liver function and disease etiology [40, 41]. Patients in an intermediate stage showed a 3-year survival rate of 50% compared with patients at a more advanced stage, which showed a 3-year survival rate of 8% [42]. Resection may still be a valid option in selected patients [43]. Radical resection can be considered in patients with large single HCC nodules with well-compensated liver function and adequate remnant liver volume and in selected patients with multi nodular HCC or in patients with limited macroscopic vascular invasion; the 5-year survival is 46% in patients with multifocal HCC and is 20% in patients with macroscopic vascular invasion [43-45]. Nevertheless, trans-arterial chemo embolization (TACE), particularly selective or super selective TACE, is considered the standard treatment of patients with compensated liver function (Child-Pugh A and Child B up to 7 points), with large single nodules (>5 cm) or multifocal HCC that does not occluding the portal venous vessels and in those without extra hepatic spread [43]. The literature has reported survival benefits of TACE when compared to symptomatic treatment, with a 2-year survival rate of 30% [46]. TACE-associated adverse events, although usually transient and manageable, occur in a significant proportion (35–90%) of patients: they include post-embolization syndrome (fever, abdominal pain), relevant liver function deterioration, ascites and gastrointestinal bleeding [46]. Selective/super selective TACE may determine a higher rate of tumor necrosis than the standard TACE, with fewer reported adverse events [47].

Embolization using drug-eluding beads (DEB-TACE) is a recent technique that allows to deliver high dose of doxorubicine directly into the tumor, thus decreasing systemic toxicity. an RCT comparing DEB-TACE with conventional TACE, showed no difference between the two techniques regarding response and disease control rates with significantly reduced liver toxicity ($P < .001$) and doxorubicin-related side effects ($P < .0001$) [48]. Further large-scale prospective trials are required to further ascertain this survival benefit [49].

Radio embolization is a form of brachytherapy in which intra-arterially injected radioactive microspheres loaded with yttrium 90 (^{90}Y) are used for internal radiation purposes. Its aim is to deliver tumoricidal doses of radiation to tumors sparing the normal liver tissue. All of the evidence that supports the use of radio embolization in cases of HCC is based on retrospective series or non-controlled prospective studies, but some evidence has been provided that radio embolization can prolong survival over non-specific therapy in patients who are not amenable to TACE. This evidence is further supported by the comparison of numerous studies that have reported survival rates in the range of 9–16 months [49, 50]. In a retrospective study of 245 patients, Y-90 radio embolization compared with TACE showed similar median survival (20.5 months vs. 17.4 months, respectively; P<.232), and mortality, with less toxicity (P<.05) and a longer time to progression (13.3 months vs. 8.4 months; P<.046) [49, 51].

Advanced HCC

Patients with advanced stage HCC (macroscopic vascular invasion, lymph-node or distant metastases) are candidate to palliative treatment. In a large-scale retrospective analysis of 403 patients with HCC the presence of distant metastases at the time of diagnosis were present in 148 patients (37%). In this cohort of patients the site of extra hepatic metastases were the lung (55%), abdominal lymph nodes (41%), and bone (28%) [52].

Sorafenib is an oral molecular-targeted multi-kinase inhibitor of the vascular endothelial growth factor receptor and the platelet-derived growth factor receptor. It is the only chemotherapeutic agent that has demonstrated a significant improvement in the time to progression and in the overall survival of patients with advanced HCC. The adverse effects are easily managed without treatment-related mortality [35, 53, 54]. Its use is recommended for patients with HCC who demonstrate good performance status (PS) and Child-Pugh class A advanced HCC and patients for whom other treatments are not indicated [55]. The reported median overall survival in these patients is 10.7 months [53]. There is not conclusive data about the usefulness of sorafenib in patients with Child-Pugh class B [49]. It has been reported a shorter time to progression (3 months vs. 5 months), poorer median overall survival (3.2 months vs. 9.5 months), and an increased incidence of toxicity (13% vs. 3% incidence of encephalopathy) in these patients compared to patients with Child- Pugh class A [56], that confirmed the subgroup analyses from two large randomized trials (SHARP and Asia-Pacific trials). Another ongoing, global, prospective, observational study (the GIDEON trial, Global Investigation of Therapeutic Decisions in HCC and of its Treatment with Sorafenib) showed that adverse effects of sorafenib forced to interrupt treatment in a larger amount of patients with Child- Pugh class B (38% vs. 23%), that also showed worse survival (5 months vs. 10.5 months) compared with the patients in Child-Pugh class A [57, 58].

End-Stage HCC

Patients with end-stage disease present as Okuda stage III or with a Performance Status of 3–4 that reflects a severe tumor-related disability. Similarly, patients with tumors with a Child-Pugh score of C also account for a very poor prognosis. The 6-month survival rate in these patients is 5% [45]. In these patients is recommended only best supportive care and at this time there are no specific treatment option available.

HCC in Human Immunodeficiency Virus Infected Patients

The survival rates of patients infected by human immunodeficiency virus (HIV) has dramatically increased after the introduction of highly active antiretroviral therapy (HAART) [59]. In these patients, cancer has become the most important factor related with survival and it represents the first cause of death [60]. Although it is not known whether HIV infection alone is a risk-factor for HCC [61], in HIV patients the associated infection with HCV or HBV is very common due to the shared routes of transmission: 25% of HIV positive persons in the Western world has HCV co-infection, up to 75% when considering only intravenous drug users [62]. Besides, HAART is known to have some direct hepato toxic effects, which are amplified among HIV-positive patients chronically infected with HBV or HCV [63]. In HIV positive patients HCC prevalence rate is higher compared to HIV-negative population (82/10,000 according to the Data Collection on Adverse Events of Anti HIV Drugs) [64].

HIV can have a direct role in carcinogenesis due to HIV-tat protein inducing growth signals and enhancing HCC cell proliferation and antitumor immune response [65]. However several epidemiological studies did not demonstrated a higher rate of HCC HIV mono-infected patients compared to general population [61]. Although there are clear evidences that HIV can accelerate the progression of HCV- and HBV-liver disease to cirrhosis and HCC. In fact, the presence of HIV alters the natural history of HCV infection: it increases the likelihood of chronic liver disease (over 90%) due to the lack of critical $CD4^{+}$ T-cell responses against HCV [66]. Furthermore, once chronic HCV infection is established, liver disease progression is faster, resulting in a higher frequency of cirrhosis and its complications compared to HCV mono-infected patients [67]. The molecular mechanisms of accelerated fibrosis in co-infected patients are still not fully understood.

Among HIV positive patients cumulative clinical data suggest a more aggressive course of HCC: [65, 68, 69] patients with HIV seem to be younger and more frequently symptomatic than HIV-negative patients, with an higher median alfa-fetoprotein levels, a more advanced and infiltrating HCC type, a more advanced stage of cirrhosis and a reduced survival rate in comparison with HIV negative patients. HCCs in HIV patients are often advanced at presentation and not amenable of curative treatment [65].

Until a few years ago, the presence of HIV infection was an exclusion criterion for liver transplantation. The main concern was the risk of HIV progression after OLT with a poor post-transplantation prognosis. Nevertheless, several studies demonstrated that most HIV positive transplanted patients have a good long-term survival [70]. Di Benedetto et al. [70] showed a series of 7 HIV positive patients with HCC that, by fulfilling the Milan criteria, underwent OLT with an overall survival rate was 85.7% and only one patient died of a myocardial infarction with a functioning graft and no HCC recurrence. Also Radecke et al. [71] reported that out of 5 cases of OLT in HIV-infected cirrhotic subjects, two had stable liver function and non-progressive HIV infection under HAART, 61 and 23 months after OLT, respectively; unfortunately, in this report, three out of five patients died due to graft failure. Another recent multicenter comparative study [72] involving three transplant centers in Italy, comparing 125 non-HIV infected patients to 30 HIV-infected patients submitted to liver transplantation for HCC, the investigators did not found differences between HIV-infected and -uninfected patients in terms of overall and recurrence free survival. The 1 and 3 years overall survival post-LT was 77% and 65% versus 86.4% and 70%, respectively

(p = 0.32), for HIV-infected and HIV-negative patients. In this report the HCC recurrence rates for HIV-infected and HIV-negative patients were 6.7% (2 out of 30 patients) and 14.4% (18 out of 125 patients), respectively (p = 0.15). Time to HCC recurrence onset was 27.1 months and 9.9, respectively (p = 0.003). One- and 3-year HCC-disease-free survival for patients with and without HIV infection was 100% and 95.2% and 91.4% and 83.6%, respectively (p = 0.32) [72] Clinical post-transplant management of OLT in HIV positive patients is more complex than in the HIV negative counterpart. The main reported problem in these patients has been an earlier and more aggressive HCV recurrence, fast occurrence of hepatic fibrosis, a greater rate of acute rejection (from 33% to 38%) and a higher incidence of tacrolimus toxicity [73]. The outcome of HIV-positive liver recipients depends on the immunological status of the patient at the time of OLT. There is a considerable agreement about the necessity of a full virological control of the underlying HIV infection before OLT: in fact, transplanted patients with higher CD4+ cell count and undetectable HIV viral load display clinical courses similar to HIV negative recipients [74]. It is very important to have an early HAART resumption post-LT. This should prevent the CD4 cell count decline secondary to HIV replication as well as decrease the risk of hepatitis C virus recurrence resulting to reduced cellular immune function [72]. Di Benedetto et al. [72] proposed some criteria to select HIV positive patients with HCC eligible to OLT: firstly, patients must completely fulfill the Milan criteria, they should also have an undetectable HIV viral load (<50 copies/mL) and a $CD4^{+}$ cell count more than 200/mmc. Secondly, after OLT, HAART needs re-introduced as soon as clinically possible according to the opinion of a multidisciplinary transplant team (surgeons, infectivologist and oncologists) with great experience in the management of pharmacologic interactions between HAART and immunosuppressive agents [75].

Regarding the other treatments, in several papers patients are equally treated according to their liver function and tumor stage, with no differences between HIV-infected and HIV negative patients [65, 76, 77].

The study of Berretta et al. [65] considering 97 patients in the HIV-infected group and 338 in the non–HIV-infected group, reported a median survival time was significantly shorter in HIV-infected patients than in HIV-uninfected patients, 35 months versus 59 months, respectively (p = 0 .048). The 1- and 5-year survival rates were 81.5% versus 85.8% and 34% versus 49.1%, for HIV-infected patients versus HIV-uninfected patients, respectively. Anyway, the median survival time was not different between HIV infected and uninfected patients treated with potentially curative therapy: 52 months in HIV-infected patients versus 62 months in uninfected patients (p = 0 .901) Stratifying by specific treatment type, the median survival time also was not different between groups. In particular, the survival in patients treated with surgery were 53 months versus 59 months (p = 0.575), respectively, for HIV-infected and uninfected patients. In patients treated with RFA/PEI, these were 51 months versus 53 months (p = 0 .673). Conversely, a significant difference was observed in survival between groups when considering patients who did not receive potentially curative therapies (i.e., TACE): 35 months versus 65 months (p = 0.051) for HIV-infected versus uninfected patients, respectively. Interestingly, the recurrence rate after therapy was similar between the two groups, regardless of the treatment option (70.7% versus 61.8%; p = 0 .135). However, the rate of retreatment at recurrence was dramatically higher in the HIV-uninfected group than in their HIV-infected counterparts (86.2% versus 61.01%; p = 0.001).

Few data are available on the safety and efficacy of sorafenib in HIV-infected patients with unresectable HCC and concomitant HAART. An Italian study [78] reported 27 consecutive HIV patients treated with sorafenib and concomitant HAART for advanced HCC. Three patients achieved a partial response, 12 achieved a stable disease, and 12 showed progression. The median time to progression and overall survival was 5.1 (range 0.5–13.3) and 12.8 (range 1.1–23.5) months, respectively. No significant differences in time to progression and overall survival were found between patient groups with different severities of liver dysfunction (according to the Child–Pugh classification) or between patient groups with different severities of HIV infection (according to the CDC staging of the disease). Grades 3–4 toxicities included diarrhea (four patients, 14.8%), hypertension (three patients, 11%), and hand-and-foot skin reaction (four patients, 14.9%). The role of concomitant use of HAART in the HIV setting is not clear. Anyway, adverse events occurring in this group of patients were mostly low grade. On the basis of the information currently available, the administration of sorafenib in combination with the specific HAART is not expected to cause increased toxicity. Studies on pharmacokinetics and drug interactions between HAART and sorafenib are needed to better clarify this feature.

Conclusion

Treatment of HCC is complex because it is related both to the stage of tumor and to the degree of liver impairment. Also long term results are closely linked to these two different aspects of this disease.

BCLC treatment allocation system can be utilized to guide the selection of different options, although final decision should be individualized and tailored to the patient. Moreover new prognostic markers would be useful to identify different categories of risk and to guide treatment selection.

References

[1] Llovet JM and Bruix J. Systematic review of randomized trials for unresectable hepatocellular carcinoma: Chemoembolization improves survival. *Hepatology*. 2003; 37: 429-42.

[2] EASL-EORTC clinical practice guidelines: management of hepatocellular carcinoma. *Journal of hepatology*. 2012; 56: 908-43.

[3] Chen MS, Li JQ, Zheng Y, et al. A prospective randomized trial comparing percutaneous local ablative therapy and partial hepatectomy for small hepatocellular carcinoma. *Annals of surgery*. 2006; 243: 321-8.

[4] Feng K, Yan J, Li X, et al. A randomized controlled trial of radiofrequency ablation and surgical resection in the treatment of small hepatocellular carcinoma. *Journal of hepatology*. 2012; 57: 794-802.

[5] Xu G, Qi FZ, Zhang JH, Cheng GF, Cai Y and Miao Y. Meta-analysis of surgical resection and radiofrequency ablation for early hepatocellular carcinoma. *World journal of surgical oncology*. 2012; 10: 163.

[6] Sato M, Tateishi R, Yasunaga H, et al. Mortality and morbidity of hepatectomy, radiofrequency ablation, and embolization for hepatocellular carcinoma: a national survey of 54,145 patients. *Journal of gastroenterology*. 2012; 47: 1125-33.

[7] Bruix J and Sherman M. Management of hepatocellular carcinoma: an update. *Hepatology*. 2011; 53: 1020-2.

[8] Fitzmorris P, Shoreibah M, Anand BS and Singal AK. Management of hepatocellular carcinoma. *Journal of cancer research and clinical oncology*. 2014.

[9] Mazzaferro V, Chun YS, Poon RT, et al. Liver transplantation for hepatocellular carcinoma. *Annals of surgical oncology*. 2008; 15: 1001-7.

[10] Ioannou GN, Perkins JD and Carithers RL, Jr. Liver transplantation for hepatocellular carcinoma: impact of the MELD allocation system and predictors of survival. *Gastroenterology*. 2008; 134: 1342-51.

[11] Park CW, Tsai NT and Wong LL. Implications of worse renal dysfunction and medical comorbidities in patients with NASH undergoing liver transplant evaluation: impact on MELD and more. *Clinical transplantation*. 2011; 25: E606-11.

[12] Cucchetti A, Cescon M, Bertuzzo V, et al. Can the dropout risk of candidates with hepatocellular carcinoma predict survival after liver transplantation? *American journal of transplantation : official journal of the American Society of Transplantation and the American Society* of *Transplant Surgeons*. 2011; 11: 1696-704.

[13] Yao FY, Ferrell L, Bass NM, et al. Liver transplantation for hepatocellular carcinoma: expansion of the tumor size limits does not adversely impact survival. *Hepatology*. 2001; 33: 1394-403.

[14] Duffy JP, Vardanian A, Benjamin E, et al. Liver transplantation criteria for hepatocellular carcinoma should be expanded: a 22-year experience with 467 patients at UCLA. *Annals of surgery*. 2007; 246: 502-9; discussion 9-11.

[15] Ravaioli M, Grazi GL, Piscaglia F, et al. Liver transplantation for hepatocellular carcinoma: results of down-staging in patients initially outside the Milan selection criteria. *American journal of transplantation : official journal of the American Society of Transplantation and the American Society of Transplant Surgeons*. 2008; 8: 2547-57.

[16] Yao FY, Kerlan RK, Jr., Hirose R, et al. Excellent outcome following down-staging of hepatocellular carcinoma prior to liver transplantation: an intention-to-treat analysis. *Hepatology*. 2008; 48: 819-27.

[17] Clavien PA, Lesurtel M, Bossuyt PM, Gores GJ, Langer B and Perrier A. Recommendations for liver transplantation for hepatocellular carcinoma: an international consensus conference report. *The lancet oncology*. 2012; 13: e11-22.

[18] Oliveri RS, Wetterslev J and Gluud C. Transarterial (chemo)embolisation for unresectable hepatocellular carcinoma. *The Cochrane database of systematic reviews*. 2011: CD004787.

[19] Ni JY, Liu SS, Xu LF, Sun HL and Chen YT. Meta-analysis of radiofrequency ablation in combination with transarterial chemoembolization for hepatocellular carcinoma. *World journal of gastroenterology: WJG*. 2013; 19: 3872-82.

[20] Mazzaferro V, Llovet JM, Miceli R, et al. Predicting survival after liver transplantation in patients with hepatocellular carcinoma beyond the Milan criteria: a retrospective, exploratory analysis. *The lancet oncology*. 2009; 10: 35-43.

[21] Ravaioli M, Ercolani G, Neri F, et al. Liver transplantation for hepatic tumors: a systematic review. *World journal of gastroenterology: WJG*. 2014; 20: 5345-52.

[22] Guglielmi A, Ruzzenente A, Conci S, Valdegamberi A and Iacono C. How much remnant is enough in liver resection? *Digestive surgery*. 2012; 29: 6-17.
[23] Ruzzenente A, Valdegamberi A, Campagnaro T, et al. Hepatocellular carcinoma in cirrhotic patients with portal hypertension: is liver resection always contraindicated? *World journal of gastroenterology: WJG*. 2011; 17: 5083-8.
[24] Guglielmi A, Ruzzenente A, Valdegamberi A, et al. Radiofrequency ablation versus surgical resection for the treatment of hepatocellular carcinoma in cirrhosis. *Journal of gastrointestinal surgery: official journal of the Society for Surgery of the Alimentary Tract*. 2008; 12: 192-8.
[25] Yamazaki S and Takayama T. Surgical treatment of hepatocellular carcinoma: evidence-based outcomes. *World journal of gastroenterology: WJG*. 2008; 14: 685-92.
[26] Llovet JM, Fuster J and Bruix J. Prognosis of hepatocellular carcinoma. *Hepato-gastroenterology*. 2002; 49: 7-11.
[27] Huan-Wei C, Shan L, Wan-Yee L, et al. Prognostic impact of hepatic resection for hepatocellular carcinoma: The role of the surgeon in achieving R0 resection - A retrospective cohort study. *Int. J. Surg*. 2014.
[28] Imamura H, Seyama Y, Kokudo N, et al. One thousand fifty-six hepatectomies without mortality in 8 years. *Arch. Surg*. 2003; 138: 1198-206; discussion 206.
[29] Shah SA, Cleary SP, Wei AC, et al. Recurrence after liver resection for hepatocellular carcinoma: risk factors, treatment, and outcomes. *Surgery*. 2007; 141: 330-9.
[30] Nagao T, Inoue S, Yoshimi F, et al. Postoperative recurrence of hepatocellular carcinoma. *Annals of surgery*. 1990; 211: 28-33.
[31] Shah SA, Cleary SP, Tan JC, et al. An analysis of resection vs transplantation for early hepatocellular carcinoma: defining the optimal therapy at a single institution. *Annals of surgical oncology*. 2007; 14: 2608-14.
[32] Pedica F, Ruzzenente A, Bagante F, et al. A re-emerging marker for prognosis in hepatocellular carcinoma: the add-value of fishing c-myc gene for early relapse. *PloS one*. 2013; 8: e68203.
[33] Ruzzenente A, Guglielmi A, Sandri M, et al. Surgical resection versus local ablation for HCC on cirrhosis: results from a propensity case-matched study. *Journal of gastrointestinal surgery : official journal of the Society for Surgery of the Alimentary Tract*. 2012; 16: 301-11; discussion 11.
[34] Cucchetti A, Piscaglia F, Cescon M, Ercolani G and Pinna AD. Systematic review of surgical resection vs radiofrequency ablation for hepatocellular carcinoma. *World journal of gastroenterology*: WJG. 2013; 19: 4106-18.
[35] Llovet JM, Ricci S, Mazzaferro V, et al. Sorafenib in advanced hepatocellular carcinoma. *The New England journal of medicine*. 2008; 359: 378-90.
[36] Giorgio A, Tarantino L, de Stefano G, Coppola C and Ferraioli G. Complications after percutaneous saline-enhanced radiofrequency ablation of liver tumors: 3-year experience with 336 patients at a single center. *AJR American journal of roentgenology*. 2005; 184: 207-11.
[37] Cho YK, Kim JK, Kim MY, Rhim H and Han JK. Systematic review of randomized trials for hepatocellular carcinoma treated with percutaneous ablation therapies. *Hepatology*. 2009; 49: 453-9.

[38] Eisele RM, Denecke T, Glanemann M and Chopra SS. [Minimal-invasive microwave coagulation therapy for liver tumours: laparoscopic and percutaneous access]. *Zentralblatt fur Chirurgie*. 2014; 139: 235-43.

[39] Chen X, Liu HP, Li M and Qiao L. Advances in non-surgical management of primary liver cancer. *World journal of gastroenterology:* WJG. 2014; 20: 16630-8.

[40] Lencioni R, Chen XP, Dagher L and Venook AP. Treatment of intermediate/advanced hepatocellular carcinoma in the clinic: how can outcomes be improved? *The oncologist*. 2010; 15 Suppl 4: 42-52.

[41] Piscaglia F and Bolondi L. The intermediate hepatocellular carcinoma stage: Should treatment be expanded? *Digestive and liver disease: official journal of the Italian Society of Gastroenterology and the Italian Association for the Study of the Liver*. 2010; 42 Suppl 3: S258-63.

[42] Yuen MF, Chan AO, Wong BC, et al. Transarterial chemoembolization for inoperable, early stage hepatocellular carcinoma in patients with Child-Pugh grade A and B: results of a comparative study in 96 Chinese patients. *The American journal of gastroenterology*. 2003; 98: 1181-5.

[43] Zhang ZM, Guo JX, Zhang ZC, Jiang N, Zhang ZY and Pan LJ. Therapeutic options for intermediate-advanced hepatocellular carcinoma. *World journal of gastroenterology: WJG*. 2011; 17: 1685-9.

[44] Ruzzenente A, Capra F, Pachera S, et al. Is liver resection justified in advanced hepatocellular carcinoma? Results of an observational study in 464 patients. *Journal of gastrointestinal surgery: official journal of the Society for Surgery of the Alimentary Tract*. 2009; 13: 1313-20.

[45] Bruix J and Sherman M. Management of hepatocellular carcinoma. Hepatology. 2005; 42: 1208-36.

[46] Lopez RR, Jr., Pan SH, Hoffman AL, et al. Comparison of transarterial chemoembolization in patients with unresectable, diffuse vs focal hepatocellular carcinoma. Arch Surg. 2002; 137: 653-7; discussion 7-8.

[47] Dufour JF, Bargellini I, De Maria N, De Simone P, Goulis I and Marinho RT. Intermediate hepatocellular carcinoma: current treatments and future perspectives. *Annals of oncology: official journal of the European Society for Medical Oncology / ESMO*. 2013; 24 Suppl 2: ii24-9.

[48] Lammer J, Malagari K, Vogl T, et al. Prospective randomized study of doxorubicin-eluting-bead embolization in the treatment of hepatocellular carcinoma: results of the PRECISION V study. *Cardiovascular and interventional radiology*. 2010; 33: 41-52.

[49] Fong ZV and Tanabe KK. The clinical management of hepatocellular carcinoma in the United States, Europe, and Asia: a comprehensive and evidence-based comparison and review. *Cancer*. 2014; 120: 2824-38.

[50] Salem R, Lewandowski RJ, Mulcahy MF, et al. Radioembolization for hepatocellular carcinoma using Yttrium-90 microspheres: a comprehensive report of long-term outcomes. *Gastroenterology*. 2010; 138: 52-64.

[51] Salem R, Lewandowski RJ, Kulik L, et al. Radioembolization results in longer time-to-progression and reduced toxicity compared with chemoembolization in patients with hepatocellular carcinoma. *Gastroenterology*. 2011; 140: 497-507 e2.

[52] Katyal S, Oliver JH, 3rd, Peterson MS, Ferris JV, Carr BS and Baron RL. Extrahepatic metastases of hepatocellular carcinoma. *Radiology*. 2000; 216: 698-703.

[53] Cheng AL, Kang YK, Chen Z, et al. Efficacy and safety of sorafenib in patients in the Asia-Pacific region with advanced hepatocellular carcinoma: a phase III randomised, double-blind, placebo-controlled trial. *The lancet oncology*. 2009; 10: 25-34.

[54] Di Benedetto F, Tarantino G, Montalti R, et al. Sorafenib before liver transplantation for hepatocellular carcinoma: risk or give up. *Transplant international: official journal of the European Society for Organ Transplantation*. 2011; 24: e97; author reply e8-9.

[55] Kaneko S, Furuse J, Kudo M, et al. Guideline on the use of new anticancer drugs for the treatment of Hepatocellular Carcinoma 2010 update. *Hepatology research: the official journal of the Japan Society of Hepatology*. 2012; 42: 523-42.

[56] Abou-Alfa GK, Amadori D, Santoro A, et al. Safety and Efficacy of Sorafenib in Patients with Hepatocellular Carcinoma (HCC) and Child-Pugh A versus B Cirrhosis. *Gastrointestinal cancer research: GCR*. 2011; 4: 40-4.

[57] Yau T, Chan P, Ng KK, et al. Phase 2 open-label study of single-agent sorafenib in treating advanced hepatocellular carcinoma in a hepatitis B-endemic Asian population: presence of lung metastasis predicts poor response. *Cancer*. 2009; 115: 428-36.

[58] Chiu J, Tang YF, Yao TJ, et al. The use of single-agent sorafenib in the treatment of advanced hepatocellular carcinoma patients with underlying Child-Pugh B liver cirrhosis: a retrospective analysis of efficacy, safety, and survival benefits. *Cancer*. 2012; 118: 5293-301.

[59] Nunnari G, Leto D, Sullivan J, et al. Seminal reservoirs during an HIV type 1 eradication trial. *AIDS research and human retroviruses*. 2005; 21: 768-75.

[60] Diamond C. Malignancy-related causes of death in human immunodeficiency virus-infected patients in the era of highly active antiretroviral therapy. *Cancer*. 2005; 103: 650; author reply 1.

[61] Giordano TP, Kramer JR, Souchek J, Richardson P and El-Serag HB. Cirrhosis and hepatocellular carcinoma in HIV-infected veterans with and without the hepatitis C virus: a cohort study, 1992-2001. *Archives of internal medicine*. 2004; 164: 2349-54.

[62] Buffet-Janvresse C, Peigue-Lafeuille H, Benichou J, et al. HIV and HCV co-infection: situation at six French university hospitals in the year 2000. *Journal of medical virology*. 2003; 69: 7-17.

[63] Sulkowski MS, Thomas DL, Chaisson RE and Moore RD. Hepatotoxicity associated with antiretroviral therapy in adults infected with human immunodeficiency virus and the role of hepatitis C or B virus infection. *Jama*. 2000; 283: 74-80.

[64] Weber R, Sabin CA, Friis-Moller N, et al. Liver-related deaths in persons infected with the human immunodeficiency virus: the D:A:D study. *Archives of internal medicine*. 2006; 166: 1632-41.

[65] Berretta M, Garlassi E, Cacopardo B, et al. Hepatocellular carcinoma in HIV-infected patients: check early, treat hard. *The oncologist*. 2011; 16: 1258-69.

[66] Danta M, Semmo N, Fabris P, et al. Impact of HIV on host-virus interactions during early hepatitis C virus infection. *The Journal of infectious diseases*. 2008; 197: 1558-66.

[67] Smukler AJ and Ratner L. Hepatitis viruses and hepatocellular carcinoma in HIV-infected patients. *Current opinion in oncology*. 2002; 14: 538-42.

[68] Zanet E, Berretta M, Benedetto FD, et al. Pancreatic cancer in HIV-positive patients: a clinical case-control study. *Pancreas*. 2012; 41: 1331-5.

[69] Brau N, Fox RK, Xiao P, et al. Presentation and outcome of hepatocellular carcinoma in HIV-infected patients: a U.S.-Canadian multicenter study. *Journal of hepatology*. 2007; 47: 527-37.

[70] Di Benedetto F, De Ruvo N, Berretta M, et al. Hepatocellular carcinoma in HIV patients treated by liver transplantation. *European journal of surgical oncology : the journal of the European Society of Surgical Oncology and the British Association of Surgical Oncology*. 2008; 34: 422-7.

[71] Radecke K, Fruhauf NR, Miller M, et al. Outcome after orthotopic liver transplantation in five HIV-infected patients with virus hepatitis-induced cirrhosis. *Liver international: official journal of the International Association for the Study of the Liver*. 2005; 25: 101-8.

[72] Di Benedetto F, Tarantino G, Ercolani G, et al. Multicenter italian experience in liver transplantation for hepatocellular carcinoma in HIV-infected patients. *The oncologist*. 2013; 18: 592-9.

[73] Di Benedetto F, Berretta M, De Ruvo N, et al. Is advanced hepatocellular carcinoma amenable of cure by liver transplantation with sorafenib as a neoadjuvant approach plus m-TOR inhibitors monotherapy? *Journal of surgical oncology*. 2012; 105: 111-2.

[74] Tavio M, Grossi P, Baccarani U, et al. HIV-infected patients and liver transplantation: who, when and why. *Current HIV research*. 2011; 9: 120-7.

[75] Nunnari G, Berretta M, Pinzone MR, et al. Hepatocellular carcinoma in HIV positive patients. *European review for medical and pharmacological sciences*. 2012; 16: 1257-70.

[76] Lim C, Goutte N, Gervais A, et al. Standardized care management ensures similar survival rates in HIV-positive and HIV-negative patients with hepatocellular carcinoma. *J. Acquir Immune Defic. Syndr*. 2012; 61: 581-7.

[77] Yopp AC, Subramanian M, Jain MK, et al. Presentation, treatment, and clinical outcomes of patients with hepatocellular carcinoma, with and without human immunodeficiency virus infection. *Clinical gastroenterology and hepatology : the official clinical practice journal of the American Gastroenterological Association*. 2012; 10: 1284-90.

[78] Berretta M, Di Benedetto F, Dal Maso L, et al. Sorafenib for the treatment of unresectable hepatocellular carcinoma in HIV-positive patients. *Anti-cancer drugs*. 2013; 24: 212-8.

In: Hepatocellular Carcinoma in the 3rd Millennium
Editors: M. Berretta and B. Cacopardo
ISBN: 978-1-63484-025-5

Chapter 10

Hepatocellular Carcinoma: Palliative and Supportive Treatment

***Ottaviano M. Tomassi*[1] *and Daniele Bernardi*[2,*]**
[1]Senior Assistant, Medical Oncology Unit, Ospedale Civile, San Donà di Piave (VE), Italy
[2]Director, Medical Oncology Unit, Ospedale Civile, San Donà di Piave (VE), Italy

Abstract

In the recent years the management of locoregional and systemic symptoms of advanced Hepatocellular Carcinoma has improved. Although the mortality induced by the extrahepatic diffusion of the tumor is limited, treatment is necessary because of the severity of symptoms and the impact on quality of life. The therapeutic goal in patients with End-Stage Liver Disease is symptom control and maintenance of the best possible quality of life. In this setting, best supportive care consists of a broad spectrum of services and interventions aimed at improving patient's ability to tolerate treatments and better facing the impact with cancer. Active control of symptoms, by means of integrated medical interventions and multidisciplinary approaches (psychosocial, palliative, nutritional), must not be confined to the very end stage of the disease but must be part of a global approach to cancer patients.

Introduction

In Western countries, large-scale ultrasound surveillance has contributed to increase the number of patients with an early diagnosis of hepatocellular carcinoma (HCC), allowing a better understanding of the natural history and therapeutic approach of this disease. In recent years, the management of loco regional and systemic symptoms of advanced HCC has

[*] Corresponding author: Correspondence to: Daniele Bernardi, Medical Oncology Unit, OspedaleCivile, 30027 San Donà di Piave (VE). E-mail: Daniele.Bernardi@ulss10.veneto.it.

improved, with particular regard to the extra hepatic metastases, that in the past were rarely detected due to the rapid death of the patients.

Two studies on patient populations that were followed until death showed super imposable data on the percentage of patients developing extra hepatic metastases (13.5% and 15.2% respectively) and the sites of disease more frequently involved: lungs (53.8% vs. 43%), bone (35.5% vs. 37%) and lymph nodes (33.8% vs. 45%) with a median survival of 5-7 months and with 21.7% vs. 24.9% of patients surviving at 1 year [1, 2]. Although the mortality induced by the extra hepatic diffusion of the tumor is limited (11%), treatment is necessary because of the severity of symptoms, particularly bone pain, and the impact on quality of life (Health-Related Quality of Life, HRQoL). Most of the patients with HCC have cirrhosis and in the late phase of HCC may develop clinical decompensation (jaundice, ascites, hepatic encephalopathy, gastrointestinal bleeding). This means that the late phase of HCC may be represented as an End-Stage Liver Disease (ESLD) where the relevance of cirrhosis depends on the clinical course of the disease.

The National Consensus Project for Quality Palliative Care defines the goal of palliative care as to "prevent and relieve suffering and to support the best possible quality of life for patients and their families, regardless of the stage of the disease or the need for other therapies . Palliative care involves a multidisciplinary approach to optimize symptom management and health status without excluding medical therapies to achieve these goals. The concept of palliative care is integrated easily into standard medical management of ESLD.

In a study by Lin and co-workers [3], the majority of patients with end-stage HCC in a hospice program (77.3% out of 110 total patients) had cirrhosis, but only in 38 patients (34.5%) this was decompensated (Child-Plough class C). This subgroup of patients required more clinical assistance as compared to the patients with end-stage HCC without cirrhosis or with compensated cirrhosis.

The number, prevalence and severity of symptoms in a patient with advanced stage cancer is relevant, and, generally, increases as approaching death. In a program of palliative care on 1000 cancer patients, the median number of symptoms per patient was 11, with a range between 1 and 27 [4]. The therapeutic goal in patients with ESLD is symptom control and maintenance of the best possible quality of life. In this setting, best supportive care means a broad spectrum of services and interventions aimed at improving patient's ability to tolerate treatments and better facing the impact with cancer. Active control of symptoms, by means of integrated medical interventions and multidisciplinary approaches (psychosocial, palliative, and nutritional), must not be confined to the end stage of the disease but must be part of a global approach to cancer patients. Treatments directed against the disease and directed against symptoms must be simultaneously administered, as a support of the clinical and psychosocial situation both of the patient and his family.

Pain

As in the case of other tumors, pain in advanced HCC is present in almost 75% of patients and is favored by the abdominal tension caused by ascites, hepatomegaly and, in one third of patients, bone metastases [5]. Patients very often complain of a visceral, dull pain. Pharmacologic treatment relies on specific pain-drugs and adjuvant drugs (NSAIDs or corticosteroids) and treatment strategy consists of NSAIDs in the case of light pain, minor opioids in moderate pain, and major opioids in severe pain, as in the advice of the WHO three-step analgesic scale. NSAIDs can be associated to drugs used for moderate-intense pain and either opioids or NSAIDs can be associated to adjuvants.

In the approach to pain, drugs must be administered at given times throughout the day but also providing the possibility of occasional administrations, whenever needed, tailoring the treatment to the patient, in order to prevent collateral effects.

Recently, the three-step scale has been modified with the inclusion of both rotation of opioids and the administration route. Moreover, treating pain by means of invasive procedures is now an increasingly used chance. Neuropathic and bone metastases-related pain are the most difficult to manage, and the spine is frequently involved (56%) [6].

Patients affected by neuropathic pain are more frequently treated with tricyclic antidepressants (TCAs) and serotonin/norepinephrine reuptake inhibitors (SNRIs), GABA (Gamma-amino-butyric acid)-ergic drugs, such as gabapentin and pregabalin, opioids and tramadol [7]. Bone pain, instead, can be actively controlled by radiotherapy [8] and the administration of bisphosphonates [9] that can reduce the dose and the frequency of administration of major opioids.

A recent review concerning the efficacy of radiotherapy in controlling bone metastasis-induced pain has shown that the conventional approach or hypo fractionation of the dose (single dose 8 Gy) can reduce pain in almost 60% of patients with a complete response in about 25%. Due to the shorter duration of the effect, single dose must be reserved to patients with an expected short survival time [8].

New drugs showing efficacy in the treatment of pain are endotelin 1-receptor antagonists (i.e., atratensan), anti-RANK-L (Receptor Activator of Nuclear factor Kappa-B Ligand) antibodies that mimic the action of osteoprotegerin (i.e., denosumab), anti-NGF (Nerve Growth Factor) antibodies.

In selected cases, spinal metastases can be treated with vertebral reconstruction or intraspinal infusion of analgesics. Breakthrough pain, also including motion-related pain, can be treated with immediate-release opioids using a route of administration that can guarantee a rapid effect and a short duration, such as trans-mucosal, or with a preemptive administration, when a situation that could trigger pain is foreseen, such as patient moving around for personal hygiene or a radiotherapy session.

Fatigue

Fatigue is a very common symptom in cancer patients, in particular in those with advanced HCC, and can cause intense distress [10]. It is essential that physicians research actively this symptom [11] using questions assessing the physical (using the word “weakness”) and cognitive (using the word “fatigue”) dimensions and by means of multidimensional questionnaires.

A recent and effective definition of fatigue is "subjective feeling of tiredness, weakness or lack of energy" [10]. The main causes of fatigue include psychological distress (anxiety and depression), insomnia or hypersomnia, physical inactivity, resulting in muscular and cardio-respiratory deconditioning, anemia, emaciation, fever, infections, metabolic, hormonal and hydro-electrolytic disorders, direct consequences of the primary treatment of the tumor, chronic inflammatory response, abnormalities in the hypothalamic-pituitary-adrenal axis.

In HCC the correlation between TACE (Transcatheter hepatic Arterial ChemoEmbolizzation) and the onset of fatigue has been reported, as well as the correlation between such symptoms and treatments with diuretics and beta-adrenergic antagonists.

To date, a number of studies on the etiopathogenetic treatment of fatigue by using anti-cytokines and anti-inflammatory agents have shown no effects.

Symptomatic treatments can be pharmacologic or not; among the first ones we include growth factors, psychostimulants, bisphosphonates, anti-TNF (Tumor Necrosis Factor) antibodies and antagonists, antidepressants and progestins. Clinically relevant results have been achieved only with erythropoietin and darbepoietin in anemia and the psychostimulant methylphenidate [12].

Non-pharmacologic treatments are exercise (aerobic) and rehabilitation, psychosocial interventions (stress management, support groups, relaxation techniques), but their effectiveness has not been definitively confirmed [13-17].

Fatigue can also occur as a result of the treatment with sorafenib, the multikinase inhibitor that in the recent years has become the standard of treatment in advanced-stage HCC, when loco-regional treatment is no longer indicated; taking care of the palliation of the adverse events caused by this drug is mandatory when dealing with the simultaneous care of these patients. According to the data of phase II and III studies, fatigue develops in approximately 20-22% (all grades) of patients, with Grade 3-4 in 3%. In addition, in patients taking sorafenib, fatigue may be exacerbated by the onset and persistence of diarrhea. In this setting, treatment of the symptoms takes place through the recognition of the symptom and the patient-physician daily relationship. This can be done by using "strength management" techniques, and also maintaining adequate hydration and scheduling “rest periods” during the day [18]. If anorexia develops, “appetite stimulants” such as dronabinol can be used in order to increase food intake [19]. Temporary discontinuation of the drug is required only in case of grade 3-4 toxicity and treatment has to be restarted at lower dosage only after resolution or clear reduction (back to grade 1) of toxicity. Definitive discontinuation must be considered only when a new episode of severe and/or persistent fatigue occurs.

In the last days/hours of life, fatigue may also be considered as a defense and protection from physical and mental suffering. Therefore, in this case, aggressive treatment should be avoided.

Pruritus and Other Skin Symptoms

The onset of pruritus depends on the occurrence of cholestasis due to the intra hepatic infiltration or the biliary tree obstruction caused by HCC. Cholestatic pruritus is also centrally mediated by endogenous opioids [20-22]. Pruritus can be monitored by means of visual analogs tools or questionnaires exploring patient’s personal perception. Medical treatment of the symptom should be aimed at neutralizing the etiopathogenetic pathways that are not always completely understood [23, 24].

Initial treatment in cirrhotic patients consists of the oral administration of cholestyramine, 2-16 g/day (usually 4 g four times per day), making cholesterol and biliary acids unabsorbable. In fact, cholestyramine is a non-absorbable anyonic-exchange resin which is capable of binding biliary acids in the intestine preventing their absorption in the terminal ileum and favoring the formation of an insoluble complex excreted with feces. Cholestyramine can determine constipation and the lack of absorption of other drugs; therefore, the concomitant administration with other drugs should be thoroughly avoided. Whenever HCC induces jaundice, initial treatment usually consists of antihistaminic drugs that have an unspecific sedative effect facilitating night rest. In this setting, benzodiazepines, with their sedative and anxiolytic effect, can be used as well.

Although pruritus is the second level of nociception (being pain the first) mediated also by the serotoninergic system, few results exist in the literature concerning the administration of serotonin reuptake inhibitors (SSRIs), such as paroxetine, sertraline and mirtazapine. These drugs block the transformation of the precursors of endogenous opioids in the active forms that are responsible for the onset of pruritus. Efficacy has been described of the administration of serotonin-antagonists, such as ondansetron.

Small case series have shown the efficacy of some other drugs in the treatment of this symptom:

- Peripheral antagonists of opioid-receptors, such as naltrexone (dosage 37,5-50 mg/day), naloxon and nalmefene, with a gradually increasing dosage to avoid abstinence syndrome ;
- Codeine and buprenorphine, acting through a competitive mechanism on the endogenous receptors inducing pruritus;
- Hepatic enzyme inductors: rifampicin, (300-450 mg/day), upregulating cytochrome p450 metabolic pathway, with the result of a higher metabolism of endogenous opioids. The use of this drug is limited in this setting, due to the high risk of hepatic toxicity, especially during long lasting administrations.
- Anecdotal results have been achieved with phenobarbital, metronidazol and anesthetics such as propofol and lidocaine
- Potentially effective, but still to be confirmed, are dronabinol (cannabinoid) and gabapentin (anticonvulsant).

Physical interventions, such as moisturizers and baths of baking soda, have also to be mentioned in the management of this symptom.

In treatment-refractory pruritus, plasmapheresis or dialysis, with the aim to remove the substances responsible for pruritus, have to be avoided, since they are inappropriate for terminal patients [25].

Other skin symptoms can occur while under treatment with sorafenib, such as skin rash (from erythema to generalized exfoliative, ulcerative or bullous dermatitis) and/or Palmo-Plantar Erythrodysesthesia (PPE), that can progress into ulcerative dermatitis, interfering with daily activities. Mild toxicity can occur in about 70% of patients, whereas more severe can sum up to 10% of treated patients. When cutaneous rash occurs, neutral detergents for body hygiene or moisturizers can be used, paying attention to avoid hot water; synthetic fabrics should not be worn.

Topical steroids seem to be effective in mild rash, while antihistaminics have shown limited efficacy. In severe skin rash reactions, oral steroids are claimed to lead to a complete resolution, but data in the literature are not strongly in favor of this approach [26].

The onset of PPE should be prevented by removing cutaneous thickness and applying urea 10% cream three times per day. While undergoing treatment with sorafenib, patients should wear cotton gloves and try to avoid hot water. In case of grade 1 toxicity, urea 20-40% treatment cream is generally used, whereas, in case of grade 2 toxicity, topical steroids (i.e., clobetasol propionate) or oral antinflammatory drugs (i.e., Ibuprofen 600-800 mg tid) are required, together with pain drugs such as codein, when needed. In this case, a reduction of the dose of sorafenib should also be considered. In grade 3 cutaneous toxicity, a reduction of the dose of sorafenib or a temporary discontinuation are mandatory; treatment should be then restarted at reduced dosage, but, in case of recurrent episodes of grade 3 toxicity, treatment should be definitively interrupted [18, 27].

Hepatic Encephalopathy

Hepatic encephalopathy is an alteration of the central nervous system as a result of hepatic insufficiency, after the exclusion of other known metabolic, infectious, intracranial vascular events, or space-occupying lesions which may present with similar symptomatology [28].

It appears as a neuropsychiatric syndrome which may result in impairment of the sleep-wake cycle, cognition, memory, consciousness, personality changes, motor-sensory abnormalities and decreased energy levels representing a continuum of manifestations of hepatic encephalopathy that can be experienced by the patient or elicited by the physician on history taking or physical examination [29]. The broad spectrum of neuropsychiatric manifestations reflects the range of pathophysiological mechanisms, for example impairment of neurotransmitter system, impaired cerebral perfusion and cerebral edema, and/or atrophy that interplay with one another. The challenge remains to dissect these purported mechanisms singularly for possible pharmacological intervention to improve treatment.

The full-blown framework of hepatic encephalopathy may arise as a result of the following factors:

- increased ammonia levels as a result of increased production of circulating ammonia from kidney, intestinal or muscular causes;
- reduction of ammonia elimination due to worsening liver failure, hypokalemia;
- central sedation due to analgesics and sedative-hypnotics together with the development of GABA-receptor hypersensitivity to benzodiazepines;
- concomitant presence of hypovolemia, hypoxia, hypoglycemia, and acid-base balance and electrolytic alterations.

The clinical picture of advanced hepatic encephalopathy is characterized by a form of delirium with confusion, ataxia, flapping tremor, inappropriate behaviors and personality changes, worsening sleepiness leading to stupor and coma.

Initial treatment is a cathartic, most often a non-absorbable disaccharide (lactulose or lactilol) with the aim to obtain few evacuations per day of soft feces [30]. Cathartics reduce intestinal ammonia load by its work as a cathartic and by acidification of the gut lumen which inhibits ammoniagenic coliform bacteria, leading to increased levels of nonammoniagenic lactobacilli. The acidification process results in retention of ammonia (NH_3) in the colon as ammonium (NH_4^+), thus trapping it and preventing its absorption. The trapped ammonium is then expelled in the stool. Diarrhea has to be avoided to prevent dehydration and electrolyte balance disorders with sudden worsening of encephalopathy [31].

In patients refractory or intolerant to lactulose, a non-absorbable antibiotic can be administered, such as rifaximin 1-2 g/day, paromomycin 4 g/day or metronidazole 250 mg 2-3 times a day. In fact, modulation of the gut microbiota may represent a good therapeutic target for the prevention and treatment of hepatic encephalopathy. In particular, due to its low rate of systemic bioavailability and good tolerability profile, the non-absorbable antibiotic rifaximin could be an "ideal" antimicrobial for selective targeting at the gastrointestinal tract in this kind of patients [32]. Neomycin should be avoided, given it's virtually nefrotoxic effect that makes this drug not recommended for a prolonged treatment in these patients.

At all times during the treatment it is necessary to promote a veggie-rich diet, to administer branched-chain amino acids and to prevent the occurrence of precipitating factors such as constipation and dehydration.

Cancer Anorexia-Cachexia Syndrome

The Cancer Anorexia-Cachexia Syndrome (CACS) is one of the characterizing aspects in patients affected by HCC in which, similarly to other tumors in advanced stages, it has a negative prognostic value. About half of all cancer patients show a syndrome of cachexia that can have a profound impact on quality of life, symptom burden and patient's sense of dignity [33]. There is loss of lean body mass with or without a loss of body fat.

Primary cachexia is associated with biochemical abnormalities or metabolic disorders caused by the cytokines produced by the tumor mass and the monocyte-macrophage system in response to cancer. Secondary cachexia is favored by the reduced food intake due to an obstacle to the natural way of feeding and, therefore, is predominant in gastro-intestinal and head and neck tumors.

Numerous cytokines have been postulated to play a role in the etiology of cancer cachexia. Cytokines can elicit effects that mimic leptin signaling and suppress orexigenic ghrelin and neuropeptide Y (NPY) signaling, inducing sustained anorexia and cachexia not accompanied by the usual compensatory response. Furthermore, cytokines have been implicated in the induction of cancer-related muscle wasting. Cytokine-induced skeletal muscle wasting is probably a multifactorial process, which involves a protein synthesis inhibition, an increase in protein degradation, or a combination of both.

The clinical signs of cancer cachexia include weight loss, anorexia, nausea, weakness, deterioration of the Performance Status, modification of the body image.

The presence of ascites causes early satiety, protein loss secondary to frequent paracentesis, autonomic nervous system failure resulting in gastroparesis.

In fact, HCC represents a contributory cause for the onset of symptoms of the upper gastrointestinal tract due to mechanical (hepatomegaly, bleeding varices) and metabolic causes (liver failure, hepato-renal syndrome, hydroelectrolytic disorders).

There is evidence that both the turnover of total body protein mass and the oxidation rate of proteins are higher in patients with advanced HCC as compared to patients with chronic liver disease or suffering from tumors with liver metastases. In particular, in these patients amino acids derived from muscle mass catabolism are reintegrated in plasma proteins such as immunoglobulins G, transferrin and fibrinogen, without a restoration of the body mass due to the very low food intake [34].

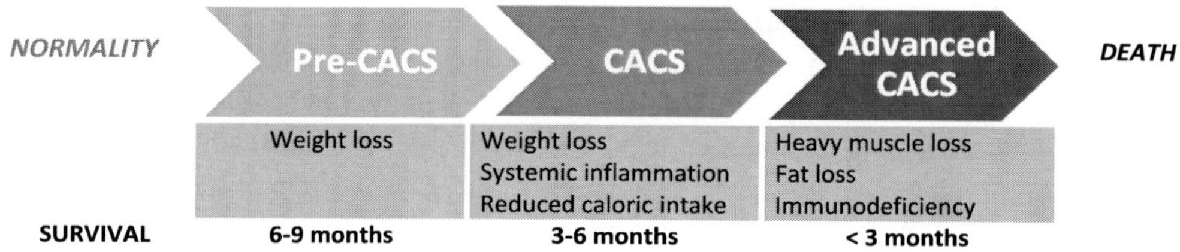

Figure 1. Cancer anorexia-cachexia syndrome (CACS): dietary counselling is necessary from phase 1 (pre-CACS); CACS therapy is urgent in phase 2 (CACS) because of its limited effectiveness during phase 3 (Advanced CACS) (modified from Fearon) [40].

Management of cachexia must take into account the patient's prognosis, as it may take several weeks for patient to respond to anti-cachectic treatment [35]. For patients with a short life expectancy, treatment options for cachexia may add to the disease burden without offering adequate symptom relief and thus may not be appropriate. Health care professionals should discuss all treatment options with the patient and ensure that they are well informed about available treatments and expected treatment outcomes. All patients should have equal access to appropriate assessment and management of cachexia, whether they are receiving home care, day care or are hospital inpatients.

Pharmacologic treatment of cachexia in HCC should intervene in the complex metabolic and cytokine pathways as well as on the symptoms by stimulating appetite and weight gain [36].

Among the many drugs studied, only corticosteroids, in the short run, and high-dose progestins, in the long run, have shown efficacy and, therefore, their use is suggested [19, 37, 38].

Progestational drugs, cannabinoids and cyproheptadine are used in the clinic as appetite stimulants in the therapy of CACS [39]. These drugs have be shown to be partially effective in reversing or maintaining the symptom of body weight loss in patients with chronic illness.

Clearly, it is necessary to treat CACS right after the diagnosis of advanced, incurable disease, when decreased appetite and weight loss are not evident yet (Figure 1) [40]. Only in this way we can reduce the chances of therapeutic failure. Body weight must be accurately monitored, frequent nutritional assessments must be performed in order to promptly snatch a body weight loss >10% or the reduction of caloric income (less than 1500 kcal/day) or the sharp increase of systemic inflammation markers (C-Reactive Protein, CRP). In fact, individualized dietary counseling is very effective in improving patient's food intake and nutritional status [41, 42]. However, the influence of counseling in reducing psychological distress in patients with a palliative care setting remains to be established [35]. Adequate education and counseling should also address the concerns of family members who may worry that their relative appears to be "starving to death" by underscoring the difference between starvation and cachexia.

Protein restriction, which in the past was often encouraged in patients with advanced HCC to prevent hepatic encephalopathy, today must be carefully evaluated: supplementation with branched-chain amino acids seems to delay the progression of the disease and significantly reduce anorexia.

Ascites

Neoplastic ascites is caused in 50% of cases by peritoneal carcinomatosis, in 15% by liver invasion and portal vein compression, in 15% by the combination of the two and in 20% by lymphatic invasion with subsequent chylous ascites [43]. This symptom is responsible for 6% of the hospice admissions [44].

Ascites causes a mass effect with subsequent occurrence of abdominal distension, nausea and vomiting, early satiety and, in the late phase, dyspnea and lower limb swelling.

Paracentesis is the main and more effective procedure in the management of the symptoms of ascites [45]. Hypotension following paracentesis is less frequent in cancer patients due to the different etiopathogenetic mechanism of accumulation as compared to cirrhotic ascites.

In cirrhotic patients affected by HCC, cirrhosis is the main cause of the development of ascites. Nevertheless, in these patients the administration of diuretics and sodium restriction is more effective than in cancer patients with ascites due to peritoneal carcinomatosis.

In fact, these treatments affect the natural history of cirrhosis even if, in the advanced phase of the disease, with a life expectancy of only few weeks, every therapeutic approach consisting in a “sacrifice” for the patients must be accurately evaluated with an eye on the risk/benefit ratio.

Medical treatment consists in the association between spironolactone (initial dose 100 mg/day) and a loop-acting diuretic such as furosemide (40 mg/day, administered once daily, usually in the morning to avoid nocturia) [46, 47]. Furosemide can be added also later on, when it is necessary to obtain a stronger diuretic effect. The dosage of diuretics should be increased in a gradual manner. Moreover, the administration of diuretics should be accompanied with sodium restriction and NSAIDs should not be used in order to avoid resistance to diuretics and aggravate ascitic fluid accumulation via prostaglandin inhibition [45].

Conversely, attention should be paid to diuretic-induced dilutional hyponatremia with subsequent development of cerebral edema and multiorgan failure.

Periodic paracentesis is effective in the palliation of symptoms in diuretic-refractory ascites. The frequency of paracentesis is determined upon the need of the management of the symptoms: body weight should be checked every 2 weeks and paracentesis should be performed when a weight gain higher than 3 kg occurs. Albumin should be administered after paracentesis when more than 4 liters of abdominal fluid have been removed, dextran poligeline for lower volumes [45, 48]. There is some controversy, however, regarding the use of albumin infusion given its high cost, and it has not been uniformly recommended after large-volume paracentesis. In selected cases, when frequent paracenteses are required, a permanent peritoneal drainage catheter can be used, allowing the patient itself, or the caregiver, to remove the ascitic fluid when abdominal tension is present. Due to the possible complications associated with the management of these catheters, they should be used only during home-based or hospice-based palliative programs [44].

Table 1. Therapeutic approaches to obstructive jaundice (modified from Baron [49])

	Advantages	Disadvantages
Surgery	Long term palliation Contemporary palliation of pain and gastrointestinal occlusions	More invasive Morbidity and mortality
Percutaneous	Non surgical	Pain Bleeding External drainage
Endoscopic	Non surgical Less painful Feasible on outpatient basis	Stent occlusion Expertise required Complications (perforation, pancreatitis, bleeding)

Obstructive Jaundice

The progressive development of obstructive jaundice is responsible for a rapidly deteriorating quality of life, due to the onset of pruritus and recurrent cholangitis.

Obstructive jaundice, due to both hilar and non-hilar bile duct compression, is rare in HCC but more frequent in cholangiocarcinoma, carcinoma of the gallbladder and metastatic cancers. Symptoms most frequently associated with jaundice are coagulation disorders (impaired absorption of vitamin K), pruritus and cholangitis [25]. Jaundice can be surgically managed with a bypass or through interventional procedures such as the insertion of a stent (percutaneously or endoscopically) (Table 1) [49, 50].

Surgical approach is contraindicated in patients with a low Performance Status and in patients whose life expectancy is lower than 6 months. Laparoscopic or laparotomic surgery can overcome the obstruction through a bilio-enteric bypass: choledocic or hepatic enterostomy (generally with jejunum). The connection of the hepatic ducts with jejunum has lower chances of success with higher possibility of relapse and complications in comparison to the bypass with the extra hepatic bile ducts that is used in pancreatic cancer.

The placement of a percutaneous or endoscopic or combined stent has substituted surgery. Stents can be plastic or metallic, with the latter ones (covered and uncovered and self-expandable) having the best chances of medium-long term success.

The endoscopic approach has higher chances of success and lower adverse effects but requires a high grade of expertise. On the contrary, percutaneous transhepatic cholangiography (PTHC) can determine an external, external-internal or internal drainage by placing a definitive endoprosthesis; the latter result is desirable, since the management of an external drainage is difficult, due to the infectious-hemorrhagic complications and the psychological distress for the patient. Therefore, the percutaneous approach is applied in case of failure of the endoscopic approach or when the latter is not technically feasible due to the type of obstruction (generally intra hepatic). Moreover, a multidisciplinary management is necessary, so that the right approach can be undertaken based upon several parameters: Performance Status, life expectancy, patient's preference, site of obstruction and choice of the treating centre.To date no randomized studies are present in the literature comparing stent and percutaneous trans-hepatic catheter. In patients with a life expectancy higher than six months there seems to be an advantage, in terms of costs, in favor of metallic in comparison to plastic stents [51]. Furthermore, a fully covered metallic stent has been shown to be useful in controlling hemobilia secondary to HCC with bile duct invasion [52].

In addition to that, biliary drainage allows, in a second time, to treat some patients with TACE. A recent prospective study has shown that 39 out of 60 patients that had undergone a percutaneous or endoscopic biliary drainage achieved an adequate reduction of the bilirubin values (defined as a 70% reduction of the initial value or a reduction <2 mg/dl within 15 days after the procedure) with a median survival of 147 days vs 38 (p<0.001); among these 39 patients, those undergoing TACE as well (22 patients) achieved a longer median survival as compared to the patients undergoing only symptomatic palliative therapy (410 vs. 77 days, p<0.001) (Figure 2) [53].

Another retrospective study has evaluated the efficacy of the Percutaneous Transhepatic Biliary Drainage (PTBD) in 16 patients with obstructive jaundice due to neoplastic embolization of the biliary ducts in patients with HCC. The success rate of the procedure was 100%: 2 patients had an external drainage positioned, 7 an internal drainage and in 7 patients a covered internal stent was used with the removal of the external drainage. Symptoms and quality of life improved in 75% of patients (12 out of 16) [54].

According to a review by Minami and Kudo [51], the resolution of jaundice, by means of a biliary drainage, can facilitate the administration of specific anticancer treatments, increasing life expectancy and decreasing mortality.

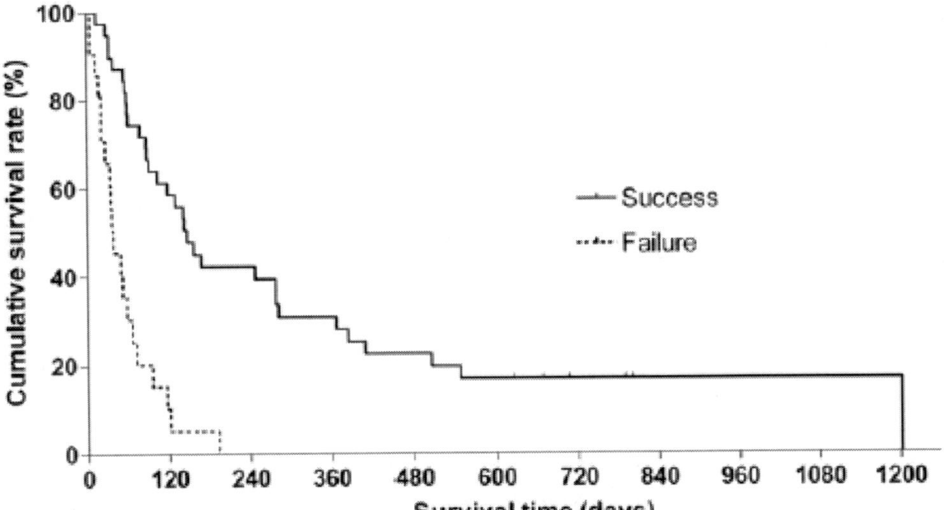

Figure 2. Cumulative survival rates in patients with unresectable hepatocellular carcinoma and obstructive jaundice according to successful drainage. Among 60 patients (39 achieved successful drainage and 21 did not), the median overall survival was 147 days in the successful drainage group, as compared with 38 days in the unsuccessful drainage group (P < .001, log-rank test). From Choi J, et al. [53].

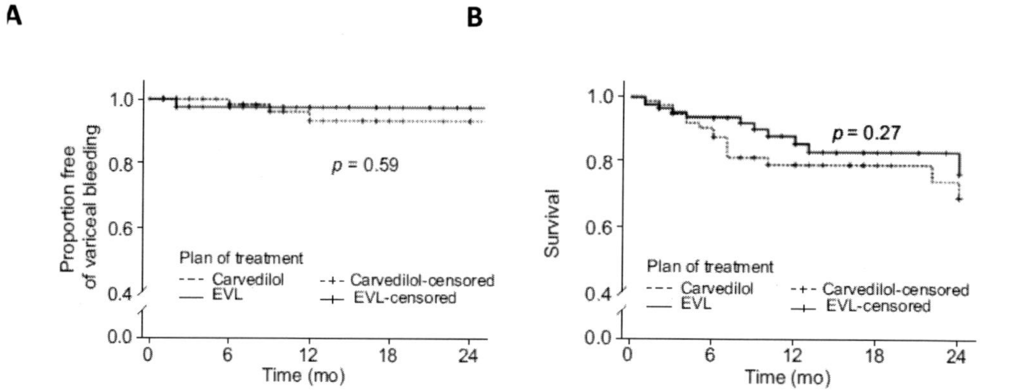

GI bleed (mo)	0	6	12	18	24
Carvedilol	82	82	55	28	17
EVL	86	84	57	30	19

Mortality	0	6	12	18	24 (mo)
Carvedilol	82	54	27	18	15
EVL	86	53	31	25	12

EVL: endoscopic variceal ligation.

Figure 3. A) Kaplan Meier survival curve estimating time to variceal bleeding; B) Overall mortality by plan of treatment. From Shah HA, et al. [57].

Hemorrhage

Hemorrhage can take place at the very end of life of these patients or during the metastatic period of the disease. In this last situation, endoscopy needs to be performed in order to be able to recognize the cause of bleeding and treat it by ligation or sclerosis of bleeding vessels.

At the end of life, on the contrary, bleeding must be regarded as the final event in the clinical history of the patient and treated as a "refractory" symptom by "palliative sedation." This result can be achieved by the administration of 5 mg Midazolam induction dose and subsequent infusion of the same medication subcutaneously or intravenously (0.2-0.5 mg per kg body weight in 24 hours or 1-4 mg/hour) to keep sedation.

Bleeding mortality in patients affected by HCC associated with cirrhosis is higher than in cirrhotic only patients [55].

The mortality rate of the first episode of bleeding from esophageal varices is high (20-35%) and the bleeding itself is a very traumatic event for the patient. The development of the "red-color" esophageal varices is a predictor of imminent bleeding, and its appearance is considered, in Japan, an indicator for the beginning of prophylactic therapy. There are two independent risk factors for the appearance of "red esophageal" varices and therefore the possibility of imminent hemorrhage: the detection of a tumoral thrombus in the portal vein and an HCC with a diameter greater than 5 cm; in these circumstances, a more aggressive therapy should be started to manage portal hypertension and prevent bleeding of esophageal varices [56].

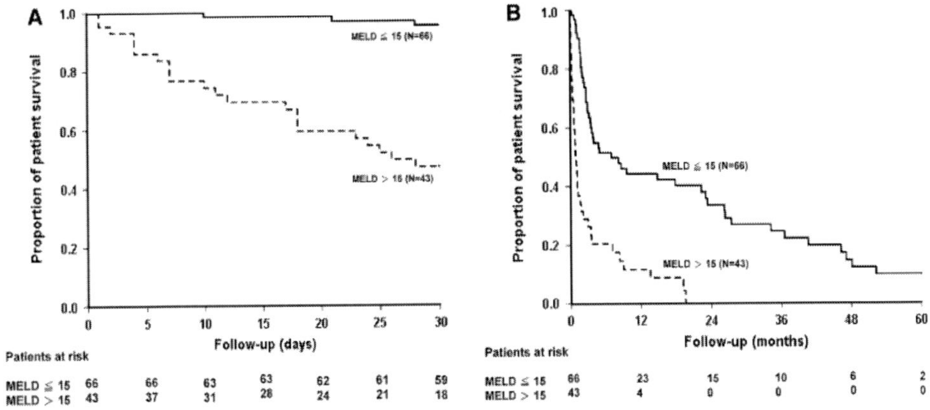

Figure 4. comparison of gastric variceal bleeding patients with Model for End stage Liver Disease (MELD) score >15 vs MELD <15. A) 30-day cumulative survival ($p < .0019$), B) 5-year cumulative survival ($p < 0.001$). From Chang CJ et al. [58].

A recent multicenter randomized trial, albeit with inadequate statistical power, suggests that, in cirrhotic patients, prophylactic therapy with carvedilol is no better than prophylactic variceal ligation to prevent first bleeding (Figure 3) [57].

The risk of developing a second variceal bleeding is increased in patients with newly diagnosed HCC (diagnosed two months before the first bleeding). The recent diagnosis of HCC, a high score (>15) according to the "Model for End-stage Liver Disease (MELD)," and active bleeding are prognostic factors of bleeding recurrence. The advanced stage of disease, a high MELD score and high levels of alanine aminotransferase (ALT) values are predictors of mortality (Figure 4) [58].

A recent Chinese study, conducted in only 11 patients, showed that a Trans-jugular Intrahepatic Portosystemic Shunt (TIPS) is technically feasible with good short-term efficacy in the management of complications: gastrointestinal bleeding was stopped in nine patients and in six patients encephalopathy was readily controlled with medical therapy [59].

Fever and Infections

Cirrhotic patients affected by HCC are susceptible to infections and fever is a common symptom. A number of contributing factors, such as the presence of ascites, immunosuppression, portal hypertension, gastrointestinal bleeding and invasive treatments, can facilitate bacterial infections. These involve in 25-50% the genitourinary tract, in 20% the respiratory system and 10-30% are represented by spontaneous bacterial peritonitis in the apparent absence of any intra-abdominal source of infection [60-64]. Genitourinary and upper respiratory tract infections can be managed at home with the administration of oral mono or poliantibiotic therapy; in case of peritonitis, endocarditis or pneumonia, the patient should be admitted to the hospice to facilitate the administration of intravenous antibiotic therapy and the monitoring of the clinical course.

Table 2. Reported cases of pulmonary oil embolism after TACE, from WU GC, et al. [65]

	Tumor Characteristics				Respiratory Symptoms		
Case (Reference)	Age/Sex	Size (cm)	AV Shunt (in Angiography)	IO (mL)	Symptoms	Onset	Outcome
1 (Chung et al.)	44/M	15 x 17	-	40	C, H, D, T	4th d	Recovered
2 (Chung et al.)	56/M	13 x 18	-	30	C, H	5th d	Recovered
3 (Chung et al.)	31/F	15 x 20	-	30	C, H, D, T	2nd d	Recovered
4 (Chung et al.)	61/M	12 x 18	-	26	C, D	4th d	Died
5 (Chung et al.)	57/M	17 x 20	-	25	C, H, D, T	2nd d	Recovered
6 (Chung et al.)	55/M	12 x 14	-	22	C, H, D	2nd d	Recovered
7 (Yamaura et al.)	7/child		-	14			Recovered
1 (Czauderna et al.)	7/girl	9 x 9	-	< 10	D,T	Immediately	Died
1 (Xia et al.)			-	25	C, D	6^{th}hr	Died
1 (Kwok et al.)	63/M	15	-	17	D	2nd d	Died

-, absent; AV shunt, arteriovenous shunting in the hepatocellular carcinoma; C, Cough; D, dyspnea; H, hemoptysis; IO, iodized oil; T, tachypnea.

Dyspnea

Dyspnea is present in 40% of patients with very advanced stage of the HCC; the etiology of is multifactorial: anemia, paralysis, and/or compression of the diaphragm by hepatomegaly and ascites, respiratory muscle weakness from cachexia.

The symptom may be also, as reported in the literature, a complication of interventional therapeutic procedures such as chemoembolization (TACE) or as a result of pulmonary embolism by lipiodol contrast medium (Table 2) [65].

Treatment implies an action on several factors favoring the development of the symptom and consists of: the reduction of the abdominal compression by means of paracentesis, the use of anabolic steroids to reduce muscle weakness, symptomatic treatment with glucocorticoid, opioids, and benzodiazepines, oxygen therapy, functional-rehabilitative and cognitive-behavioral interventions.

Rarely, but always to be considered, dyspnea may be caused, in advanced stages of disease, even by pleural localization, intrabronchial metastases or peribronchial lymph node involvement; in such circumstances, it is possible to manage symptoms with thoracentesis and subsequent chemical pleurodesis, intracavitary laser therapy, or placement of endobronchial stents in order to achieve a good clinical control for several weeks or even a few months [66, 67].

Finally, some case-reports describe patients with rapid onset of dyspnea caused by intracardiac metastases in which a clinical benefit was achieved by the surgical removal of the secondary localization [68, 69].

Depression

Depression is common in patients with ESLD; prevalence rate is 30 to 40% [70]. A more precise estimate is difficult to assess based on the inability to exclude hepatic encephalopathy as a cause of mood disturbance in terminally ill patients [71]. Depression in patients with ESLD has been shown to be associated with poor outcome compared with non-depressed patients with ESLD. Although an approach similar to managing depression in patients with advanced cancer seems applicable, there is need for more data regarding the management of depression in patients with ESLD. Treatment of depression in patients with HCC is a goal of palliative care because, associated with other mood disorders, depression has a correlation with the deterioration of the quality of life and the decreased adaptability.

In a study including 101 patients with hepatobiliary neoplasm, vascular invasion and level of depression were independent predictors of prognosis. The number of NK cells was significantly lower in patients with major depression than in the general population and correlated with survival. Therefore, a mediating role of NK cells was hypothesized between depressive symptoms and survival [20]. Should this hypothesis be confirmed, it would be necessary to seek actively, from the very beginning of the disease, depressive symptoms; early therapy would lead to an improvement in the effectiveness of the immune system with a possible gain in terms of survival time and quality of life.

Physicians, therefore, should learn to distinguish between the existential distress and clinical depression (carefully consider the sadness and anticipated mourning in terminal stage of the disease). Early detection of depression will allow a combined psychologic and pharmacologic approach, both often effective in other cancer settings.

Depression is often associated with sleep disorders (about 25% of patients with depression show sleep disorders); these are present in approximately 50% of patients with HCC and persist a month after palliative treatments such as TACE. This invasive procedure, in fact, can be responsible for symptoms such as pain and chest tightness that, if not properly controlled, can cause or induce the persistence of sleep disorders [72].

In a study by Huang and Lin, the authors suggest that depression, sleep disorders and fatigue are closely interrelated in patients suffering from HCC and that depression is a mediator between sleep disorders and fatigue [73]. Longitudinal studies show that sleepless subjects and patients with persistence of insomnia, at a second revaluation, have a higher risk of developing depression. Moreover, the onset of insomnia in adolescence is related to an increased chance of developing depression in adulthood. Furthermore, epidemiological studies that have assessed fatigue without clear etiology have shown that depression is a strong predictor of chronic and newly diagnosed fatigue; fatigue is, in turn, a predictor and a result of depression.

In patients suffering from HCC these three symptoms are often simultaneously present and should therefore be evaluated and treated at the same time (Figure 5) [74].

Renal Failure and Hepatorenal Syndrome

Hepatorenal syndrome (HRS) is a severe functional renal failure occurring in patients with cirrhosis and ascites. It develops as a consequence of the severe reduction in the renal perfusion secondary to splanchnic arterial vasodilation. Arterial vasodilation leads to a decrease in the effective blood volume, homeostatic activation of vasoactive systems such as rennin-angiotensin-aldosterone system (RAAS), antidiuretic hormone (ADH) and sympathetic nervous system, and, consequently, renal vasoconstriction [75]. HRS is sub-classified into types 1 and 2. Type 1 HRS is characterized by rapid progressive renal failure, usually accompanied by multiorgan failure. Type 2 HRS manifests itself as a slowly progressive functional renal failure associated with refractory ascites. A 40% premature mortality rate has been reported in type 1 HRS [76], but may be as high as 83% [77]. Mortality associated with type 2 HRS ranges from 20% to 60%.

ESLD is often associated with renal failure that may be due to pre-renal causes such as hypovolaemia after bleeding, diarrhea, vomiting, and inadequate diuretic therapy.

Sometimes it is the result of iatrogenic causes such as drugs that reduce renal perfusion (NSAIDs, ACE-inhibitors) or nephrotoxic drugs (aminoglycosides).

Finally, glomerulonephritis and viral or immune-mediated nephropathy can occur in cirrhotic patients. Treatment consists in removing the toxic drug and in expanding plasma volume (both in renal and pre-renal kidney failure).

The therapeutic approach consists in the management of ascites and the administration of perfusion-increasing drugs such as dopamine at sub-pressor doses and albumin.

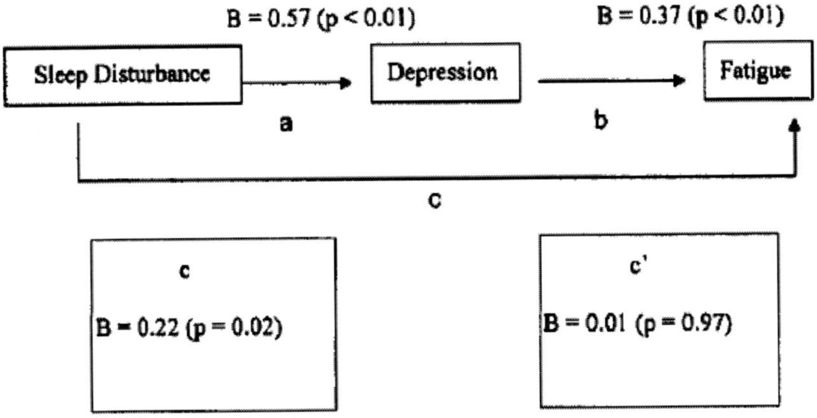

B: Bivariate Pearson Correlation;
a: correlation between independent variable "sleep disturbance" and presumed mediator "depression"
b: correlation between presumed mediator "depression" and outcome variable "fatigue"
c: correlation between outcome variable "fatigue" and independent variable "sleep disturbance"
c': correlation between fatigue with both independent variable "sleep disturbance" and presumed mediator "depression."

Figure 5. Depression is a mediator between sleep disorders and fatigue in hepatocellular carcinoma. Results of the mediation model. Modified from Huang TW et al. [73].

REFERENCES

[1] Natsuizaka, M; Omura, T; Akaike, T; et al. Clinical features of hepatocellular carcinoma with extrahepatic metastases. *J GastroenterolHepatol*, 2007, 20(11), 1781-1787.

[2] Uka, K; Aikata, H; Takaki, S; et al. Clinical features and prognosis of patients with extrahepatic metastases from hepatocellular carcinoma. *World J Gastroenterol*, 2007, 13(3), 414-420.

[3] Lin, M-H; Wu, P-Y; Tsai, S-T; et al. Hospice palliative care for patients with hepatocellular carcinoma in Taiwan. *Palliat Med*, 2004, 18, 93-99.

[4] Walsh, D; Donnelly, S; Rybicki, I. The symptoms of advanced cancer. Relationship to age, gender and performance status in, 1000 patients. *Support Care Cancer*, 2000, 8, 175-179.

[5] Itoh, Y; Ohkubo, K; Iuchi, H; et al. Chronological changes of causes of death and distant metastasis in hepatocellular carcinoma. *Oncol Rep*, 2002,9, 331-335.

[6] Kim, SU; Kim, do Y; Park, JY;et al. Hepatocellular carcinoma presenting with bone metastasis: clinical characteristics and prognostic factors. *J Cancer Res ClinOncol*, 2008, 134(12), 1377-1384.

[7] Dworkin, RH; O'Connor, A; Backonja, M; et al. Pharmacologic management of neuropathic pain: evidence-based recommendations. *Pain*, 2007, 132(3), 237-251.

[8] Chow, E; Harris, K; Fan, G; et al. Palliative radiotherapy trials for bone metastases: a systematic review. *J ClinOncol*, 2007, 25, 1423-1436.

[9] Wong, R; Wiffen, PJ. Bisphosphonates for the relief of pain secondary to bone metastases. *Cochrane Database Systematic Reviews.*, 2002, (2) CD002068.

[10] Radbruch, L; Strasser, F; Elsner, F; et al. Fatigue in palliative cancer patients – an EAPC approach. *Palliat Med*, 2008, 22, 13-32.

[11] Dy, SM; Lorenz, KA; Naeim, A; et al. Evidence-based recommendations for cancer fatigue, anorexia, depression and dyspnea. *J ClinOncol*, 2008, 26(23), 3886-3895.

[12] Bruera, E; Valero, V; Driver, L; et al. Patient-controlled methylphenidate for cancer fatigue: a double-blind, randomized, placebo-controlled trial. *J ClinOncol*, 2006, 24(13), 2073-2078.

[13] Courneya, KS; Mackey, JR; Bell, GJ; et al. Randomized controlled trial of exercise training in postmenopausal breast cancer survivors: cardiopulmonary and quality of life outcomes. *J ClinOncol*, 2003, 21(9), 1660–1668.

[14] Dimeo, FC; Stieglitz, RD; Novelli-Fischer, U; et al. Effects of physical activity on the fatigue and psychologic status of cancer patients during chemotherapy *Cancer*, 1999, 85(10), 2273–2277.

[15] Mock V. Evidence-based treatment for cancer-related fatigue. *J Natl Cancer InstMonogr*, 2004, (32), 112–118.

[16] Schwartz, AL; Mori, M; Gao, R; et al. Exercise reduces daily fatigue in women with breast cancer receiving chemotherapy. *Med Sci Sports Exerc*, 2001, 33(5), 718–723.

[17] Segal, RJ; Reid, RD; Courneya, KS; et al. Resistance exercise in men receiving androgen deprivation therapy for prostate cancer. *J ClinOncol*, 2003, 21(9), 1653–1659.

[18] Walko, CM; Grande, C. Management of common adverse events in patients treated with sorafenib: nurse and pharmacist perspective. *Seminars in Oncology*, 2014,41(S2), S17-28.

[19] Pascual, López A;Roqué, i Figuls M;Urrútia, Cuchi G; et al. Systematic review of megestrol acetate in the treatment of anorexia-cachexia syndrome. *J Pain Symptom Manage*, 2004,27(4), 360-369.

[20] Steel, JL;Geller, DA;Gamblin, TC;et al. Depression, immunity, and survival in patients with hepatobiliary carcinoma. *J ClinOncol*, 2007, 25 (17), 2397-2405.

[21] Kremer, AE; Martens, JJ; Kulik, W; et al. Lysophosphatidic acid is a potential mediator of cholestatic pruritus. *Gastroenterology*, 2010, 139, 1008-1018.

[22] Oude, Elferink RP; Kremer, AE; Beuers, U. Mediators of pruritus during cholestasis. *CurrOpinGastroenterol*, 2011,27, 307-312.

[23] Levy, C. Management of pruritus in patients with cholestatic liver disease. GastroenterolHepatol (NY) 2011, 7(9), 615-617.

[24] Kremer, AE; Bolier, R; van Dijk, R; et al. Advances in pathogenesis and management of pruritus in cholestasis. *Dig Dis.*, 2014, 32(5), 637-645.

[25] Sanchez, W; Talwalkar, JA. Palliative care for patients with end-stage liver disease ineligible for liver transplantation. *GastroenterolClin North Am*, 2006, 35(1), 201-2019.

[26] Pérez-Soler, R; Delord, JP; Halpern, A; et al. HER1/EGFR inhibitor-associated rash: future directions for management and investigation outcomes from the HER1/EGFR inhibitor rash management forum. *Oncologist*, 2005, 10(5), 345-56.

[27] Brose, MS; Frenette, CT; Keefe, SM; et al. Management of sorafenib-related adverse events: a clinician's perspective. *Seminars in Oncology*, 2014,41 (S2), S1-16.

[28] Poh, Z; Chang, PEJ. A current review of the diagnostic and treatment strategies of hepatic encephalopathy. *Int J Hepatol*, 2012, 2012, 480309.

[29] Ferenci, P; Lockwood, A; Mullen, K; et al. Hepatic encephalopathy – definition, nomenclature, diagnosis, and quantification: final report of the working party at the,

11th World Congress of Gastroenterology, Vienna, 1998. *Hepatology*, 2002, 35(3), 716-721.
[30] Blei, AT; Cordoba, J. Hepatic encephalopathy. *American J Gastroenterol*, 2001, 96(7), 1968-1976.
[31] Bass, NM. Review article: The current pharmacological therapies for hepatic encephalopathy. *Aliment PharmacolTher*, 2007, 25, 23-31.
[32] Garcovich, M; Zocco, MA; Roccarina, D; et al. Prevention and treatment of hepatic encephalopathy: focusing on gut microbiota. *World J Gastroenterol*, 2012, 18(46), 6693-6700.
[33] Suzuki, H; Asakawa, A; Amitani, H; et al. Cancer cachexia – pathophysiology and management. *J Gastroenterol*, 2013, 48, 574-594.
[34] O'Keefe, SJ; Ogden, J; Ramjee, G; Rund, J. Contribution of elevated protein turnover and anorexia to cachexia in patients with hepatocellular carcinoma. *Cancer Research*, 1990, 50(4), 1226-1230.
[35] Radbruch, L; Elsner, F; Trottenberg, P; et al. Clinical practice guidelines on cancer cachexia in advanced cancer patients. 2010, Aachen, Department of Palliative Medicinen/European Palliative Cancer Research Collaborative.
[36] Yavuzsen, T; Davis, MP;Walsh, D; et al. Systematic review of the treatment of cancer-associated anorexia and weight loss. *J ClinOncol*, 2005, 23(33), 8500-8511.
[37] Nelson, KA. The cancer anorexia-cachexia syndrome. *SeminOncol*, 2000, 27(1), 64-68.
[38] Argiles, JM; Meijsing, SH; Pallarés-Trujillo, J; et al. Cancer cachexia: a therapeutic approach. *Med Res Rev*. 2000, 21(1), 83-101.
[39] Inui, A. Cancer anorexia-cachexia syndrome: current issues in research and management. *CA Cancer J Clin*, 2002, 52(2), 72-91.
[40] Fearon, KCH. Cancer cachexia: developing multimodal therapy for a multidimensional problem. *Eur J Cancer*, 2008, 44, 1124-1132.
[41] Ravasco, P; Monteiro-Grillo, I; Vidal, PM;Camilo, ME. Dietary counselling improves patient outcomes: a prospective, randomized, controlled trial in colorectal cancer patients undergoing radiotherapy. *J ClinOncol*, 2005, 23(7), 1431–1438.
[42] Strasser, F. Eating-related disorders in patients with advanced cancer. *Support Care Cancer*, 2003, 11(1), 11-20.
[43] Rosenberg, SM. Palliation of malignant ascites. *GastroenterolClin North Am*, 2006,25, 189-99.
[44] Mercadante, S; Intravaia, G; Ferrera, P;et al. Peritoneal catheter for continuous drainage of ascites in advanced cancer patients.*Support Care Cancer*, 2008, 16(8), 975-78.
[45] Runyon, BA. Management of adult patients with ascites caused by cirrhosis. *Hepatology*, 1998, 27, 264-272.
[46] Fogel, MR; Sawhney, VK; Neal, EA; et al. Diuresis in the ascitic patient: a randomized controlled trial of three regimens. *J ClinGastroenterol*, 1981, 3(1), 73-80.
[47] Perez-Ayuso, RM; Arroyo, V; Planas, R; et al. Randomized comparative study of efficacy of furosemide versus spironolactone in nonazotemic cirrhosis with ascites: relationship between the diuretic response and the activity of the renin-aldosterone system. *Gastroenterology*, 1983, 84(5 Pt 1), 961-968.
[48] Sola-Vera, J; Minana, J; Ricart, E; et al. Randomized trial comparing albumine and saline in the prevention of paracentesis-induced circulatory dysfunction in cirrhotic patients with ascites. *Hepatology*, 2003, 37, 1147-1153.

[49] Baron, TH. Palliation of malignant obstructive jaundice. *Gastroenterol Clin North Am*, 2006, 35, 101-112.

[50] Bergasa, NV. Medical palliation of the jaundiced patients with pruritus. *GastroenterolClin North Am*, 2006, 35, 113-123.

[51] Minami, Y; Kudo, M. Hepatocellular carcinoma with obstructive jaundice: endoscopic and percutaneous biliary drainage. *Dig Dis.*, 2012, 30(6), 592-597.

[52] Kawaguchi, Y; Ogawa, M; Maruno, A; et al. A case of successful placement of a fully covered metallic stent for hemobilia secondary to hepatocellular carcinoma with bile duct invasion. *Case Rep Oncol*, 2012, 5, 682–686.

[53] Choi, J; Ryu, JK; Lee, SH; et al. Palliative treatment of unresectable hepatocellular carcinoma with obstructive jaundice using biliary drainage with subsequent transarterial chemoembolization. *J Palliat Med.*, 2013, 16(9), 1026-33.

[54] Lu, Z; Sun, W; Wen, F; et al. Clinical application of percutaneous drainage in treating hepatocellular carcinoma with bile duct tumor thrombus. *ContempOncol (Pozn)*, 2013,17(2), 176-183.

[55] Singal, AK; Jampana, SC;Singal, V;Kuo, YF. Hepatocellular carcinoma predicts in-hospital mortality from acute variceal hemorrhage among patients with cirrhosis. *J ClinGastroenterol*, 2012, 46(7), 613-619.

[56] Kadouchi, K; Higuchi, K; Shiba, M; et al. What are the risk factors for aggravation of esophageal varices in patients with hepatocellular carcinoma? *J GastroenterolHepatol.*, 2007, 22(2), 240-6.

[57] Shah, HA; Azam, Z; Rauf, J; et al. Carvedilol vs. esophageal variceal band ligation in the primary prophylaxis of variceal hemorrhage: a multicentre randomized controlled trial. *J Hepatol.*, 2014, 60(4), 757-64.

[58] Chang, CJ; Hou, MC; Liao, WC; et al. Risk factors of early re-bleeding and mortality in patients with ruptured gastric varices and concomitant hepatocellular carcinoma. *J Gastroenterol*, 2012, 47(5), 531-9.

[59] Zhao, JB; Feng, C; Zhu, QH; et al. Transjugular intrahepatic portosystemic shunt with covered stents for hepatocellular carcinoma with portal vein tumor thrombosis. *World J Gastroenterol*, 2014, 20(6), 1602-1607.

[60] Johnson, DH; Cunha, BA. Infections in cirrhosis. *Infect Dis Clin North Am.*, 2001, 15, 363-371.

[61] Borzio, M; Salerno, F; Piantoni, L; et al. Bacterial infection in patients with advanced cirrhosis: a multicentre prospective study. *Dig Liver Dis*, 2001, 33(1), 41-48.

[62] Goulis, J; Patch, D; Borroughs, AK. Bacterial infection in the pathogenesis of variceal bleeding. *Lancet*, 1999, 353, 139-142.

[63] Navasa, M; Rimola, A; Rodés, J. Bacterial infections in liver disease. *Semin Liver Dis*, 1997, 17(4)323-333.

[64] Garcia-Tsao, G. Bacterial infection in cirrhosis: treatment and prophylaxis. *J Hepatol*, 2005, 42S:85-92.

[65] Wu, GC; Peng, WC; Chen, CW; et al. Acute respiratory distress syndrome after transcatheter arterial chemoembolization of hepatocellular carcinomas. *Am J Med Sci.*, 2009, 338(5), 357-60.

[66] Weng, MT; Wong, JM; Wei, SC. Dyspnea and shoulder pain in a patient with hepatocellular carcinoma. *ClinGastroenterolHepatol.*, 2013 Jun, 11(6), e41.

[67] Hamai, Y; Hihara, J; Aoki, Y; et al. Airway stenting for tracheal obstruction due to lymph node metastasis of hepatocellular carcinoma. *Anticancer Res.*, 2013, 33(4), 1761-1764.

[68] Ulus, T; Birdane, A; Dündar, E; Tünerir, B. Asymptomatic course of a metastatic mass completely filling the right atrium in a patient with hepatocellular carcinoma. *Turk Kardiyol Dern Ars.*, 2012, 40(1), 52-54.

[69] Seo, JB; Kim, JS; Jeong, DS; et al. A case of left atrial metastasis from hepatocellular carcinoma: life-saving palliative resection using cardiopulmonary bypass. *Korean Circ J.*, 2011, 41(9), 542-545.

[70] Singh, N; Gayowski, T; Wagener, MM; Marino, IR. Depression in patients with cirrhosis: impact on outcome. *Dig Dis Sci*, 1997, 42, 1421-1427.

[71] Lin, MH; Wu, PY; Tsai, ST; et al. Hospice palliative care for patients with hepatocellular carcinoma in Taiwan. *Palliat Med*, 2004, 18, 93-99.

[72] Chu, TL; Yu, WP; Chen, SC; et al. Comparison of differences and determinants between presence and absence of sleep disturbance in hepatocellular carcinoma patients. *CancerNurs.*, 2011, 34(5), 354-360.

[73] Huang, TW; Lin, CC. The mediating effects of depression on sleep disturbance and fatigue: symptom clusters in patients with hepatocellular carcinoma. *CancerNurs.*, 2009, 32(5), 398-403.

[74] Jozuka, H; Jozuka, E; Suzuki, M; et al. Psycho-neuro-immunological treatment of hepatocellular carcinoma with major depression--a single case report. *CurrMed Res Opin.*, 2003, 19(1), 59-63.

[75] Arroyo, V; Fernandez, J. Management of hepatorenal syndrome in patients with cirrhosis. *NatRevNephrol*, 2011, 7, 517–526.

[76] Salerno, F; Cazzaniga, M; Merli, M; Spinzi, G; Saibeni, S; et al. Diagnosis, treatment and survival of patients with hepatorenal syndrome: a survey on daily medical practice. *J Hepatol*, 2011, 55,1241–1248.

[77] Carvalho, GC; Regis, Cde A; Kalil, JR; Cerqueira, LA; Barbosa, DS; et al. Causes of renal failure in patients with decompensated cirrhosis and its impact in hospital mortality. *Ann Hepatol*, 2012, 11, 90–95.

In: Hepatocellular Carcinoma in the 3rd Millennium
Editors: M. Berretta and B. Cacopardo
ISBN: 978-1-63484-025-5

Chapter 11

New Entities in the Treatment of Hepatocellular Carcinoma: HIV-Positive and Elderly Patients

Massimiliano Berretta[1,2], Valli De Re[3], Paolo De Paoli[4], Vincenzo Canzonieri[5], Raffaele Di Francia[2,6], Fabrizio Di Benedetto[7] and Umberto Tirelli[1]

[1]Medical Oncology A Unit, National Cancer Institute, IRCCS, Aviano (PN), Italy
[2]GORI, Gruppo Oncologico Ricercatori Italiani, Pordenone (PN), Italy
[3]Facility of Bio-Proteomics/BIT, National Cancer Institute, IRCCS, Aviano (PN), Italy
[4]Scientific Directorate, National Cancer Institute, IRCCS, Aviano (PN), Italy
[5]Pathology Unit, National Cancer Institute, IRCCS, Aviano (PN), Italy
[6]Department of Haematology, National Cancer Institute, Fondazione "G. Pascale," IRCCS, Naples, Italy
[7]Liver and Multivisceral Transplant Center, Univeristy of Modena and Reggoi Emilia, Modena, Italy

Abstract

The hepatocellular carcinoma (HCC) is the most common primary cancer of the liver and, according to the WHO report, the fourth commonest cause of death. The estimated incidence of new cases worldwide is about 500,000-1,000,000 per year, causing 600,000 deaths globally per year. The incidence of HCC has been rising in developed western countries in the last two decades, along with the emergence of hepatitis C virus infection and to the rise of immigration rates from HBV-endemic countries.

In addition, even though the incidence of HCC reaches its highest peak among persons over 65 years, an increased incidence among younger individuals has been noted in the last two decades both in USA and Europe. In the last decades two kinds of HCC patients are more interesting, for clinical characteristics, than typical patients with HCC: elderly and HIV-positive patients.

In fact due to the increase of the life expectancy in many countries, HCC represents a new challenge in this particular setting of patients.

INTRODUCTION

The hepatocellular carcinoma (HCC) is the most common primary cancer of the liver [1] and, according to the WHO report [2], the fourth commonest cause of death. The estimated incidence of new cases worldwide is about 500,000-1,000,000 per year, causing 600,000 deaths globally per year [3] Although there are large areas of the world where the incidence of HCC is still unknown [4-6], several countries like East Asia and some Sub-Saharan African regions result to be affected by a very high prevalence of HCC (over 20 cases/100,000 population) [7].

Areas with moderately high risk (11-20 cases/100,000 population) include Italy, Spain and Latin America; conversely France, Germany and the United Kingdom have an intermediate risk (5-10 cases/ 100,000 population). A relatively low prevalence (less than 5 cases/100,000 population) is found in United States, Canada and Scandinavia.

The incidence of HCC has been rising in developed western countries *during* the last two decades [1-8] along with the emergence of hepatitis C virus infection and to the *increase* of immigration rates from HBV-endemic countries. In addition, even though the incidence of HCC reaches its highest peak among persons over 65 years [9], an increased incidence among younger individuals has been noted in the last two decades both in USA and Europe.

In the last decades two kinds of HCC patients are more interesting, for clinical characteristics, than typical patients with HCC: elderly and HIV-positive patients. In fact due to the increase of the life expectancy in many countries, HCC represents a new challenge in this particular setting of patients.

HCC IN HIV-POSITIVE PATIENTS

The survival rates of patients with human immunodeficiency virus (HIV) have been dramatically improved after the advent of highly active antiretroviral treatment (HAART), and HIV related morbidity and mortality have been remarkably decreased [10, 11]. At the same time, the morbidity and mortality related to many different non–HIV-related diseases, such as chronic liver diseases (CLDs) has shown a significant increase [12, 13]. In fact, up to 50% of deaths among people with HIV infection now accounts for end-stage liver diseases (ESLDs), which are primarily related to complications of chronic hepatitis B virus (HBV) or hepatitis C virus (HCV) co infection, as well as hepatotoxicity associated with antiretroviral therapy and alcohol use [14-16].

Mortality associated with HCV infection is expected to continue to increase over the next 25 years [17, 18]. In a national survey on deaths among HIV-infected patients, liver diseases represented the third most frequent underlying cause of death [18].

HIV-infected patients have a sevenfold higher risk for HCC than the general population [19, 20]. Since the introduction of HAART, no decrease in the incidence of HCC has been observed, unlike for other HIV-associated cancers [20-22].

In the general population, HCC occurs several decades after the initial infection with HCV or HBV [21, 23, 24]. Large retrospective cohort studies *have* also excluded that HIV infection alone may be a risk factor for HCC [22]. The HIV co infection with HCV or HBV is common and a significantly higher risk for developing HCC, as a result of chronic viral hepatitis, is well documented.

Little is known about the HIV and HBV and/or HCV interaction over the long term. HIV co infection seems to accelerate disease progression and to reduce the efficacy of anti-HCV and anti-HBV treatments.

Conversely, it is uncertain whether HIV infection directly increases the likelihood of HCC in patients with viral hepatitis [25-28]. HAART, besides its potential indirect effects on HCC risk through improvements in immune reconstitution and survival, is known to have some direct hepatotoxic effects, especially among HIV-infected patients with chronic HBV or HCV infections [16, 29]. A large retrospective cohort study on US veterans demonstrated that HIV positive persons had a higher risk to develop HCC than HIV negative ones but, after adjusting for HCV and alcohol abuse, HIV status was not independently associated with cancer [30].

Also the 2001 French Mortavic study [31], a prospective 1-year cohort study involving 25,178 HIV positive patients (enrolled between 1995 to 1997), showed a significant increase in death from ESLD and HCC. Death due to ESLD rose from 1.5% to 14.3% whereas HCC-related mortality rose 5-fold, from 4.7% to 25%; interestingly, all HCC deaths were in patients HCV co-infection. Throughout the same period, AIDS-related mortality rate fell from 91.6% (in 1995) to 48.7%, suggesting that the increased HCC rate in the 2001 cohort could be due to the increased longevity of patients in the HAART era.

In a prospectively followed cohort of HIV-infected individuals, HCC deaths related to HCV infection raised from 10% in 2000 to 25% in 2005 [32]. In contrast, the incidence of HCC development and related deaths among HIV-HBV co-infected individuals seemed to be stable [32]. A retrospective study conducted between 1991 and 2000 on a cohort of US veterans with hepatitis C [33] showed that the incidence of HCC did not differ between HIV/HCV co-infected and HCV mono-infected patients in the HAART era, whereas it was significantly lower among HIV/HCV co-infected individuals previously to HAART introduction, demonstrating that, in the pre-HAART-era, HIV patients' deaths occurred before the development of HCC. Furthermore, in countries where HAART is largely unavailable, other retrospective studies confirmed the incidence of HCC to be lower or equal to that of the average population [34, 35].

In 2004, the Italian Cooperative Group on AIDS and Tumours (GICAT) [36], identified a total of 41 consecutive patients with HCC (from a joint Italian and Spanish database) and retrospectively investigated their main epidemiological characteristics comparing them with those of 384 HIV negative controls, diagnosed over the same period. The GICAT study emphasized the younger age of HIV positive patients at the diagnosis of HCC (age 40-46 vs. 60-70 in HIV negatives).

In most studies HCV infection was the main risk factor for HCC development in both HIV positive and negative subjects.

The median time to develop HCC after HCV infection was found to be around 22 years in HIV positive patients: 10 years shorter than that reported among HIV negative patients that acquired HCV infection with transfusion [37].

Alcohol abuse (a risk behaviour often associated with HIV) and insulin resistance (which causes non alcoholic fatty liver disease and frequently occurs in HIV-infected individuals submitted to protease inhibitors) are other potential risk factors for HCC development among the HIV-positive population [38, 39].

HIV-HBV and HIV-HCV Co-Infection: Prevalence and Significance of a Complex Interaction

HIV-infected persons are often HCV and/or HBV co-infected, because of shared routes of transmission. The prevalence of co-infection differs according to the demographic characteristics of infected patients and their geographic origin [40]. In the Western countries around 25% of patients are HIV-HCV co-infected [41]; in Europe, for instance, the prevalence of HIV/HCV co-infection ranges from 33% to 75% when considering intravenous drug users (IVDUs) according to the European SIDA cohort data on 3,048 HIV positive patients [42]. Also in the USA, the highest rates of HIV/HCV co-infection can be seen among IVDUs [43]. In Europe, up to 9% of HIV positive patients are also HBsAg positive [44, 45]; e.g., in Italy, between 3% and 4% of HIV positive individuals carry HBsAg [46]. The data might be inaccurate, due to a large number of occult HBV infections, associated to detectable HBV DNA on quantitative polymerase chain reaction (PCR) [47, 48].

HCV typically develops in HCC through the stage of cirrhosis, occurring in about 28-30 years [49, 50]. Cirrhosis leads to the development of HCV-related HCC. HCV do not integrate into the host genome and probably hepatocarcinogenesis in patients with HCV relate to the immune-mediated inflammation and hepatocellular damage. HBV chronic infection represents another major cause for HCC [51] but, unlikely HCV, it may occur in HBsAg carriers without cirrhosis, because the direct involvement of many viral-related factors such as viral proteins, BCP mutation in the viral genome, and Pre-S deletion mutants [52, 53]. Furthermore, HBV can integrate its DNA into the host genome, with several mutagenic consequences, including large inverted duplications, deletions, amplifications and translocation, resulting in chromosomal instability [53-55]. As expected, patients with both HCV-HBV infections are more likely to develop HCC than those mono-infected, therefore, HBV vaccination should be highly recommended to all patients with chronic hepatitis C [56]. The role of HIV on cancer has been long investigated. Murine models in vivo studies have revealed a possible role of the HIV Tat gene in liver tumorigenesis [53-55]. A higher incidence of HCC and other extra-hepatic malignancies has been found in transgenic mice expressing this gene emphasizing that the oncogenic effect of Tat gene is not potentially liver-specific. Tat gene seems to be able to stimulate cell proliferation, because of its anti-apoptotic activity [57, 58] angiogenic functions [59, 60] and ability to induce expression of growth factors [61], cytokines [62, 63] and transcription factors [64]. This experimental datum contrasts with many epidemiological studies that deny any particular role of HIV itself on HCC development. In large retrospective study by Giordano et al. [27], it has been shown that HCC rate among HIV mono-infected patients is similar to that in the general population.

Despite the missing demonstration that HIV itself might be the cause for HCC, it has been *proved* that the progression of HCV- and HBV-liver disease to cirrhosis and HCC could be accelerate by HIV. In fact, the co-infection with HIV alters the natural history of HCV increasing the probability of chronicity (over 90%) because the significant lack of CD4+ T-cell responses against HCV [65, 66]. Moreover, in the HIV setting, when the chronic HCV infection is established, the liver disease progression results more rapid, ensuing a higher incidence of cirrhosis and its complications, than in patients with only HCV infection [67-70]. The molecular mechanisms of accelerated fibrosis in co-infected patients are yet to be understood. Bruno et al. [71], studied the HIV-gp120 capability to exert multiple effects on human hepatic stellate cells (HSCs), modulating their phenotype in a profibrogenic way.

Incubation of HSCs with gp120 significantly increased HSCs migration and expression of proinflammatory cytokines, as well as monocyte chemo attractant protein-1 (MCP-1) and type 1 procollagen. Recent data suggest that HIV gp-120 binding to CXCR4 receptor, expressed on the surface of hepatocytes and HSCs, is able to up regulate tumour necrosis factor (TNF)-related apoptosis, inducing ligand (TRAIL) R2 expression. Results indicated that HIV infection makes hepatocytes more susceptible to liver injury [72]. During HIV co-infection, the hepatotoxicity of antiretroviral drugs and immune reconstitution syndrome may also indirectly increase the liver damage [32].

Further prospective studies are recommended to further evaluate the role of HIV in co-infected subjects with HCC. It would be necessary to avoid common bias, quite frequent in some of the quoted retrospective cohort studies. For example, the prevalence of HCV-HBV-HIV co-infections could be underestimated because not all HCV-HBV patients have been tested for HIV. Furthermore, time of viral hepatitis infection is often unknown, making it difficult to correlate HCC rates to mono- or co-infection. In fact, patients with isolated HCV or HBV may just have acquired infection earlier than co-infected patients and this different period of exposure to viral insult may obviously influence HCC incidence. Considering these evaluations, an ideal prospective study should include cross-testing for co-infections before individual allocation to groups, standardized screening for HCC and regular evaluation of HIV viral load in the co-infected cohort, in order to evaluate the potential effect of HAART-induced viral suppression on HCC pathogenesis.

Clinical Characteristics

HCC is generally asymptomatic during its initial stage, then, in more advanced phases, hepatomegaly, jaundice and abdominal pain may appear. However, HCC clinical presentation and prognosis vary considerably according to the number and size of tumoral lesions.

Liver cancer may appear either as a single nodular or infiltrating lesion with an eccentric growth or as a multinodular widespread tumour *ab initio*. In some patients HCC lesions have a slow growth rate, with a two-fold increase in 20 months, in other cases it could double in less than one month [73-75]. Multinodular HCC is more common in patients with more than one risk factor [76] and is classified in primitive multicentric HCC or metastatic cancer from a primitive HCC. This distinction has important clinical implications because primitive multicentric HCC are less aggressive and recur less frequently after ablation than metastatic cancers from a primitive HCC [77, 78]. Among HIV positive patients cumulative clinical data suggest a more aggressive course of HCC [79-81]. Data from the HIV-HCC Italian-Spanish Group [82] showed a more advanced and infiltrating HCC (also with extra nodal metastases), a more advanced stage of cirrhosis at presentation and a reduced survival rate in HIV-positive patients compared with the general population. A 2007 US-Canadian multicenter retrospective study [83] identified 63 HIV-infected patients affected by HCC from 1992 to 2005 and compared them to 226 HIV-negative HCC controls. The HIV positive group was younger and more frequently symptomatic than controls and showed higher median alpha-fetoprotein levels. In contrast with other studies, in this case tumour staging and survival were similar between cases and controls. In untreated HCC cases, the presence of undetectable HIV-RNA was an independent predictor of a better survival. In a recent, large, multicenter, observational study, Berretta et al. [84], confirmed HIV-positive HCC subjects to be younger and to have a shorter survival time after treatment than HIV-negative patients.

HCC: Treatment Options

The curative therapeutic strategies' for HCC in patients with HIV are often compromised because the advanced stage at presentation. Until a few years ago, HIV infection was an exclusion criterion for liver transplantation. The main concerns were the risk of HIV progression after orthoptic liver transplantation (OLT), a poor post-transplantation prognosis and eventually a waste of graft [85]. In 2003, Ettorre et al. [86] demonstrated that about 50% of HIV-positive patients with HCC were not suitable for surgical treatment and only 28% of these patients were more likely to receive a successful surgical treatment.

Later, the GICAT cohort reported on a series of 41 HIV positive patients affected by HCC, 15 (35%) of whom fulfilled the Milan criteria and could potentially be treated with OLT as a curative intent. Despite these results, none of them received liver transplantation and only two underwent surgical resection resulting in a 2-year survival of 41% in treated patients and 0% in untreated cases [36].

The introduction of HAART has significantly changed the outcome of HIV infection, increasing patients' long-term survival. Liver transplantation should then be taken in consideration in the treatment of HCC. Many studies have proved that the majority of HIV positive transplanted patients have a good long-term survival [87, 85]. A 2008 report of Di Benedetto et al. [85] has shown a series of 7 HIV positive patients with HCC and fulfilling the Milan criteria, who have received OLT. After a mean follow up of 232 days, the overall survival rate was 85.7%; only one patient died of a myocardial infarction with a functioning graft and no HCC recurrence. Radecke et al. [88] reported that out of 5 cases of OLT in HIV-infected cirrhotic subjects. In this study, 2 patients achieved stable liver function and non-progressive HIV infection under HAART, 61 and 23 months after OLT, respectively; unfortunately, three out of five patients died because of graft failure.

The liver post-transplant clinical management in the HIV-positive setting is definitely more complex than in the general population. These patients report an earlier and more aggressive HCV recurrence (about 33% of patients) [89], fast occurrence of hepatic fibrosis, a higher rate of rejection (from 33% to 38%) [85, 87-90] and a greater incidence of tacrolimus toxicity [91].

The outcome of HIV-positive liver recipients depends on the immunological status of the patient at the time of OLT [92]. A full virological control of the underlying HIV infection before OLT is considered necessary; in fact, the clinical course of HIV-positive patients transplanted patients with higher CD4+ cell count and undetectable HIV viral load is similar to that of HIV negative recipients. Di Benedetto et al. proposed some criteria to select HIV positive patients with HCC eligible to OLT: the completely fulfil of the Milan criteria is mandatory, patients should also have an undetectable HIV viral load (< 50 copies/mL) and a CD4+ cell count greater than 200/mmc. After OLT, HAART needs to be reinstituted as soon as clinically possible according to the opinion of a multidisciplinary transplant team (surgeons, infectivologists and oncologists) with great experience in the management of pharmacologic interactions between HAART and immunosuppressive agents (see also Table 1). In conclusion, OLT should be considered as an opportunity for patients with HIV and HCC: even if accurate selection protocols are mandatory, with regards to HIV status and HCC stage, now the key question is not "if" but "who" should be referred to liver transplantation.

Medical Treatment

Two large phase III trials, although restricted to patients with well-preserved liver function (Child–Pugh class A/B) and with no HIV infection, have shown the effectiveness of orally active multikinase inhibitor sorafenib in improving the median OS and TTP in patients with unresectable HCC [93, 94].

Table 1. Criteria of considering liver transplantation in HIV-patients (according to Di Benedetto 2008 and O'Grady 2005)

Liver disease criteria • Child-Turcotte-Pugh score ≥B7; MELD score ≥14 Milan criteria:* • No more than 3 tumour nodules • No nodule greater than 5 cm in diameter • Absence of macroscopic portal vein invasion • Absence in recognizable extra hepatic disease
HIV infection criteria Immunological criteria • None of AIDS-defining opportunistic infections in the previous year • CD4 cell count >200 cells/µL or >100/µL in case of therapy intolerance Virological criteria • Undetectable HIV viral load (<50 copies/mL) in the last 12 months or effective therapeutic options for HIV infection during the post-transplant period
General criteria • Favourable psychiatric evaluation • Social stability • N alcohol abuse for at least six months • No drug consumption for at least two years (patients who are on stable methadone maintenance programs can be included and can continue on the maintenance programmers after the procedure) • No extra hepatic malignancy • No pregnancy

*Patients with HCC who are being considered for liver transplantation should not have a needle biopsy due to the significant rate of needle-track seeding leading to post-transplant recurrence.

Sorafenib has considerably changed the treatment and prognosis of unresectable HCC, offering a therapeutic opportunity for some patients, for whom no effective treatment had been available. Despite the emerging role of HCC as a major cause of morbidity and mortality in HIV-infected patients, no large pivotal trials have been reported the safety and efficacy of sorafenib in this particular setting, which is often discriminated against in clinical trials or for standard oncologic treatment, solely because of their HIV infection.

In the past few years, four case reports have described the safety and efficacy of sorafenib in HIV-infected patients, but they are merely anecdotal [95-98]. The Italian Cooperative Group on AIDS and Tumours (GICAT) has reported on the safety and efficacy of sorafenib in HIV-infected patients with unresectable HCC. In this study, the patient population included patients with Child–Pugh class A–C cirrhosis, BCLC tumour stage B–D, and receiving HAART concomitantly. Despite this study being the first of its kind, and therefore potentially useful, its retrospective nature is a limiting factor, which should be considered if outcomes are to be compared with the prospective trials above mentioned [93, 94]. The analysis of the intention-to-treat group showed a median OS of 12.8 months. A subgroup analysis with respect to Child–Pugh class, BCLC stage, and CDC stage showed a tendency toward improved survival only according to the BCLC stage (Figures 1–3). Indeed, for patients with BCLC stage A–B or C–D, the median TTP were 8.7 and 2.1 months, respectively, and the median OS were 14.7 and 5.6 months, respectively. These data suggest that in sorafenib-treated patients with unresectable HCC, HIV infection, and a good viroimmunological profile, survival outcomes depend on the BCLC tumour stage, which is also the determining factor for survival in the general patient population.

The evidence supports the suggestion that, to date, because of the use of HAART and its beneficial effects on viroimmunological profile, HIV-positive patients with HCC should be considered similar to the general population. In fact, no significant differences in TTP and OS were found between patient groups with different severities of liver dysfunction (according to the Child–Pugh classification) or between patient groups with different severities of HIV infection (according to the CDC staging of the disease).

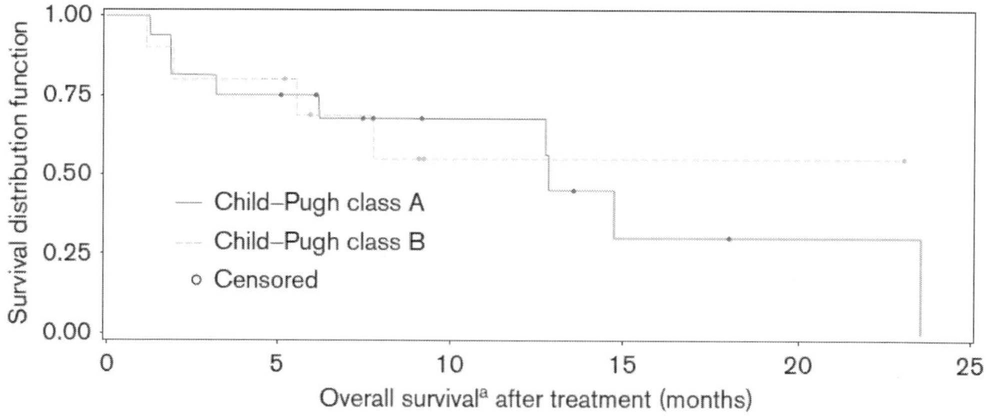

Figure 1. Kaplan–Meier curves representing overall survival after the start of treatment according to the Child–Pugh classification [A (N = 16) and B (N = 10)]. [a]Wilcoxon's test indicates no significant difference between groups.

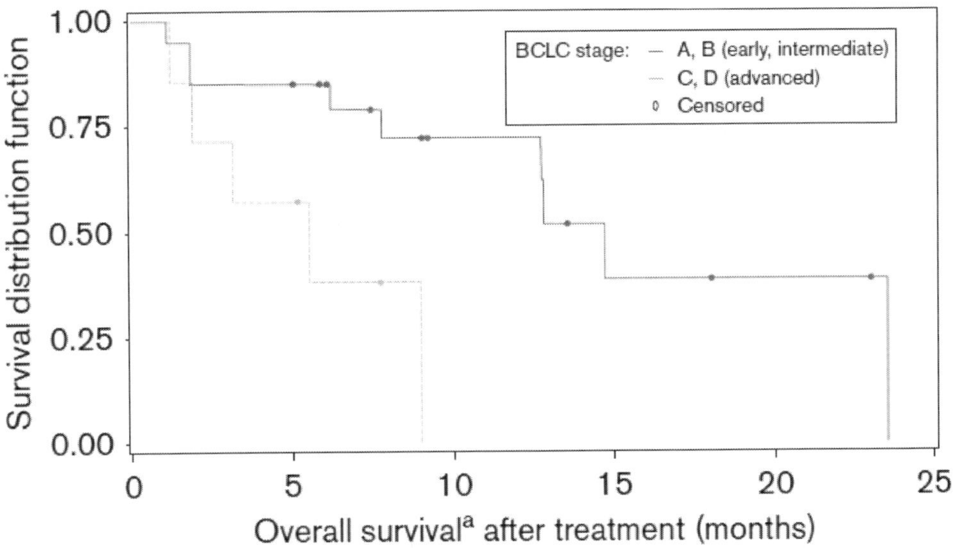

Figure 2. Kaplan–Meier curves representing survival after the start of treatment according to Barcelona Liver Clinic Cancer (BCLC) staging [A or B (N = 20) and C or D (N = 7)]. [a]Wilcoxon's test (P = 0.04) indicates a significant difference between groups.

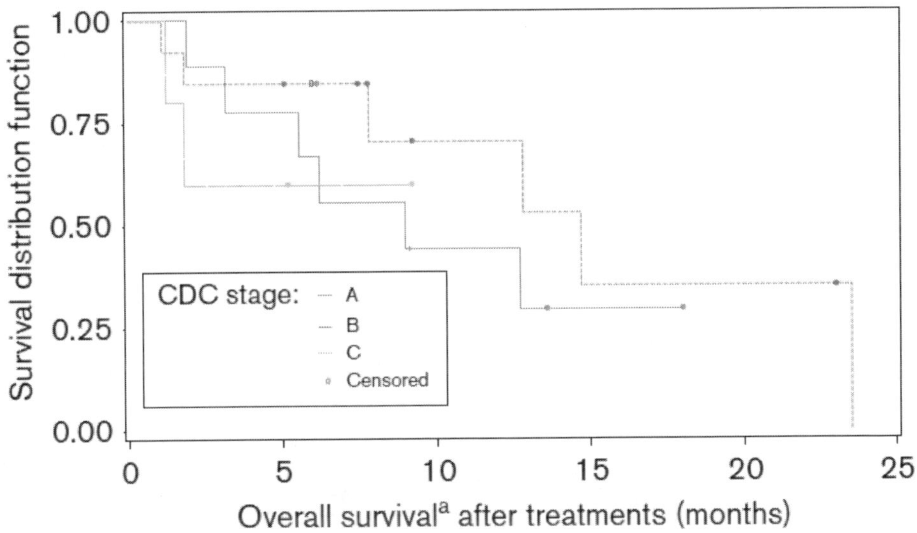

Figure 3. Kaplan–Meier curves representing survival after the start of treatment for Centres for Disease Control and Prevention (CDC) staging of HIV infection [A (N = 9), B (N = 13), and C (N = 5)]. [a]Wilcoxon's test indicates no significant difference between groups.

Conclusion

The management of HCC in HIV-positive patients lack of universally approved guidelines [23, 24, 39, 99]. Recent data have demonstrated that there are no differences in the outcome of HIV-infected and HIV-uninfected patients in terms of HCC response to the available therapy; different therapeutic strategies for HCC in the HIV setting should be advocated in order to integrate HIV and HCC treatments.

HCC therapeutic trials specifically designed for HIV-infected patients are also necessary. Early diagnosis of HCC and retreatment for HCC recurrence have a key role in the survival of patients, therefore, regular screening programs for HCC should be extended to HIV-infected patients according to proposed guidelines [23, 39, 99-102], together with a greater proclivity for treatment and retreatment options in cases of an HCC diagnosis or recurrence. This may be an important and needed breakthrough for this rising problem.

HCC in Elderly Patients

Management of malignant disease in the elderly has become a global clinical issue, due to the increase of life expectancy in many countries [103]. In the past years, many elderly patients have been considered less effectively responsive to treatments compared to younger patients, due to their lifetime addition of different illnesses [104-106]. This hypothesis has been reviewed by some studies and the need for a careful selection of patients has been strengthened, thus implying the possibility to offer elderly patients the same treatment options than younger ones with acceptable results [107-110]. Accordingly, OLT in the old age has now been reconsidered by some authors, even if it was once banned to elderly patients because of ethical reasons and for lack of available organs, rising different debates if consider it as a therapeutic option for elderly patients [111-113]. Of great importance is to define who is old. A person chronological age is scarcely correlated to physiological age, but it may be used as a frame of reference. The age of 70 years is the threshold for this analysis; in fact, many studies have described the 70 years of age landmark as the lower limit after which physiological senescence, the incidence of organ dysfunction and the development of co-morbidities begin to increase [114, 115]. Co-morbidities should be assessed when describing elderly patients; however, there is some controversy about how to define it and to stratify the risk of death secondary to the number and the severity of associated conditions [116, 117]. The World Health Organization-Eastern Cooperative Oncology Group Performance Status (PS) [118, 119], the Charlson's scale [120], and the Cumulative Illness Rating Scale-Geriatrics (CIRS-G) [121], are some of the co-morbidity scales that have been proposed in order to achieve a comorbidity index to quantify the risk of death in each case.

Several reports have outlined significant differences in the cohort of aged patients with HCC. Elderly patients are less frequently HBsAg positive and more often anti-HCV positive [114, 122-124]. Some authors suggest a changing pattern of male/female ratio, reporting a high frequency of old female patients with HCC [114, 124, 125], and it is recognized that the peak age for women is postponed by 5 years compared to men [121]. However, there is some disagreement among authors [122, 123]. This could be explained in younger males with an earlier viral infection due to behavioural risk factors; alcohol abuse may increase the incidence of HCC in males earlier than in females [114, 125].

It is also important to mention the impact of non-alcoholic steatohepatitis (NASH) as a risk for HCC onset in elderly patients. The phenomenon of hepatic steatosis and non-alcoholic fatty liver disease (NAFLD) has been recognized as a part of the metabolic syndrome. It is associated with obesity, dyslipidemia, hypertension, sleep apnoea, and diabetes mellitus type 2 [126-129].

The visceral fat accumulation recurrent in patients with NAFLD/NASH is cause of insulin resistance and hyperinsulinemia that can accelerate hepatocarcinogenesis [130, 131]. This event can have an import role in patients as they get older. Elderly NAFLD patients, especially with diabetes, should be therefore monitored carefully during follow-up screening for HCC [132].

Liver Resection

A debate on the safety use of hepatic resection for the treatment of HCC in the elderly patients has been raised in the past decades. Several authors [133, 134] reported high morbidity and mortality rates especially after major hepatic resection in elderly patients compared to younger patients, discouraging the use of this procedure for these patients. Instead, other authors described this treatment as safe and effective in both elderly and younger patients [104, 135-137]. There is, therefore, a common misconception that all elderly patients are at high surgical risk only due to their advanced age, consequently a curative treatment has often been denied to them. Nowadays, the vast majority of authors do not consider age itself as a contraindication to surgical treatment anymore and a different approach has been developed in the management of these patients. The patient is considered in toto, with all his/her co morbidities, performance status and functional reserve. Thus both well-selected elderly patients and younger patients are often offered the same treatment options.

Huang J. et al. [122] reported in 2009 the long-term outcomes and prognostic factors of elderly patients with HCC undergoing hepatectomy. The authors evaluated 67 HCC patients older than 70 years of age, compared with 268 younger patients as controls. More preoperative co morbidities ($P<0.001$) were found in the elderly, but no significant difference in the incidence of postoperative complications ($P = 0.220$). In their experience the OS rates after hepatectomy at 1-, 3-, and 5-years were 83.3%, 54.6%, and 43.2% in the elderly group and 71.6%, 39.9%, and 31.4% in the control group, respectively. The disease-free survival (DFS) rates after hepatectomy at 1, 3, and 5 years were 66.8%, 57.7%, and 47.0% in the elderly group, and 65.2%, 40.8%, and 36.2% in the control group, respectively. The survival of the elderly group appeared to be better than that of the control group, but the difference was not significant ($P = 0.157$). They also found, even if not statistically significant, a lower recurrence rate in the elderly group (55.3% vs. 63.5%); Interestingly, no differences were found in the kind of treatment after the recurrence in both groups (repeated hepatic resection, TACE, RFA, PEI, percutaneous microwave coagulation therapy, systemic chemotherapy, radiotherapy). Elderly patients were, in fact, fully included in a comprehensive approach for the treatment of HCC, regardless of their age. pTNM staging was the only independent prognostic factor for the postoperative survival of the elderly patients with HCC. Huang et al. concluded that liver resection for HCC is safe in elderly patients without preoperative co morbidities or with well-controlled preoperative co morbidities.

In 2009 Kaibori M et al. [108] compared the results of hepatectomy for HCC in patients older than 70 years with the results of younger patients. These authors, as well as the previous ones, evidenced a higher incidence of associated diseases, but, in contrast, in their analysis the older group showed a better preoperative liver function. They also found no significant differences in DSF and OS between the younger and elderly groups. Interestingly in this study, alcohol abuse was identified as one of the independent prognostic indicators for DFS and OS in patients older than 70 years. In fact, the recurrence rate for elderly patients with a high alcohol intake was significantly higher than that of younger patients with alcohol abuse. Therefore, they concluded that, in particular for elderly patients with HCC, it is fundamental to stop drinking because preoperative alcohol abuse was a factor indicating a poor prognosis for DSF and OS after resection. They also reported a higher incidence of postoperative delirium in the elderly group. Some papers previously reported older age as a risk factor for postoperative delirium [137-139]. This may be due to a higher frailty and a reduced capacity of self-regulation in response to stresses like those imposed by surgery and anaesthesia; furthermore, age related changes of pharmacodynamics and pharmacokinetics increase the side effects of drugs that can lead to postoperative delirium. The same data is deduced by Cho SW et al. [140] who reported only confusion as an age-specific postoperative complication that was far more common in the elderly than the young. They investigated whether advanced age was associated with a higher rate and severity of postoperative complications after hepatic resection for primary and secondary liver malignancies, through a paired matched analysis. A total of 75 patients aged less than 70 years were compared to 75 patients older than 70 years. They found that advanced age led to longer hospital stay and more frequent discharge to a rehabilitation institution. Thus it can be assumed that elderly patients need a more intense monitoring and greater nursing care and physical therapy, but that they can benefit from liver resection as much as younger individuals. It is important to inform elderly patients of the possibilities of their postoperative hospital course and prepare them for possible rehabilitation required after major liver resection. Nanashima A et al. [141] recently examined the features and survival of 188 HCC patients who underwent hepatectomy. They divided the patients into four groups according to age: young patients <50 years of age, patients between 50-69 years, patients between 70-79 and finally patients aged more than 80 years, thus giving an insight also of extremely old patients. The physiologic ability and surgical stress (E-PASS) score, including preoperative risk score (PRS), surgical stress score (SSS), and comprehensive risk score (CRS) were assessed [142]. They found a higher frequency of preoperative systemic complications in the elderly patients, particularly in the group of patients aged more than 80 years of age. PS and American Society of anaesthesiologists (ASA) score were also significantly increased in the elderly patients ($p<0.05$). The tumour recurrence and DFS rates were similar among the four groups. In line with the other studies they reported that comorbidity and lower general status were significantly higher in the elderly patients. They also found a higher rate of systemic postoperative complications in the elderly patients, in agreement with previous papers, even though the duration of hospitalization did not differ among the four groups. Thus they recorded age >70 and PRS >0.32 as significantly associated with post-operative complications; therefore they concluded that accurate follow-up and proper decision on treatment modality upon assessment of PRS are fundamental for these patients.

In 2009 Oishi K et al. analyzed 502 patients aged less than 75 versus 64 patients aged more than 75 undergoing hepatic resection. The incidence of cirrhosis in the older group was 31%, whereas that in the younger group was 52% ($p = 0.03$). Preoperative laboratory tests also showed that the older group had better liver function than the younger group. On the other hand pathological features showed that the older group was characterized by a higher tumour burden in terms of size (p = 0.057) and microscopic vascular invasion (p = 0.04) compared to the younger group. Different studies have reported that elderly patients with HCC have a preserved liver function and a lower rate on liver cirrhosis [124, 143]. It may be due to the precocious death of patients with cirrhosis and HCC before reaching the age of 70 years and that those who survive have a good hepatic function. In accordance with other authors they assert that hepatectomy in patients with good liver function is feasible, and that the prognosis after surgery for elderly patients is comparable to that for younger patients.

Similar results in terms of post-operative complications, DFS and OS were previously reported by Ferrero A et al. [107] and Kondo K et al. [144] respectively in 2005 and 2008. Both groups suggest that hepatic resection is justified for HCC in selected patients aged 70 years or older.

De Benedetto et al. [145], from the Hepato-Biliary-Pancreatic Surgery and Liver Transplantation Unit - Italy, have evaluated 198 HCC patients between January 2001 and November 2010. The 68.2% (135/198) of patients has been younger than 70 years of age and 63 (31.8%) patients have been 70 years of age or older. The 42.9% of the younger group of patients (85 patients) have undergone liver resection compare to the 48 (24.5%) of the elderly group. On a pair-matched basis 48 patients aged over 70 have been compared to 48 younger ones, according to sex, aetiology and stage of liver disease, tumour burden and infiltration of cut margin. OS and DFS in the two groups have been similar. The survival rates in the younger group have resulted, at 1, 3- and 5-years, 83.3%, 61.1% and 26.1%, respectively, in comparison with the 78%, 62.2% and 45.6% of the elderly group (p=0.48). DFS rates at 1-, 3- and 5-years have been 69.9%, 43.6% and 30.6%, respectively, in the younger group and 71%, 44.1% and 24.5% in the elderly group (p = 0.74). The incidence of post-operative complications has been similar in both groups (37.5% vs. 50%, p = 0.3). As concerns Dindo's classification [146], similar minor procedures (grade 3) have been required by both groups. Furthermore, a significant reduction in performance status calculated using the classification of Karnofsky [147] has been found in the senior patients' group, compared to the younger group (respectively 71 ± 8% vs. 74 ± 7% p = 0.013). In the elderly group, the ECOG PS score appeared worse than the younger group, although not statistically significant. These data have confirmed that well selected older-patients can safely undergo hepatic resection with satisfactory results [148].

Ablative Treatments

The differences in features and outcomes after ablative treatments between elderly and young patients have been treated in few papers [149-155], and most of them are mainly focused on radiofrequency ablation (RFA).

RFA presents excellent results in tumours ≤2cm (90-100% complete necrosis) [156], but for bigger nodules the probability of achieving a complete necrosis is higher when combined or repeated treatments are performed. Currently, RFA is considered the best loco-regional treatment, but it has some limitations. Some contraindications may arise when considering the possible procedure-related damage when tumours are located close to other organs (kidney, colon, or gallbladder). Moreover, the treatment may also not been effective when the lesions are nearby large vessels thus they may not be completely ablated due to the heat sink effect [157].

Two studies evaluated the efficacy, the safety and the results of RFA in the elderly HCC population [148, 151]. Different results were seen; while no difference in terms of cumulative OS and RFS after RFA comparing 107 patients older than 75 to 354 younger patients have been recorded by Takahashi et al. suggesting that RFA should be used for elderly patients even in cases of comorbidity, Kao WY et al. did not present encouraging results in the group of elderly patients (158 vs. 100 patients aged more or less than 65). Noteworthy, Kao et al. have found that, particularly for patients with very early stage of disease (tumour size of 2 cm or less or in BCLC stage 0), the younger group presented a significantly higher OS than the elder one due to their better liver functional reserve. If considering the low cut-off age (65 years) of this study, these findings are in contrast with other studies, maybe because the higher tumoral burden found in the elderly group. Tateishi et al. [149]. have not shown any difference in the 3-year survival rate between patients aged over 68 years (76%) and under 68 years (79.2%) in 1,000 patients treated with RFA, even though a detailed analysis of specific risk factors on age has not been performed. The only paper describing the effect of age on the outcome after trans-arterial chemoembolization (TACE) is by Thornton RH et al. [153]. The authors have analyzed 200 patients aged more than 70 versus 168 younger patients undergoing TACE. The distribution and severity of complications have resulted similar between the two groups. Similarly to other reports, the elderly group had significantly more cardiovascular and cardiopulmonary co morbidities at baseline. Of great interest is that when these data have been adjusted for the presence of cardiovascular comorbidity, the association between age and the likelihood of a cardiopulmonary complication has lost significance, meaning that older patients without a cardiovascular comorbidity have had the same probabilities than younger patients to have from cardiopulmonary complication, whereas an older patient with such a comorbidity has been more likely to suffer a cardiopulmonary complication. In this series, other measurements of morbidity, including severity of complications, need for intensive care unit admission, and length of hospitalization have been not different between the younger and older groups.

Liver Transplantation

An interesting matter of debate is whether elderly HCC patients deserve OLT, and the current shortage of available organs makes the question even harder to solve. This is, however, nowadays more an ethical issue, it regards a very small percentage in the worldwide casuistry. Schwartz J. J. et al. [110] in 2012 examined the post-transplant overall survival of elderly HCC patients (aged 70 years or old) versus younger patients. In this study 6,320 liver transplants were analyzed, 143 were 70 years old or older (42% of whom were affected by HCC). Thus, as also noted by Perkins J. D. [111], this issue concerns a very small percentage of patients, only 0.91% of the population in Schwartz's study.

All the same time these results cannot be underestimated and some considerations are also needed. As reported by Schwartz et al. in the group of older recipients, a decreased OS after OLT has been observed, with an actuarial survival rate of 54.5%. Therefore, even though the OS rates in elderly patients with HCC are far more poorly after OLT in comparison with younger patients, the results have been comparable to the rates associated with other indications for transplantation in this age group, regardless of the HCC diagnosis. In particular, the difference in survival appeared after 18 months and became accentuated 5 years after OLT when the difference between the older and younger groups was almost 15%. They sadly concluded that OLT in older patients should not be supported, even though the presence of HCC does not affect the post-OLT outcome as compared to OLT for other indications. It is of interest to reflect on the elegant comment of Perkins J. D. [111] on this matter, he asserts that patients with adequate functional liver reserve (mainly Child-Pugh status A or even B patients), with a resectable tumour, should undergo liver surgery or otherwise ablative treatments sparing the patients from the possibility of early mortality, pain, discomfort and various liver transplant complications, with an extreme gap in terms of cost-effectiveness and sparing of organs. An open debate concerns decompensated cirrhotic patients with HCC who are amenable to neither resection nor loco regional treatments. In a particular age when disparity between demand and available organs keeps on growing, it is important to wonder how to streamline the actual resources.

Targeted Treatments

Generally, elderly patients with HCC are less intensively investigated and more conservatively treated despite similar tumour stages at diagnosis, leading to significantly worse survival outcomes [158]. On the other hand, HCC in elderly patients may have more favourable tumour biology than in younger patients.

A study on hepatitis C infection-related HCC patients demonstrated that, overall, elderly patients presented with more favourable tumour characteristics and had better overall prognosis [159]. In the literature, data on the optima management of HCC in elderly patients is rare. In fact, Although age did not seem to influence treatment options or preclude patients from treatment [160, 161], most studies included heterogeneous cohorts with variable underlying liver function and tumour stages.

Most of these studies were also performed prior to the era of sorafenib, which is now the recommended treatment for advanced HCC [162].

Sorafenib, a bi-aryl urea [163], is a small molecular inhibitor of several Tyrosine protein kinases (VEGFR and PDGFR) and Raf kinases (more avidly C-Raf than B-Raf) [164, 165]. It inhibits tumour angiogenesis and increases the rate of apoptosis in a wide range of tumour models [166].

Protein kinases are overactive in many of the molecular pathways that cause cells to become cancerous. These pathways include Raf kinase, PDGF (platelet-derived growth factor), VEGF receptor 2 and 3 kinases and c Kit the receptor for Stem cell factor.

Cellular signalling that is mediated by Raf-1 and vascular endothelial growth factor (VEGF) pathways have been implicated in the molecular pathogenesis of HCC [165-168], providing a rationale for investigating sorafenib for this indication. In the phase III registrative SHARP trial [93], the median age of treated patients was 64.9 years and thus it is difficult to draw further considerations on this treatment in elderly patients.

The first report on the outcome and safety of the use of sorafenib in elderly patients affected by advanced HCC is by Wong H et al. [161]. Analyzing the 35 older patients treated with sorafenib they concluded that the "the survival benefits and overall treatment-related adverse events of sorafenib are comparable in elderly and younger advanced HCC patients."

This was the first paper reporting, even if within a limited series of data, the feasibility of this approach in elderly patients.

Conclusion

A multidisciplinary approach should be taken when assessing elderly patients with HCC; stage of HCC and liver disease should be taken into account and regardless of the chronological age, the best treatment should be offered. Co morbidities have to be clearly defined, and when possible, the functional reserve of the patient should be known.

Table 2. Patient Characteristics

	HIV positive (n=104)	HIV negative (n=484)	*P*
Age at HCC diagnosis (years), mean ± SD	48.03 (± 7.4)	67.54 (±9.6)	<.001
Age at HIV diagnosis (years), mean ± SD	33.70 (±10.1)	--	
Patients with age >70 (%)	3 (2.8%)	101 (20.8%)	<.001
Male Sex	99 (95.2%)	358 (73.9%)	<.001
Aetiology of Chronic Liver Disease			
HCV	56 (53.8%)	307 (63.4%)	
HBV	11 (10.6%)	71 (14.6%)	
HCV+HBV	36 (34.6%)	18 (3.7%)	
Cryptogenic	1 (1.0%)	43 (8.9%)	.000*
Alcohol	0	41 (8.6%)	
Other	0	4 (0.8%)	
Alcohol Abuse (in viral aetiology)	11 (10.5%)	59 (13.3%)	.517
HIV parameters			
Risk factors			
IVDU	76%	--	
MSM	11,5%	--	
Hetero	8,7%	--	
Others	3,8%	--	
CD4 cells <200 per ml	25 (24.1%)	--	
HIV RNA copies <50/ml	61 (58.6%)	--	
CDC group			
A	46 (44.3%)	--	
B	37 (35.5%)	--	
C	21 (20.2%)	--	
HAART (yes/no)**	89/15		
Performance status (0-1/ ≥ 2)**	87/17	339/145	.005
Characteristics of Liver Function			
Child Turcotte-Pugh (CTP) score , mean ± SD	7.35 (±1.7)	7.55 (±2.0)	.343
CTP stage A	45 (43.2%)	243 (50.2%)	
CTP stage B	33 (31.8%)	161 (33.2%)	.105*
CTP stage C	26 (25.0%)	79 (16.3%)	

*chi-square; **at HCC diagnosis HCC = hepatocellular carcinoma; SD = Standard Deviation; HIV = human immunodeficiency virus. IVDU = Intravenous Drug User.

Table 3. Tumour Characteristics

	HIV positive (n=104)	HIV negative (n=484)	*P*
Diagnosis under screening program	58 (55.7%)	371 (76.7%)	<.001
Diagnosis made by			
Biopsy	31 (29.8%)	128 (26.4%)	.468
Imaging	73 (70.2%)	356 (73.6%)	
Hepatic lesions			
Single	53 (50.9%)	202 (41.7%)	.101
Multiple	51 (49.1%)	282 (58.3%)	
Median size single lesion (cm), [range]	3.5 [1.1-9]	3.7 [1-12]	.151
Portal Vein Thrombosis	19 (18.2%)	84 (17.3%)	.887
Extra hepatic Metastases	4 (3.8%)	26 (5.3%)	.630
One site	3	20	
Multiple sites	1	6	
Stage at diagnosis (BCLC)			
A	29 (27.9%)	64 (13.3%)	
B	40 (38.5%)	141 (29.1%)	<.001*
C	11 (10.5%)	223 (46.0%)	
D	24 (23.1%)	56 (11.6%)	
AFP serum levels (ng/ml)	420 [1.3-25120]	478 [1.0-7800]	.716
(median)[range]	68 (65.3%)	284 (58.6%)	.227
Number with AFP >200 ng/ml	53 (50.9%)	185 (38.2%)	.371
Number with AFP >400 ng/ml			
Time from HIV infection to	18.6(±6.9)	--	
HCC, mean (years)	15.2(±3.6)	24.5(±5.8)	<.001
Time from CLD to HCC mean (years)			

CLD = Chronic Liver Disease; AFP = Alpha-fetoprotein*chi-square for trend.

Liver resection and ablative treatments should never be denied to these patients only because of their advanced age, and curative procedures should be performed in tertiary hepato-biliary-pancreatic Centres. Each elderly HCC patient has to be evaluated singularly, stratifying each time the risk for the procedure so as to determine which the best treatment is, analyzing all the possibilities that can be offered. This similar approach showed a good efficacy and safety in another "frail" patients' category with HCC and HIV infection [84, 85, 87, 90, 92, 94, 169-171].

A consideration can be made from this review of the literature: the vast majority of the patients studied in the papers analyzed, derive from a group of already selected patients, thus no clear data can be obtained about the patients considered not eligible for curative treatment because of their co-morbidities or medical unfit status. In the forthcoming years physicians should aim to understand the critical points and the boundaries beyond which the risk of an operative procedure becomes too high for the latter patients. Furthermore, the applicability, the safety and the outcome after aggressive treatments in patients with advanced HCC, such as portal vein embolization, prior extended hepatectomies, combined loco regional treatments and/or chemotherapy protocols, should be assessed. In a constantly aging society it appears to be mandatory.

REFERENCES

[1] Gomaa A. I., Khan S. A., Toledano M. B., Waked I., Tayiorrobinson S. D. Hepatocellular carcinoma: epidemiology, risk factors, and pathogenesis. *World J. Gastroenterol.*, 2008; 14: 4300-4308.

[2] Jong-Wook L. Global health improvement and WHO: Shaping the future. *Lancet*, 2003; 362: 2083-2088.

[3] Parkin D. M., Pisani P., Ferlay J. Estimates of the worldwide incidence of 25 major cancers in 1990. *Int. J. Cancer*, 1990; 80: 827-841.

[4] Montalto G., Cervello M., Giannitrapani L., Dantona F., Terranova A., Castagnetta L. A. Epidemiology, risk factors and natural history of hepatocellular carcinoma. *Ann. N Y Acad. Sci.*, 2002; 963: 13-20.

[5] Ferlay J., Parkin D. M., Pisani P. Globocan Graphical Package 1: Cancer incidence and mortality worldwide. Iarc Press, Lyon, 1998.

[6] Bosch F. X., Ribes J., Diaz M., Cleries R. Primary liver cancer: Worldwide incidence and trends. *Gastroenterology,* 2004; 127: S5-S16.

[7] Nunnari G., Pomerantz R. J. Il-7 as a potential therapy for HIV-1-infected individuals. *Expert Opin. Biol. Ther.*, 2005; 5: 1421-1426.

[8] El-Serag H. B., Mason A. C. Rising incidence of hepatocellular carcinoma in the United States. *N Engl. J. Med.,* 1999; 340: 745-750.

[9] Parikh S., Hyman D. Hepatocellular cancer: A guide for the internist. *Am. J. Med.,* 2007; 120: 194-202.

[10] UNAIDS: Global summary of the HIV and AIDS epidemic. Available at http://www.unAIDS.org, 2007.

[11] Murphy E. L., Collier A. C., Kalish L. A., Assmann S. F., Para M. F., Flanigan T. P., Kumar P. N., Mintz L., Wallach F. R., Nemo G. J.; Viral Activation Transfusion Study Investigators. Highly active antiretroviral therapy decreases mortality and morbidity in patients with advanced HIV disease. *Ann. Intern. Med.,* 2001; 135:17–26.

[12] Palella F. J. Jr., Delaney K. M., Moorman A. C., Loveless M. O., Fuhrer J., Satten G. A., Aschman D. J., Holmberg S. D. Declining morbidity and mortality among patients with advanced human immunodeficiency virus infection. HIV Outpatient Study Investigators. *N Engl. J. Med.,* 1998; 338: 853–860.

[13] Bica I., Mcgovern B., Dhar R., Stone D., McGowan K., Scheib R., Snydman D. R. Increasing mortality due to end-stage liver disease in patients with human immunodeficiency virus infection. *Clin. Infect. Dis.,* 2001; 32:492– 497.

[14] Macías J., Melguizo I., Fernández-Rivera F. J., García-García A., Mira J. A., Ramos A. J., Rivera J. M., Pineda J. A. Mortality due to liver failure and impact on survival of

hepatitis virus infections in HIV-infected patients receiving potent antiretroviral therapy. *Eur. J. Clin. Microbiol. Infect. Dis.*, 2002; 21:775–781.
[15] Koziel M. J., Peters M. G. Viral hepatitis in HIV infection. *N Engl. J. Med.*, 2007; 356:1445–1454.
[16] Sulkowski M. S., Thomas D. l., Chaisson R. E., Moore R. D. Hepatotoxicity associated with antiretroviral therapy in adults infected with human immunodeficiency virus and the role of hepatitis C or B virus infection. *JAMA*, 2000; 283:74–80.
[17] Sulkowski M. S. Viral hepatitis and HIV coinfection. *J. Hepatol.*, 2008; 48: 353–367.
[18] Deuffic-Burban S., Poynard T., Sulkowski M. S., Wong J. B. Estimating the future health burden of chronic hepatitis C and human immunodeficiency virus infections in the United States. *J. Viral Hepat.*, 2007; 14:107–115.
[19] Clifford G. M., Rickenbach M., Polesel J., Dal Maso L., Steffen I., Ledergerber B., Rauch A., Probst-Hensch N. M., Bouchardy C., Levi F., Franceschi S.; Swiss HIV Cohort. Influence of HIV-related immunodeficiency on the risk of hepatocellular carcinoma. *AIDS,* 2008; 22:2135-2141.
[20] Smukler A. J., Ratner L. Hepatitis viruses and hepatocellular carcinoma in HIV-infected patients. *Curr. Opin. Oncol.*, 2002; 14:538-542.
[21] Bosch F. X., Ribes J., Díaz M., Cléries R. Primary liver cancer: Worldwide incidence and trends. *Gastroenterology,* 2004;127 Suppl. 1:S5-S16.
[22] Lewden C., Salmon D., Morlat P., Bévilacqua S., Jougla E., Bonnet F., Héripret L., Costagliola D., May T., Chêne G.; Mortality 2000 study group. Causes of death among human immunodeficiency virus (HIV)-infected adults in the era of potent antiretroviral therapy: Emerging role of hepatitis and cancers, persistent role of AIDS. *Int. J. Epidemiol.,* 2005; 34:121-130.
[23] Bruix J., Sherman M. Management of hepatocellular carcinoma. *Hepatology,* 2005; 42:1208-1236.
[24] El-Serag H. B., Marrero J. A., Rudolph L., Reddy K. R. Diagnosis and treatment of hepatocellular carcinoma. *Gastroenterology,* 2008; 134: 1752-1763.
[25] Thio C. L., Seaberg E. C., Skolasky R. Jr., Phair J., Visscher B., Muñoz A., Thomas D. L.; Multicenter AIDS Cohort Study. HIV-1, Hepatitis B virus, and risk of liver-related mortality in the Multicenter Cohort Study (MACS). *Lancet,* 2002; 360:1921-1926.
[26] Salmon D., Robain M., Rockstroh J. K., Benhamou Y. Therapeutic management of hepatitis and HIV infection in co-infected patients: Results of a survey performed before the 2005 Consensus Conference. *J. Hepatol.,* 2006; 44 1 Suppl.:S2-S5.
[27] Giordano T. P., Kramer J. R., Souchek J., Richardson P., El-Serag H. B. Cirrhosis and hepatocellular carcinoma in HIV-infected veterans with and without the hepatitis C virus: A Cohort Study, 1992–2001. *Arch. Intern. Med.*, 2004; 164:2349-2354.
[28] Pineda J. A., Romero-Gómez M., Díaz-García F., Girón-González J. A., Montero J. L., Torre-Cisneros J., Andrade R. J., González-Serrano M., Aguilar J., Aguilar-Guisado M., Navarro J. M., Salmerón J., Caballero-Granado F. J., García-García J. A.; Grupo Andaluz para el Estudio de las Enfermedades Infecciosas; Grupo Andaluz para el Estudio del Hígado. HIV coinfection shortens the survival of patients with hepatitis C virus-related decompensated cirrhosis. *Hepatology*, 2005; 41:779-789.
[29] Reisler K. High hepatotoxicity rate seen among HAART patients. *AIDS Alert,* 2001; 16:118-119.

[30] Mcginnis K. A., Fultz S. L., Skanderson M., Conigliaro J., Bryant K., Justice A. C. Hepatocellular carcinoma and non-Hodgkin's lymphoma: The roles of HIV, hepatitis C infection and alcohol abuse. *J. Clin. Oncol.,* 2006; 24: 5005-5009.

[31] Rosenthal E., Poiree M., Pradier C., Perronne C., Salmon-Ceron D., Geffray L., Myers R. P., Morlat P., Pialoux G., Poi S., Cacoub P. Mortality due to hepatitis C-related liver disease in HIV infected patients in France (Mortavic 2001 Study). *AIDS*, 2003; 17: 1803-1809.

[32] Bonnet F., Lewden C., May T., Heripret L., Jougla E., Bevilacqua S., Costagliola D., Salmon D., Chene G., Morlat P. Malignancy-related causes of death in human immunodeficiency virus infected patients in the era of highly active antiretroviral therapy. *Cancer,* 2004; 101: 317-324.

[33] Kramer Jr., Giordano T. P., Souchek J., Richardson P., Hwang L. Y., El-Serag H. B. The effect of HIV coinfection on the risk of cirrhosis and hepatocellular carcinoma in U.S. Veterans with hepatitis C. *Am. J. Gastroenterol.,* 2005; 100: 56-63.

[34] Mbulaiteye S. M., Parkin D. M., Rabkin C. S. Epidemiology of AIDS-related malignancies an international perspective. *Hematol. Oncol. Clin. North Am.,* 2003; 17: 673-696.

[35] Beral V., Newton R. Overview of the epidemiology of immunodeficiency-associated cancers. *J. Natl. Cancer Inst. Monogr.,* 1998; 23: 1-6.

[36] Puoti M., Bruno R., Soriano V., Donato F., Gaeta G. B., Quinzan G. P., Precone D., Gelatti U., Asensi V., Vaccher E. Hepatocellular carcinoma in HIV-infected patients: epidemiological features, clinical presentation and outcome. *AIDS,* 2004; 18: 2285-2293.

[37] Di Benedetto F., Di Sandro S., De Ruvo N., Berretta M., Masetti M., Montalti R., Ballarin R., Cocchi S., Potenza L., Luppi M., Gerunda G. E. Kaposi's sarcoma after liver transplantation. *J. Cancer Res. Clin. Oncol.,* 2008; 134: 653-658.

[38] Fultz S., Justice A., Butt A., Rabeneck L., Weissman S., Rodriguez-Barradas M. Testing, referral and treatment patterns for hepatitis c virus coinfection in a cohort of veterans with HIV infection. *Clin. Infect. Dis.,* 2003; 36: 1039-1046.

[39] Bruno R., Puoti M., Sacchi P., Filice C., Carosi G., Filice G. Management of hepatocellular carcinoma in human immunodeficiency virus-infected patients. *J. Hepatol.,* 2006; 44: S146-S150.

[40] Macdonald D., Nelson M., Bower M., Powles T. Hepatocellular carcinoma, human immunodeficiency virus and viral hepatitis in the HAART era. *World J. Gastroenterol.*, 2008; 14: 1657-1663.

[41] Sherman K. E., Rouster S. D., Chung R. T., Rajicic N. Hepatitis C virus prevalence among patients infected with human immunodeficiency virus: a crosssectional analysis of the US adult AIDS clinical trials group. *Clin. Infect. Dis*., 2002; 34: 831-837.

[42] Buffet-Janvresse C., Peigue-Lafeuille H., Benichou J., Vabret A., Branger M., Trimoulet P., Goria O., Laurichesse H., Abbed A., Verdon R., Bouvet E., Lafon M. E., Dussaix E., Cormerais L., Dupon M., Henquell C., Josse A., Lagoutte P., Lariven S., Legac S., Riachi G., Verdon R., Vittecoq D.; HIV-HCV Cohort Study Group. HIV and HCV co-Infection: situation at six French University Hospitals in the year 2000. *J. Med. Virol.,* 2003; 69: 7-17.

[43] Thomas D. Hepatitis C and human immunodeficiency virus infection. *Hepatology,* 2002; 36: S201- 209.

[44] Konopnicki D., Mocroft A., De Wit S., Antunes F., Ledergerber B., Katlama C., Zilmer K., Vella S., Kirk O., Lundgren J. D. Eurosida Group Hepatitis B and HIV: Prevalence, AIDS progression, response to Highly Active Antiretroviral Therapy and increased mortality in the Eurosida Cohort. *AIDS,* 2005; 19: 593-601.

[45] Rockstroh J. K., Mocroft A., Soriano V., Tural C., Losso M. H., Horban A., Kirk O., Phillips A., Ledergerber B., Lundgren J. Eurosida Study Group. Influence of Hepatitis C Virus infection on HIV-1 disease progression and response to Highly Active Antiretroviral Therapy. *J. Infect. Dis.*, 2005; 192: 992-1002.

[46] De Luca A., Bugarini R., Cozzi Lepri A., Puoti M., Girardi E., Antinori A., Poggio A., Pagano G., Tositti G., Cadeo G., Macor A., Toti M., D'arminio Monforte A For The I.Co.N.A. Study Group. Coinfection with hepatitis viruses and outcome of the first antiretroviral regimen in previously naïve HIV-infected subjects. *Arch. Intern. Med.,* 2002; 162: 2125-2132.

[47] Pollicino T., Squadrito G., Cerenzia G., Cacciola I., Raffa G., Craxi A., Farinati F., Missale G., Smedile A., Tiribelli C., Villa E., Raimondo G. Hepatitis B virus maintains its pro-oncogenic properties in the case of occult HBV infection. *Gastroenterology,* 2004; 126: 102-110.

[48] Shiota G., Oyama K., Udagawa A., Tanaka K., Nomi T., Kitamura A., Tsutsumi A., Noguchi N., Takano Y., Yashima K., Kishimoto Y., Suou T., Kawasaki H. Occult hepatitis B virus infection in Hbs antigen-negative hepatocellular carcinoma in a Japanese population: Involvement of Hbx and P53. *J. Med. Virol.*, 2000; 62: 151-158.

[49] El-Serag H. B. Epidemiology of hepatocellular carcinoma in USA. *Hepatol. Res.,* 2007; 37(2): S88-S94.

[50] Ahn J., Flamm S. L. Hepatocellular carcinoma. *Dis. Mon.,* 2004; 50: 556-573.

[51] Liu C. J., Kao J. H. Hepatitis B birus-related hepatocellular carcinoma: epidemiology and pathogenic role of viral factors. *J. Chin. Med. Assoc.,* 2007; 70: 141-145.

[52] Arbuthnot P., Capovilla A., Kew M. Putative role of Hepatitis B virus X protein in hepatocarcinogenesis: Effects on apoptosis, DNA repair, miogenoactivated protein kinase and JAK/STAT pathways. *J. Gastroenterol. Hepatol.*, 2000; 15: 357-368.

[53] Nunnari G., Smith J. A., Daniel R. HIV-1 Tat and AIDS-associated cancer: Targeting the cellular anti-cancer barrier. *J. Exp. Clin. Cancer Res.*, 2008; 27.

[54] Corallini A., Altavilla G., Pozzi L., Bignozzi F., Negrini M., Rimessi P., Gualandi F., Barbanti Brodano G. Systemic expression of HIV-1 Tat gene in transgenic mice induces endothelial proliferation and tumors of different histotypes. *Cancer Res.,* 1993; 53: 5569-5575.

[55] Altavilla G., Caputo A., Lanfredi M., Piola C., Barbanti-Brodano G., Corallini A. Enhancement of chemical hepatocarcinogenesis by the HIV-1 Tat gene. *Am. J. Pathol.*, 2000; 157: 1081-1089.

[56] Sato S., Fujiyama S., Tanaka M., Yamasaki K., Kuramoto I., Kawano S., Sato T., Mizuno K., Nonaka S. Coinfection of hepatitis C virus in patients with chronic hepatitis B infection. *J. Hepatol.*, 1994; 21: 159-166.

[57] Zauli G., Gibellini D., Milani D., Mazzoni M., Borgatti P., La Placa M., Capitani S. Human immunodeficiency virus type 1 Tat protein protects lymphoid, epithelial, and neuronal cell lines from death by apoptosis. *Cancer Res.,* 1993, 53: 4481-4485.

[58] Campioni D., Corallini A., Zauli G., Possati L., Altavilla G., Barbanti, Brodano G. HIV type 1 extracellular Tat protein stimulates growth and protects cells of BK virus/Tat transgenic mice from apoptosis. *AIDS Res. Hum. Retroviruses,* 1995, 11: 1039-1048.

[59] Ensoli B., Gendelman R., Markham P., Fiorelli V., Colombini S., Raffeld M., Cafaro A., Chang H. K., Brady J., Gallo R. C. Synergy between basic fibroblast growth factor and HIV-1 Tat protein in induction of Kaposi's Sarcoma. *Nature,* 1994; 371: 674-680.

[60] Albini A., Barillari G., Benelli R., Gallo R. C., Ensoli B. Tat, The human immunodeficiency virus type regulatory protein, has angiogenic properties. *Proc. Natl. Acad. Sci. Usa*, 1995; 92: 4838-4842.

[61] Ensoli B., Barillari G., Salahaudin Z. S., Gallo R. C., Wong-Staal F. Tat protein of HIV-1 stimulates growth of cells derived from Kaposi's sarcoma lesions of AIDS patients. *Nature,* 1990; 345: 84-86.

[62] Scala G., Ruocco M. R., Ambrosino C., Mallardo M., Giordano V., Baldassare F., Dragonetti E., Quinto I., Venuta S. The expression of the interleukin 6 gene induced by the human immunodeficiency virus type 1 Tat protein. *J. Exp. Med.*, 1994; 179: 961-971.

[63] Westendorp M. O., Li-Weber M., Frank R. W., Krammer P. H. Human immunodeficiency virus type 1 upregulates interleukin secretion in activated T cells. *J. Virol.,* 1994; 68: 4177-4185.

[64] De Marchi F., D'adda Di Fagagna F., Falaschi A., Giacca M. Activation of transcription factor NF-KB by the Tat protein of human immunodeficiency virus type-1. *J. Virol.*, 1996; 70: 4427-4437.

[65] Danta M., Semmo N., Fabris P., Brown D., Pybus O. G., Sabin C. A., Bhagani S., Emery V. C., Dusheiko G. M., Klenerman P. Impact of HIV on host-virus interactions during early hepatitis C virus infection. *J. Infect. Dis.*, 2008; 197: 1558-1566.

[66] Danta M., Dusheiko G. M. Acute HCV in HIV-positive individuals - A review. *Curr. Pharm. Des.*, 2008; 14: 1690-1697.

[67] Smukler A. J., Ratner L. Hepatitis viruses and hepatocellular carcinoma in HIV-infected patients. *Curr. Opin. Oncol.*, 2002; 14: 538-542.

[68] Bruno R., Gazzaruso C., Sacchi P., Zocchetti C., Giordanetti S., Garzaniti A., Ciappina V., Maffezzini E., Maserati R., Filice G. High prevalence of metabolic syndrome among HIV-infected patients: Link with the cardiovascular risk. *J. Acquir. Immune Defic. Syndr.*, 2002; 31: 363-365.

[69] Graham C. S., Baden L. R., Yu E., Mrus J. M., Carnie J., Heeren T., Koziel M. J. Influence of human immunodeficiency virus infection on the course of hepatitis C virus infection: A metaanalysis. *Clin. Infect. Dis.*, 2001; 33: 562-569.

[70] Benhamou Y., Bochet M., Di Martino V., Charlotte F., Azria F., Coutellier A., Vidaud M., Bricaire F., Opolon P., Katlama C., Poynard T. Liver fibrosis progression in human immunodeficiency virus and hepatitis C virus coinfected patients. The Multivirc Group. *Hepatology,* 1999; 30: 1054-1058.

[71] Bruno R., Galastri S., Sacchi P., Cima S., Caligiuri A., Defranco R., Milani S., Gessani S., Fantuzzi L., Liotta F., Frosali F., Antonucci G., Pinzani M., Marra F. Gp120 modulates the biology of human hepatic stellate cells: A link between HIV infection and liver fibrogenesis. *Gut,* 2010; 59(4): 513-520.

[72] Babu C. K., Suwansrinon K., Bren G. D., Badley A. D., Rizza S. A. HIV induces trail sensitivity in hepatocytes. *Plos One,* 2009; 4: E4623.

[73] Llovet J. M., Bustamante J., Castells A., Vilana R., Ayuso Mdel C., Sala M., Brù C., Rodès J., Bruix J. Natural history of untreated non surgical hepatocellular carcinoma: Rationale for the design and evaluation of therapeutic trials. *Hepatology,* 1999; 29: 62-67.

[74] Ebara M., Ohto M., Shinagawa T., Sugiura N., Kimura K., Matsutani S., Morita M., Saisho H., Tsuchiya Y., Okuda K. Natural history of minute hepatocellular carcinoma smaller than three centimeters complicating cirrhosis. A study in 22 Patients. *Gastroenterology,* 1986; 90: 289-298.

[75] Barbara L., Benzi G., Gaiani S., Fusconi F., Zironi G., Siringo S., Rigamonti A., Barbara C., Grigioni W., Mazziotti A. Natural history of small untreated hepatocellular carcinoma in cirrhosis: A multivariate analysis of prognostic factors of tumor growth rate and patient survival. *Hepatology,* 1992; 16: 132-137.

[76] Okazaki N., Yoshino M., Yoshida T., Suzuki M., Moriyama N., Takayasu K., Makuuchi M., Yamazaki S., Hasegawa H., Noguchi M. Evaluation of the prognosis for small hepatocellular carcinoma based on tumor volume doubling time. A preliminary report. *Cancer,* 1989; 63: 2207-2210.

[77] Benvegnù L., Noventa F., Bernardinello E., Pontisso P., Gatta A., Alberti A. Evidence for an association between the aetiology of cirrhosis and pattern of hepatocellular carcinoma development. *Gut,* 2001; 48: 110-115.

[78] Di Bisceglie A. M. Epidemiology and clinical presentation of hepatocellular carcinoma. *J. Vasc. Interv. Radiol.,* 2002; 13: S169-S171.

[79] Weinig M., Hakim J., Gudza I., Tobaiwa O. Hepatitis C virus and HIV antibodies in patients with hepatocellular carcinoma in Zimbabwe: A pilot study. *Trans. R. Soc. Trop. Med. Hyg.*, 1997; 91: 570-572.

[80] Bruno R., Sacchi P., Filice C., Puoti M., Filice G. Hepatocellular carcinoma in HIV-infected patients with chronic hepatitis: An emerging issue. *J. Acquir. Immune Defic. Syndr.*, 2002; 30: 535-536.

[81] Garcia-Samaniego J., Rodriguez M., Berenguer J., Rodriguez-Rosado R., Carbo J., Asensi V., Soriano V. Hepatocellular carcinoma in HIV-infected patients with chronic hepatitis C. *Am. J. Gastroenterol.*, 2001; 96: 179-183.

[82] Viriyavejakul P., Rojanasunan P., Viriyavejakul A., Punyarit P., Punpoowong B., Khachansaksumet V., Riganti M., Pongponratn E. Opportunistic infections in the liver of HIV- infected patients in Thailand: A necropsy study. *Southeast Asian J. Trop. Med. Public Health,* 2000; 31: 663-667.

[83] Bräu N., Fox R. K., Xiao P., Marks K., Nagvi Z., Taylor L. E., Trikha A., Sherman M., Sulkowski M. S., Dieterich D. T., Rigsby M. O., Wright T. L., Hernandez M. D., Jain M. K., Khatri G. K., Sterling R. K., Bonacini M., Martyn C. A., Aytaman A., Llovet J. M., Brown S. T., Bini E. J. North American liver cancer in HIV Study Group. Presentation and outcome of hepatocellular carcinoma in HIV infected patients: A U.S.-Canadian Multicenter Study. *J. Hepatol.*, 2007; 47: 527-537.

[84] Berretta M., Garlassi E., Cacopardo B., Cappellani A., Guaraldi G., Cocchi S., De Paoli P., Lleshi A., Izzi I., Torresin A., Di Gangi P., Pietrangelo A., Ferrari M., Bearz A., Berretta S., Nasti G., Di Benedetto F., Balestreri L., Tirelli U., Ventura P. Hepatocellular carcinoma in HIV-infected patients: Check early, treat hard. *Oncologist,* 2011; 16: 1258-1269.

[85] Di Benedetto F., De Ruvo N., Berretta M., Masetti M., Montalti R., Di Sandro S., Ballarin R., Codeluppi M., Guaraldi G., Gerunda G. E. Hepatocellular carcinoma in HIV patients treated by liver transplantation. *Eur. J. Surg. Oncol.*, 2008; 34: 422-427.

[86] Ettorre G. M., Vennarecci G., Boschetto A., Giovannelli L., Antonini M., Carboni F., Santoro R., Lepiane P., Cosimelli M., Lonardo M. T., Del Nonno F., Perracchio L., Maritti M., Moricca P., D'Offizi G., Narciso P., Noto P., Boumis E., Petrosillo N., Visco G., Santoro E. Resection and transplantation: evaluation of surgical perspectives in HIV positive patients affected by end-stage liver disease. *J. Exp. Clin. Cancer Res.*, 2003 Dec.; 22(4 Suppl.):167-9.

[87] Di Benedetto F., Di Sandro S., De Ruvo N., Berretta M., Montalti R., Guerrini Gp., Ballarin R., De Blasiis Mg., Spaggiari M., Smerieri N., Iemmolo Rm., Guaraldi G., Gerunda G. E. Human immunodeficiency virus and liver transplantation: our point of view. *Transplant. Proc.*, 2008; 40: 1965-1971.

[88] Radecke K., Frühauf N. R., Miller M., Ross B., Köditz R., Malagó M., Broelsch C. E., Gerken G., Treichel U. Outcome after orthotopic liver transplantation in five HIV-infected patients with virus hepatitis-induced cirrhosis. *Liver Int.*, 2005 Feb.; 25(1): 101-8.

[89] Kumada T., Nakano S., Takeda I., Sugiyama K., Osada T., Kiriyama S., Sone Y., Toyoda H., Shimada S., Takahashi M., Sassa T. Patterns of recurrence after initial treatment in patients with small hepatocellularcarcinoma. *Hepatology,* 1997; 25: 87-92.

[90] Di Benedetto F., Berretta M., De Ruvo N., Tarantino G., D'amico G., Ballarin R., Iemmolo R. M., Gerunda G. E. Is advanced hepatocellular carcinoma amenable of cure by liver transplantation with sorafenib as a neoadjuvant approach plus m-TOR inhibitors monotherapy? *J. Surg. Oncol.*, 2012; 105: 111-112.

[91] Frassetto L. A., Browne M., Cheng A., Wolfe Ar., Roland Me., Stock Pg., Carison L., Benet Lz. Immunosuppressant pharmacokinetics and dosing modifications in HIV-1 infected liver and kidney transplant recipients. *Am. J. Transplant.*, 2007; 7: 2816-2820.

[92] Tavio M., Grossi P., Baccarani U., Scudeller L., Pea F., Berretta M., Adani G.,Vivarelli M., Riva A., Tirelli U., Bresadola V., Viale P., Risaliti A. HIV-infected patients and liver transplantation: Who, when and why. *Curr. HIV Res.*, 2011; 9: 120-127.

[93] Llovet J. M., Ricci S., Mazzaferro V., Hilgard P., Gane E., Blanc J. F., de Oliveira A. C., Santoro A., Raoul J. L., Forner A., Schwartz M., Porta C., Zeuzem S., Bolondi L., Greten T. F., Galle P. R., Seit, J. F., Borbath I., Häussinger D., Giannaris T., Shan M., Moscovici M., Voliotis D., Bruix J.; SHARP Investigators Study Group. Sorafenib in advanced hepatocellular carcinoma. *N Engl. J. Med.*, 2008; 359: 378-390.

[94] Di Benedetto F., De Ruvo N., Berretta M., Masetti M., Montalti R., Di Sandro S., Quintini C., Codeluppi M., Tirelli U., Gerunda G. E. Don't deny liver transplantation to HIV patients with hepatocellular carcinoma in the highly active antiretroviral therapy era. *J. Clin. Oncol.*, 2006, 24, e26-e27.

[95] Chelis L., Ntinos N., Souftas V., Deftereos S., Xenidis N., Chamalidou E., et al. Complete response after sorafenib therapy for hepatocellular carcinoma in an HIV-HBV co-infected patient: possible synergy with HAART? A case report. *Med. Oncol.*, 2011; 28 (Suppl. 1):S165–S168.

[96] Perboni G., Costa P., Fibbia G. C., Morandini B., Scalzini A., Tagliani A., et al. Sorafenib therapy for hepatocellular carcinoma in an HIV-HCV coinfected patient. A case report. *Oncologist,* 2010; 15:142–145.

[97] Ozenne V., Gervais A., Peytavin G., Castelnau C., Valla D. C., Degos F. Suspected interaction between sorafenib and HAART in an HIV-1 infected patient: a case report. *Hepatogastroenterology*, 2011; 58: 161–162.

[98] De Nardo P., Viscione M., Corpolongo A., Bellagamba R., Vennarecci G., Ettorre G. M., et al. Treatment of recurrent hepatocellular carcinoma with sorafenib in a HIV/HCV co-infected patient in HAART: a case report. *Infect. Agent cancer*, 2012; 7:15.

[99] Bruix J., Sherman M., Llovet J. M., et al. Clinical management of hepatocellular carcinoma. Conclusions of the Barcelona-2000 EASL conference. European Association for the Study of the Liver. *J. Hepatol.,* 2001; 35:421-430.

[100] Marrero J. A., Fontana R. J., Barrat A., et al. Prognosis of hepatocellular carcinoma: Comparison of 7 staging systems in an American cohort. *Hepatology,* 2005;41:707-716.

[101] Hoofnagle J. H. Hepatocellular carcinoma: Summary and recommendations. *Gastroenterology*, 2004; 127 suppl. 1:S319-S323.

[102] Management of hepatocellular carcinoma: From prevention to molecular targeted therapy. In: Oncology; Proceedings of the 3rd International Kobe Liver Symposium on HCC with an International Liver Cancer Association (ILCA) Scientific Session; June 6–7, 2009; Hyogo, Japan. 2010.78 suppl. 1 p. 1-190.

[103] Quaglia A., Capocaccia R., Micheli A., Carrani E., Vercelli M. A wide difference in cancer survival between middle aged and elderly patients in Europe. *Int. J. Cancer*, 2007; 120: 2196-2201.

[104] Takenaka K., Shimada M., Higashi H., Adachi E., Nishizaki T., Yanaga K., Matsumata T., Ikeda T., Sugimachi K. Liver resection for hepatocellular carcinoma in the elderly. *Arch. Surg*., 1994; 129(8): 846-850.

[105] Yanaga K., Kanematsu T., Takenaka K., Matsumata T., Yoshida Y., Sugimachi K. Hepatic resection for hepatocellular carcinoma in elderly patients. *Am. J. Surg*., 1988; 155(2): 238-241.

[106] Oishi K., Itamoto T., Kobayashi T., Oshita A., Amano H., Ohdan, H., Tashiro H., Asahara, T. Hepatectomy for hepatocellular carcinoma in elderly patients aged 75 years or more. *J. Gastrointest. Surg*., 2009; 13; 695-701.

[107] Ferrero A., Viganò L., Polastri R., Ribero, D., Lo Tesoriere, R., Muratore, A., Capussotti, L. Hepatectomy as treatment of choice for hepatocellular carcinoma in elderly cirrhotic patients. *World J. Surg.,* 2005, 29(9), 1101-1105.

[108] Kaibori M., Matsui K., Ishizaki M., Saito T., Kitade H., Matsui Y., Kwon A. H. Hepatic resection for hepatocellular carcinoma in the elderly. *J. Surg. Oncol*., 2009; 99: 154-160.

[109] Massarweh N. N., Park J. O., Yeung R. S., Flum D. R. Comparative assessment of the safety and effectiveness of radiofrequency ablation among elderly medicare beneficiaries with hepatocellular carcinoma. *Ann. Surg. Oncol.,* 2012; 19: 1058-1065.

[110] Schwartz J. J., Pappas L., Thiesset H. F., Vargas G., Sorensen J. B., Kim R. D., Hutson W. R., Boucher K., Box T. Liver transplantation in septuagenarians receiving model for end-stage liver disease exception points for hepatocellular carcinoma: The National experience. *Liver Transplantation,* 2012; 18: 423-433.

[111] Perkins J. D. Treatment of an elderly patient with hepatocellular carcinoma: Counseling from the patient's point of view. *Liver Transplantation,* 2012; 18: 391-394.

[112] Frith J., Newton J. Liver transplantation in more elderly age. *Transpl. Int.,* 2009; 22: 599-600.

[113] Balducci L. Geriatric oncology: challenges for the new century. *Eur. J. Cancer,* 2000; 36: 1741-1754.

[114] Liaw Y. F., Tai D. I., Chu C. M., Lin D. Y., Sheen I. S., Chen T. J., Pao C. C. Early detection of hepatocellular carcinoma in patients with chronic type B hepatitis. A prospective study. *Gastroenterology,* 1986; 90: 263-267.

[115] Extermann M., Aapro M. Assessment of the older cancer patient. *Hematol. Oncol. Clin. N Am.*, 2000; 14: 63-78.

[116] Extermann M. Measuring comorbidity in the older cancer patient. *Eur. J. Cancer,* 2000; 36: 453-471.

[117] Oken M. M., Creech R. H., Tormey D. C., Horton J., Davis T. E., McFadden E. T., Carbone P. P. Toxicity and response criteria of the Eastern Cooperative Oncology Group. *Am. J. Clin. Oncol.,* 1982; 5: 649-655.

[118] Di Benedetto F., Berretta M., D'Amico G., Montalti R., De Ruvo N., Cautero N., Guerrini G. P., Ballarin R., Spaggiari M., Tarantino G., Di Sandro S., Pecchi A., Luppi G., Gerunda G. E. Liver resection for colorectal metastases in older adults: A paired matched analysis. *J. Am. Geriatr. Soc.,* 2011; 59: 2282-2290.

[119] Charlson M., Szatrowski T. P., Peterson J., Gold J. Validation of a combined comorbidity index. *J. Clin. Epidemiol.*, 1994; 47: 1245-1251.

[120] Conwell Y., Forbes N. T., Cox C., Caine E. D. Validation of a measure of physical illness burden at autopsy. The cumulative illness rating scale. *J. Am. Ger. Soc.,* 1993; 41: 38-41.

[121] Jing-Lin X., Sharma D., Bing-Hui Y., Bo-Heng Z., Zeng-Chen M., Zhi-Quan W., Jia F., Xin Z. D., Lun-Xiu Q., Zhao-You X. Analysis of the clinicopathological features of hepatocellular carcinoma in elderly patients. *J. Nepal Med. Assoc.,* 2008; 47: 132-135.

[122] Huang J., Li B. K., Chen G. H., Li J. Q., Zhang Y. Q., Li G. H., Yuan Y. F. Long-term outcomes and prognostic factors of elderly patients with hepatocellular carcinoma undergoing hepatectomy. *J. Gastrointest. Surg.*, 2009; 13: 1627-1635.

[123] Tsukioka G., Kakizaki S., Sohara N., Sato K., Takagi H., Arai H., Abe T., Toyoda M., Katakai K., Kojima A., Yamazaki Y., Otsuka T., Matsuzaki Y., Makita F., Kanda D., Horiuchi K., Hamada T., Kaneko M., Suzuki H., Mori M. Hepatocellular carcinoma in extremely elderly patients: An analysis of clinical characteristics, prognosis and patient survival. *World J. Gastroenterol.*, 2006; 12: 48 -53.

[124] Arase Y., Kobayashi M., Suzuki F., Suzuki Y., Kawamura Y., Akuta N., Imai N., Kobayashi M., Sezaki H., Matsumoto N., Saito S., Hosaka T., Ikeda K., Kumada H., Ohmoto Y., Amakawa K., Hsieh S. D., Ogawa K., Tanabe M., Tsuji H., Kobayashi T. Difference in malignancies of chronic liver disease due to non-alcoholic fatty liver disease or hepatitis C in Japanese elderly patients. *Hepatol. Res.*, 2012; 42: 264-272.

[125] Kozyreva O. N., Chi D., Clark J. W., Wang H., Theall K. P., Ryan D. P., Zhu A. X. A multicenter retrospective study on clinical characteristics,treatment patterns, and outcome in elderly patients with hepatocellular carcinoma. *Oncologist,* 2011; 16: 310-318.

[126] Mirici-Cappa F., Gramenzi A., Santi V., Zambruni A., Di Micoli A., Frigerio M., Maraldi F., Di Nolfo M. A., Del Poggio P., Benvegnù L., Rapaccini G., Farinati F., Zoli M., Borzio F., Giannini E. G., Caturelli E., Bernardi M., Trevisani F., Italian Liver

Cancer Group. Treatments for hepatocellular carcinoma in elderly mpatients are as effective as in younger patients: A 20-year multicentre experience. *Gut,* 2010; 59: 387-396.

[127] Vega G. L., Chandalia M., Szczepaniak L. S., Grundy S. M. Metabolic correlates of nonalcoholic fatty liver in women and men. *Hepatology,* 2007; 46: 716-722.

[128] Van der Poorten D., Milner K. L., Hui J., Hodge A., Trenell M. I., Kench J. G., London R., Peduto T., Chisholm D. J., George J. Visceral fat a key mediator of steatohepatitis in metabolic liver disease. *Hepatology,* 2008; 48: 449-457.

[129] Alexia C., Fallot G., Lasfer M., Schweizer-Groyer G., Groyer A. An evaluation of the role of insulin-like growth factors (IGF) and of type-I IGF receptor signaling in hepatocarcinogenesis and in the resistance of hepatocarcinoma cells against drug-induced apoptosis. *Biochem. Pharmacol.,* 2004; 68: 1003-1015.

[130] Nakajima T., Nakashima T., Yamaoka J., Shibuya A., Konishi E., Okada Y., Jo M., Nishikawa T., Itoh Y., Yoshikawa T. Greater age and hepatocellular aging are independent risk factors for hepatocellular carcinoma arising from non-B non-C nonalcoholic chronic liver disease. *Pathol. Int.,* 2011; 61: 572-576.

[131] Kawamura Y., Arase Y., Ikeda K., Seko Y., Imai N., Hosaka T., Kobayashi M., Saitoh S., Sezaki H., Akuta N., Suzuki F., Suzuki Y., Ohmoto Y., Amakawa K., Tsuji H., Kumada H. Large-scale long-term follow-up study of Japanese patients with non-alcoholic fatty liver disease for the onset of hepatocellular carcinoma. *Am. J. Gastroenterol.,* 2012; 107: 253-261.

[132] de Lope C. R., Tremosini S., Forner A., Reig M., Bruix J. Management of HCC. *J. Hepatol.*, 2012; 56 Suppl. 1: S75-S87.

[133] Yanaga K., Kanematsu T., Takenaka K., Matsumata T., Yoshida Y., Sugimachi K. Hepatic resection for hepatocellular carcinoma in elderly patients. *Am. J. Surg.,* 1988; 155: 238-241.

[134] Fortner J. G., Lincer R. M. Hepatic resection in the elderly. *Ann. Surg.,* 1990; 211: 141-145.

[135] Hanazaki K., Kajikawa S., Shimozawa N., Shimada K., Hiraguri M., Koide N., Adachi W., Amano J. Hepatic resection for hepatocellular carcinoma in the elderly. *J. Am. Coll. Surg.,* 2001; 192: 38-46.

[136] Nagasue N., Chang Y. C., Takemoto Y., Taniura H., Kohno H., Nakamura T. Liver resection in the aged (seventy years or older) with hepatocellular carcinoma. *Surgery,* 1993; 113: 148-154.

[137] Fong Y., Brennan M. F., Cohen M., Heffernan N., Freiman A., Blumgart L. H. Liver resection in the elderly. *Br. J. Surg*., 1997; 84: 1386-1390.

[138] Galanakis P., Bickel H., Gradinger R., Von Gumppenberg S., Förstl H. Acute confusional state in the elderly: Incidence, risk factors and complication. *Int. J. Geriatr. Psychiatry*, 2001; 16: 349-355.

[139] Okeeffe S. T., Chonchubhari A. N. Postoperative delirium in the elderly. *Br. J. Anaesth*., 1994; 73: 673-687.

[140] Cho S. W., Steel J., Tsung, A., Marsh J. W., Geller D. A., Gamblin T. C. Safety of liver resection in the elderly: How important is age? *Ann. Surg. Oncol*., 2011; 18: 1088-1095.

[141] Nanashima A., Abo T., Nonaka T., Fukuoka H., Hidaka S., Takeshita H., Ichikawa T., Sawai T., Yasutake T., Nakao K., Nagayasu T. Prognosis of patients with

hepatocellular carcinoma after hepatic resection: are elderly patients suitable for surgery? *J. Surg. Oncol.*, 2011; 104: 284-291.

[142] Haga Y., Ikei S., Ogawa M. Estimation of Physiologic Ability and Surgical Stress (E-PASS) as a new prediction scoring system for postoperative morbidity and mortality following elective gastrointestinal surgery. *Surg. Today*, 1999; 29: 219-225.

[143] Nakamuta, M., Morizono, S., Kohjima, M., Kotoh, K., Enjoji, M. Baseline characterization of patients aged 70 years and above with hepatocellular carcinoma. *World J. Gastroenterol.*, 2005, 11, 7512-7514.

[144] Kondo, K., Chijiiwa, K., Funagayama, M., Kai, M., Otani, K., Ohuchida, J. Hepatic resection is justified for elderly patients with hepatocellular carcinoma. *World J. Surg.*, 2008, 32(10), 2223-2229.

[145] Di Benedetto F., Tarantino G., Quintini C., Tirelli U., Berretta M. Hepatocellular carcinoma: Beyond the boundaries of age. *Anti Cancer Agents Med. Chem.*, 2013; 13: 1371-1377.

[146] Dindo D., Demartines N., Clavien P. A. Classification of surgical complications: A new proposal with evaluation in a cohort of 6336 patients and results of a survey. *Ann. Surg.*, 2004; 240: 205-213.

[147] Karnofsky D. A., Burchenal J. H. In Evaluation of Chemotherapeutic Agents; MacLeod CM, Ed, Columbia University Press. 1949; Page 196.

[148] Takahashi H., Mizuta T., Kawazoe S., Eguchi Y., Kawaguchi Y., Otuka T., Oeda S., Ario K., Iwane S., Akiyama T., Ozaki I., Fujimoto K. Efficacy and safety of radiofrequency ablation for elderly hepatocellular carcinoma patients. *Hepatol. Res.*, 2010; 40: 997-1005.

[149] Tateishi R., Shiina S., Teratani T., Obi S., Sato S., Koike Y., Fujishima T., Yoshida H., Kawabe T., Omata M. Percutaneous radiofrequency ablation for hepatocellular carcinoma. An analysis of 1000 cases. *Cancer*, 2005; 103: 1201-1209.

[150] Kao W. Y., Chiou Y. Y., Hung H. H., Su C. W., Chou Y. H., Huo T. I., Huang Y. H., Wu W. C., Lin H. C., Lee S. D., Wu J. C. Younger hepatocellular carcinoma patients have better prognosis after percutaneous radiofrequency ablation therapy. *J. Clin. Gastroenterol.,* 2012; 46: 62-70.

[151] Shiina S., Tateishi R., Arano T., Uchino K., Enooku K., Nakagawa H., Asaoka Y., Sato T., Masuzaki R., Kondo Y., Goto T., Yoshida H., Omata M., Koike K. Radiofrequency ablation for hepatocellular carcinoma: 10-year outcome and prognostic factors. *Am. J. Gastroenterol.,* 2012; 107: 569-577.

[152] De Giorgio M., Vezzoli S., Cohen E., Armellini E., Luca M. G., Verga G., Pinelli D., Nani R., Valsecchi M. G., Antolini L., Colledan M., Fagiuoli S., Strazzabosco M. Prediction of progression-free survival in patients presenting with hepatocellular carcinoma within the Milan criteria. *Liver Transpl.,* 2010; 16: 503-512.

[153] Thornton R. H., Covey A., Petre E. N., Riedel E. R., Maluccio M. A., Sofocleous C. T., Brody L. A., Getrajdman G. I., D'Angelica M., Fong Y., Brown K. T. A comparison of outcomes from treating hepatocellular carcinoma by hepatic artery embolization in patients younger or older than 70 years. *Cancer*, 2009; 115: 5000-5006.

[154] Collier J. D., Curless R., Bassendine M. F., James O. F. Clinical features and prognosis of hepatocellular carcinoma in Britain in relation to age. *Age Ageing*, 1994; 23: 22-27.

[155] Di Benedetto F., Tarantino G., Montalti R., Ballarin R., D'Amico G., Di Sandro S., Gerunda G. E. Laparoscopic radiofrequency ablation in the caudate lobe for

hepatocellular carcinoma before liver transplantation. *J. Laparoendosc. Adv. Surg. Tech. A.,* 2012; 22: 400-402.

[156] Singal A., Volk M. L., Waljee A., Salgia R., Higgins P., Rogers M. A., Marrero J. A. Meta-analysis: Surveillance with ultrasound for early-stage hepatocellular carcinoma in patients with cirrhosis. *Aliment Pharmacol. Ther.,* 2009; 30: 37-47.

[157] Croswell J. M., Ransohoff D. F., Kramer B. S. Principles of cancer screening: Lessons from history and study design issues. *Semin. Oncol.,* 2010; 37: 202-215.

[158] Giannini E., Romagnoli P., Fasoli A., Botta F., Risso D., Testa R. Influence of age on clinical presentation, therapeutic options, and prognosis in anti-HCV positive cirrhotic patients with hepatocellular carcinoma. *Age Ageing*, 2002; 31; 457-462.

[159] Dohmen K., Shirahama M., Shigematsu H., Irie K., Ishibashi H. Optimal treatment strategy for elderly patients with hepatocellular carcinoma. *J. Gastroenterol. Hepatol.,* 2004; 19: 859-865.

[160] Poon R. T., Fan S. T., Lo C. M., Liu C. L., Ngan H., Ng I. O., Wong J. Hepatocellular carcinoma in the elderly: results of surgical and nonsurgical management. *Am. J. Gastroenterol.*, 1999; 94: 2460-2466.

[161] Wong H., Tang Y. F., Yao T. J., Chiu J., Leung R., Chan P., Cheung T. T., Chan A. C., Pang R. W., Poon R., Fan S. T., Yau T. The outcomes and safety of single-agent sorafenib in the treatment of elderly patients with advanced hepatocellular carcinoma (HCC). *Oncologist,* 2011; 16: 1721-1728.

[162] Keating G. M., Santoro A. Sorafenib: a review of its use in advanced hepatocellular carcinoma. *Drugs,* 2009; 69: 223-240.

[163] Smalley K. S., Xiao M., Villanueva J., Nguyen T. K., Flaherty K. T., Letrero R., Van Belle P., Elder D. E., Wang Y., Nathanson K. L., Herlyn M. CRAF inhibition induces apoptosis in melanoma cells with non-V600E BRAF mutations. *Oncogene,* 2009; 28: 85-94.

[164] Wilhelm S. M., Adnane L., Newell P., Villanueva A., Llovet J. M., Lynch M. Preclinical overview of sorafenib, a multikinase inhibitor that targets both Raf and VEGF and PDGF receptor tyrosine kinase signaling. *Mol. Cancer Ther.*, 2008; 7: 3129-3140.

[165] Wilhelm S. M., Carter C., Tang L., Wilkie D., McNabola A., Rong H., Chen C., Zhang X., Vincent P., McHugh M., Cao Y., Shujath J., Gawlak S., Eveleigh D., Rowley B., Liu L., Adnane L., Lynch M., Auclair D., Taylor I., Gedrich R., Voznesensky A., Riedl B., Post L. E., Bollag G., Trail P. A. BAY 43-9006 exhibits broad spectrum oral antitumor activity and targets the RAF/MEK/ERK pathway and receptor tyrosine kinases involved in tumor progression and angiogenesis. *Cancer Res.,* 2004; 64: 7099-7109.

[166] Ito Y., Sasaki Y., Horimoto M., Wada S., Tanaka Y., Kasahara A., Ueki T., Hirano T., Yamamoto H., Fujimoto J., Okamoto E., Hayashi N., Hori M. Activation of mitogen-activated protein kinases/extracellular signal-regulated kinases in human hepatocellular carcinoma. *Hepatology,* 1998; 27: 951-958.

[167] Villanueva A., Newell P., Chiang D. Y., Friedman S. L., Llovet J. M. Genomics and signaling pathways in hepatocellular carcinoma. *Semin. Liver Dis.,* 2007; 27: 55-76.

[168] Calvisi D. F., Ladu S., Gorden A., Farina M., Conner E. A., Lee J. S., Factor V. M., Thorgeirsson S. S. Ubiquitous activation of Ras and Jak/Stat pathways in human HCC. *Gastroenterology,* 2006; 130: 1117-1128.

[169] Berretta M., Di Benedetto F., Dal Maso L., Cacopardo B., Nasti G., Facchini G., Bearz A., Spina M., Garlassi E., De Re V., Fiorica F., Lleshi A., Tirelli U. Sorafenib for the treatment of unresectable hepatocellular carcinoma in HIV-positive patients. *Anticancer Drugs,* 2013; 24: 212-218.

[170] Nunnari G., Berretta M., Pinzone M. R., Di Rosa M., Berretta S., Cunsolo G., Malaguarnera M., Cosentino S., De Paoli P., Schnell J. M., Cacopardo B. Hepatocellular carcinoma in HIV positive patients. *Eur. Rev. Med. Pharmacol. Sci.,* 2012; 16: 1257-1270.

[171] Berretta M., Zanet E., Di Benedetto F., Simonelli C., Bearz A., Morra A., Bonanno S., Berretta S., Tirelli U. Unusual presentation of metastatic hepatocellular carcinoma in an HIV/HCV coinfected patient: Case report and review of the literature. *Tumori,* 2008; 94: 589-591.

In: Hepatocellular Carcinoma in the 3rd Millennium
Editors: M. Berretta and B. Cacopardo ISBN: 978-1-63484-025-5

Chapter 12

MULTIDISCIPLINARY APPROACH FOR THE MANAGEMENT AND THE TREATMENT OF HEPATOCELLULAR CARCINOMA (HCC): NEW PERSPECTIVES

Ferdinando Martellotta*
Department of Medical Oncology, Centro di Riferimento
Oncologico, National Cancer Institute of Aviano, Aviano PN, Italy

ABSTRACT

Hepatocellular carcinoma (HCC) is a primary cancer of the liver that is predominant in developing countries (male and female ratio: 2:1) and often develops as a consequence of underlying liver disease and is most often associated with cirrhosis, therefore, the etiologic factors of the two diseases are coincident. The risk for HCC is sevenfold higher in HIV-infected than in HIV-uninfected patients. In HIV positive patients, co infection with HCV or HBV seems to accelerate disease progression and to reduce the efficacy of anti-HCV and anti-HBV therapies. In addition individuals with HIV infection may have higher HCC-related morbidity and mortality and HAART is known to have some direct hepatotoxic effects. The treatment for HCC depends essentially on cancer stage, on patient performance status, and on liver function. It, therefore, requires a multidisciplinary team (hepatologists, infectivologists, surgeons, liver transplant teams, oncologists, and interventional radiologists) able to interact with each other and to operate in the field of common therapeutic schedules. Both hepatologist and infectivologist are responsible for the management of patients with active HBV or HCV infection, for the HCC surveillance and for the assessment of the degree of liver function impairment before, during, and after cancer therapy. The patients on the transplant waiting list should be screened for HCC because the development of HCC gives increased priority for OLT and because failure to screen for HCC means that patients may develop HCC that may progress beyond listing criteria without the physician being

* Corresponding author: Ferdinando Martellotta. Department of Medical Oncology, Centro di Riferimento Oncologico, National Cancer Institute of Aviano, via Franco Gallini1, 33081 Aviano (PN), Italy. E-mail: fmartellotta@cro.it.

aware. In this phase is determining the role of nuclear medicine physicians and radiologists because the AFP is insufficiently sensitive or specific for use as a surveillance assay. The interaction between radiologists and expert molecular pathologists is determining for pathological diagnosis of dysplasia and early HCC. If the biopsy is negative for HCC the lesion should be followed by imaging at 3-6 monthly intervals and if the lesions remains atypical a repeat biopsy is recommended to improve diagnostic accuracy. Surgery and interventional radiologist are a focal point for the curative treatments. Patients who have a single lesion can be offered surgical resection if they are non-cirrhotic or have cirrhosis but still have well preserved liver function. Liver transplantation is an effective option for patients with solitary HCC <5 cm or with up to three nodules smaller than 3 cm in according to Milano criteria and a preoperative therapy can be considered if the waiting list exceeds 6 months. Percutaneous ablation with alcohol injection or radiofrequency ablation (RFA) is the best treatment for patients who cannot undergo resection or as a bridge to transplantation. Interventional radiologists and/or oncologists are responsible of management of non-curative treatment and the palliative or symptomatic treatment. The trans arterial embolization and chemoembolization (TACE) is recommended as first line non curative therapy for non surgical patients with large/multifocal HCC who do not have vascular invasion or extra hepatic spread. Chemotherapy with Sorafenib is recommended as first line for patients who have either failed TACE or with advanced HCC and still preserved liver function (Child-Pugh A) because able to prolong the life. Finally patients at terminal stage with performance status >2 and heavily impaired liver function should receive only symptomatic treatment.

INTRODUCTION

Hepatocellular carcinoma (HCC) is a primary cancer of the liver that is predominant in developing countries (male and female ratio: 2:1). The 1-year survival rate for untreated HCC is less than 20% and improves to more than 75% for patients with limited stage disease who undergo curative treatments. HCC often develops as a consequence of underlying liver disease and is most often associated with cirrhosis; therefore, the etiologic factors of the two diseases are coincident. On a global scale the most frequent causes of cirrhosis are hepatitis HBV- or HCV-related, the alcohol abuse and metabolic causes such as diabetes and obesity. Also in the geographical areas in developing the contamination of food by aflatoxin B produced by Aspergillus flavus or fumigatus plays an important role as a cofactor in carcinogenesis by HBV [1].

The risk for HCC is sevenfold higher in HIV-infected than in HIV-uninfected patients. Since the introduction of highly active antiretroviral therapy (HAART), no decrease in the incidence of HCC has been observed, unlike for other HIV-associated cancers in HIV positive patients, co infection with HCV or HBV is common, and a significantly higher risk for developing HCC as a result of chronic viral hepatitis is well documented. HIV co-infection seems to accelerate disease progression and to reduce the efficacy of anti-HCV and anti-HBV therapies. In addition to potential indirect effects on HCC risk through improvements in immune reconstitution and survival, HAART is known to have some direct hepatotoxic effects, especially among HIV-infected patients chronically infected with HBV or HCV. In addition to the elevated risk for developing HCC, individuals with HIV infection may have higher HCC-related morbidity and mortality.

Some studies showed that HIV–HCV co-infected patients develop liver cirrhosis more quickly than HCV mono-infected individuals, and that in these patients, HCC is more aggressive [2, 3]. The treatment for HCC depends essentially on cancer stage, patient performance status, and liver function therefore requires a multidisciplinary team including physicians from different disciplines (hepatologists, infectivologists, surgeons, liver transplant teams, oncologists, and interventional radiologists) able to interact with each other and operate in the field of common therapeutic schedules (Table 1). The multidisciplinary International Liver Cancer Association (ILCA) is a step toward addressing this issue. This association aims to promote novel pathogenic, diagnostic and therapeutic interventions for liver cancer by taking a transversal approach to research and bringing together scientists, physicians and allied professionals from all interrelated fields [4].

The hepatologist and the infectivologist are a focal point around whom the multidisciplinary team revolves. They are responsible of management of patients with active infection with HBV or HCV; HCC surveillance and the assessment of the degree of liver function impairment before, during and after cancer therapy. The objective of HCC surveillance must be to decrease mortality from disease therefore should be offered in the setting of a program or a process in which screening tests and recall procedures have been standardized and in which quality control procedures are in place.

HCC surveillance is widely practiced and can generally be recommended for certain at-risk groups including Asian male and female hepatitis B carriers over age 40 and 50 respectively; hepatitis B carrier with family history of HCC; cirrhotic hepatitis B or C carriers; co infection HIV/HCV or HIV/HBV or stage 4 primary biliary cirrhosis or alcoholic cirrhosis or non-alcoholic fatty liver disease (NAFDL) or genetic hemachromatosis and autoimmune hepatitis.

Also it seems prudent to continue to offer surveillance even after therapy-induced seroconversion or therapy-induced remission of inflammatory activity because the risk of HCC in these patients probably does not decrease proportionately with the improvement in fibrosis. Also the patients on the transplant waiting list should be screened for HCC because the development of HCC gives increased priority for OLT and because failure to screen for HCC means that patients may develop HCC that may progress beyond listing criteria without the physician being aware [5].

In this phase is determining the role of nuclear medicine physicians and radiologists because the AFP is insufficiently sensitive or specific for use as a surveillance assay.

The patients should be screened using exclusively ultrasonography at 6 month intervals and the interval does not need to be shortened for patients at higher risk of HCC. Any nodule not seen on a prior study should be considered abnormal and requires the activation of recall policies that determine whether an abnormality identified on surveillance is or is not HCC [6].

The contrast-enhanced study (dynamic CT-scan or MRI) is determining for the non-invasive diagnosis of HCC. In fact the presence of arterial uptake (wash-in) followed by washout in the portal venous and/or delayed phases is highly specific for HCC. The lesions smaller than 1 cm should be followed with ultrasound at 3-month intervals, if no growth over a period of up to 2 years occurs, physician can revert to routine surveillance. For lesions above 1 cm, either dynamic CT-scan or MRI should be used and if the appearances are not typical for HCC a second contrast enhanced study with the other imaging modality (dynamic CT-scan or MRI) should be performed [7]. In this phase is determining the interaction between radiologists and expert molecular pathologists.

Table 1. Multidisciplinary team

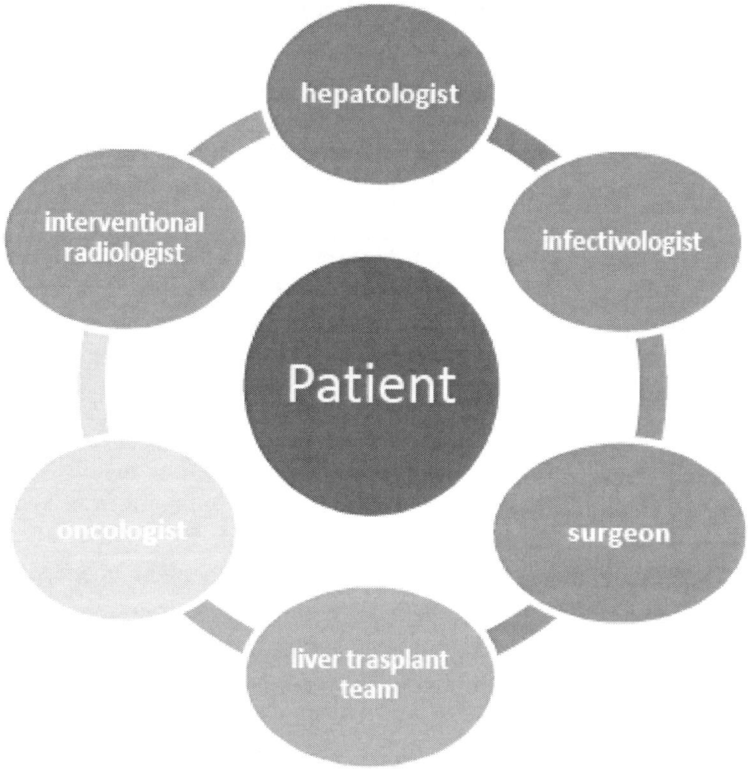

In fact if the biopsy is negative for HCC the lesion should be followed by imaging at 3-6 monthly intervals; if the lesions enlarges but remains atypical for HCC a repeat biopsy is recommended searching all the available markers (CD34, CK7, glypican 3, glutamine synthetase) to improve diagnostic accuracy [1, 5]. Oncologists and radiologists play an important role as regards the staging of HCC.

In according to the American Association for the Study of Liver disease guideline (AASLD) is essential that the staging system of HCC take into account tumor stage, liver function and physical status. The Child-Pugh classification is the gold standard for the evaluation of degree of liver dysfunction. The Barcelona Clinic Liver Cancer (BCLC) system is the only staging system that accomplishes these aims.

In fact BCLC system links staging with treatment modalities and with an estimation of life expectancy that is based on published response rates to the various treatments [8].

Surgery and interventional radiologist are a focal point for the curative treatments. Patients who have a single lesion can be offered surgical resection if they are non-cirrhotic or have cirrhosis but still have well preserved liver function, normal bilirubin and hepatic vein pressure gradient <10 mmHg. The majority of recurrences (70% at 5 years) are due to dissemination from the primary tumor during first 3 years of follow-up. Pre or post-resection adjuvant therapy is not recommended. Liver transplantation is an effective option for patients with solitary HCC <5 cm or with up to three nodules smaller than 3 cm in according to Milano criteria. The 5-year survival exceeds 70%.

Preoperative therapy can be considered if the waiting list exceeds 6 months. In this step evaluation by an infectious disease specialist and the therapy with pegylated interferon or combined therapy with pegylated interferon and ribavirin is essential to prevent the viral re-infection of the new liver that will cause significant liver damage leading to cirrhosis and will affect both graft and patient survival [5]. Percutaneous ablation with alcohol injection or radiofrequency ablation (RFA) is the best treatment for patients who cannot undergo resection or as a bridge to transplantation. The efficacy of RFA in HCC <2 cm is similar to that of ethanol but requires fewer treatment sessions while in HCC >2 cm is better that with ethanol. Post-treatment monitoring must be performed with CT or MRI indistinctly because there are no data to indicate superiority of one modality over the other. Initially a 3-4 month interval of follow-up imaging is commonly, after about 2 years of recurrence-free survival the interval can be less frequent [9, 10]. Furthermore interventional radiologists and/or oncologists are responsible of management of non-curative treatment and the palliative or symptomatic treatment. The transarterial embolization and chemoembolization (TACE) is recommended as first line non curative therapy for non surgical patients with large/multifocal HCC who do not have vascular invasion or extra hepatic spread. Patients with lobar or segmental portal vein thrombosis or Child-Pugh class B or C and/or clinical symptoms of end stage cancer are poor candidates for TACE because they have an elevated risk of liver failure and death. Chemotherapy with Sorafenib is recommended as first line for patients who have either failed TACE or with advanced HCC and still preserved liver function (Child-Pugh A) because able to prolong the life (Table 2).

In conclusion in according to the AASLD guideline for each stage there is an indicated treatment. Patients with early HCC are optimal candidates for resection (single HCC, normal bilirubin and absence relevant portal hypertension), or liver transplantation (3 nodules <3 cm or single HCC <5 cm with liver function impairment precluding resection) or percutaneous ablation (small non surgical HCC).

Table 2. Diagnostic-therapeutic flow-chart of patient with HCC

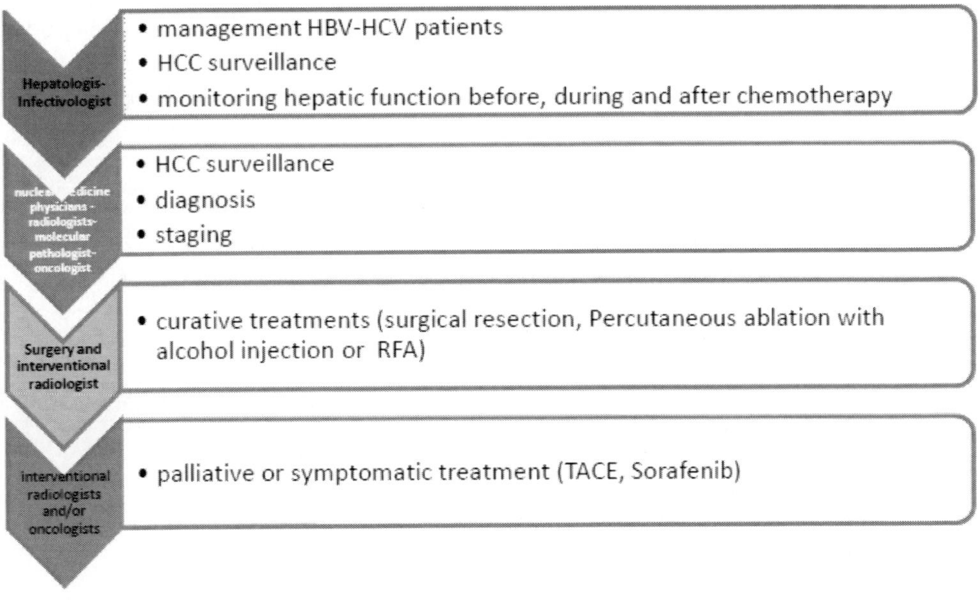

In all other cases patients have to be considered for palliative treatment with TACE (multinodular HCC and absence vascular invasion and Child-Pugh A stage) or chemotherapy (Child-Pugh A stage who fail TACE). Finally patients at terminal stage with performance status >2 and heavily impaired liver function should receive only symptomatic treatment.

REFERENCES

[1] Aravalli, N. R., Steer, C. J., Cressman, E. Molecular mechanisms of hepatocellular carcinoma. *Hepatology* 2008; 48: 2047-2063.

[2] Berretta, M., Zanet, E., Di Benedetto, F., Simonelli, C., Bearz, A., Morra, A., Bonanno, S., Berretta, S., Tirelli, U. Unusual presentation of metastatic hepatocellular carcinoma in an HIV/HCV coinfected patient: case report and review of the literature. *Tumori* 2008; 94: 589-591.

[3] Berretta, M., Garlassi, E., Cacopardo, B., Cappellani, A., Guaraldi, G., Cocchi, S., De Paoli, P., Lleshi, A., Izzi, I., Torresin, A., Di Gangi, P., Pietrangelo, A., Ferrari, M., Bearz, A., Berretta, S., Nasti, G., Di Benedetto, F., Balestreri, L., Tirelli, U., Ventura, P. Hepatocellular Carcinoma in HIV-Infected Patients: Check Early, Treat Hard. *The Oncologist* 2011; 16: 1258-1269.

[4] Gores, G. J. The emergence of a new discipline, hepatobiliary oncology. Comments from the editors. *Hepatology*. February 2008.

[5] Bruix, J., Sherman, M. Management of hepatocellular carcinoma: an update. *AASLD Practice Guideline*. July 2010.

[6] Chen, T. H., Chen, C. J., Yen, M. F., Lu, S. N., Sun, C. A., Huang, G. T., Yang, P. M. Ultrasound screening and risk factors for death from hepatocellular carcinoma in a high risk group in Taiwan. *Int. J. Cancer* 2002; 98:257-261.

[7] Burrel, M., Llovet, J. M., Ayuso, C., Iglesias, C., Sala, M., Miquel, R., Caralt, T. MRI angiography is superior to helical CT for detection of HCC prior to liver transplantation: an explants correlation. *Hepatology* 2003; 38:1034-1042.

[8] Forner, A. R. M., Rodrigruez de Lope, C., Bruix, J. Current strategy for staging and treatment: the BCLC Update and future prospects. *Semin. Liver Dis.* 2010; 30:61-74.

[9] Livraghi, T., Bolondi, L., Lazzaroni, S., Marin, G., Morabito, A., Rapaccini, G. L., Salmi, A. Percutaneous ethanol injection in the treatment of hepatocellular carcinoma in cirrhosis. A study on 207 patients. *Cancer* 1992; 69:925-929.

[10] Lin, S. M., Lin, C. J., Lin, C. C., Hsu, C. W., Chen, Y. C. Radiofrequency ablation improves prognosis compared with ethanol injection for hepatocellular carcinoma < or = 4 cm. *Gastroenterology* 2004; 127:1714-1723.

Editors' Contact Information

Dr. Massimiliano Berretta, MD, PhD
Department of Medical Oncology,
CRO Aviano National Cancer Institute IRCCS
Via Franco Gallini, 2 33081 Aviano
Tel: +390434659724
mberretta@cro.it

Dr. Bruno Cacopardo, MD
Associate Professor
Division of Infectious Disease,
"Garibaldi-Nesima" Hospital, University of Catania,
Catania Italy
Via Palermo 636, 95122 Catania
Tel: +393928020504
cacopardobruno@inwind.it

INDEX

A

B

C

D

E

F

G

H

J

K

L

M

N

Q

R

S

T

U

V

W

Y

Z